The Macrobiotic Way of Zen Shiatsu

David Sergel
The Macrobiotic Way of Zen Shiatsu

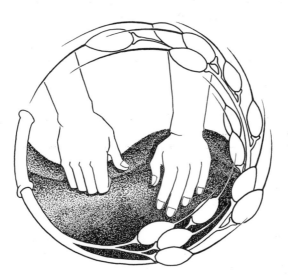

Foreword by Michio Kushi

Japan Publications, Inc.

Dedicated to
The memory of Shizuto Masunaga
Michio Kushi
The advancement of shiatsu and the realization of one peaceful world

Note to the reader: The information contained in this book is not intended to be used in the diagnosis, prescription, or treatment of disease or any health disorder whatsoever. Nor is this information intended to replace competent medical care. This book is a compendium of information which may be used as an adjunct to a rational and responsible health care plan.

Published by JAPAN PUBLICATIONS, INC., Tokyo and New York

Distributors:
UNITED STATES: *Kodansha International/USA, Ltd., 114 Fifth Avenue, New York, N. Y. 10011.* CANADA: *Fitzhenry & Whiteside Ltd., 195 Allstate Parkway, Markham, Ontario, L3R 4T8.* MEXICO AND CENTRAL AMERICA: *HARLA S. A. de C. V., Apartado 30–546, Mexico 4, D. F.* BRITISH ISLES: *Premier Book Marketing Ltd., 1 Gower Street, London WC1E 6HA.* EUROPEAN CONTINENT: *European Book Service PBD, Strijkviertel 63, 3454 PK De Meern, The Netherlands.* AUSTRALIA AND NEW ZEALAND: *Bookwise International, 54 Crittenden Road, Findon, South Australia 5007.* THE FAR EAST AND JAPAN: *Japan Publications Trading Co., Ltd., 1–2–1, Sarugaku-cho, Chiyoda-ku, Tokyo 101.*

First edition: July 1989

LCCC No. 86–81327
ISBN 0–87040–671–x

Printed in U.S.A.

Foreword

Since I began introducing shiatsu and related body energy adjustment arts to America in the mid-sixties, I wanted to see these practical healing arts distributed as widely as possible to all modern societies. Because of their simplicity and practicality, they have great value for the layman for the improvement of personal and family health.

Although several types of massage have been developed in western societies, the shiatsu system (and related body energy adjustment arts) have added a profound dimension to our understanding of the physical, mental and spiritual constitution and characteristics of humanity.

For almost thirty years I have searched for the proper person to introduce these arts to the West, both in practice and in theory. During this period Shizuko Yamamoto and Patrick McCarty, among others, have introduced the art of body adjustment very well, and we were very happy to have their perspectives and approaches which complemented and supplemented previous books which had been written. Meanwhile, I wrote the *Book of Dō-In* with the assistance of Olivia Oredson and other associates in connection with the art of body energy adjustment. As the years went by, several other fine books were published in this field by various shiatsu experts.

Olivia Oredson also authored *Macrobiotic Palm Healing: Energy at Your Finger-Tips* which also deals with the art of using physical and mental energy for healing purposes. However, many friends and associates in the field of natural health care have been waiting for the book which comprehensively introduces the art of shiatsu to the general public. Finally, the author of this book, David Sergel—who has both studied and taught at the Kushi Institute in Brookline, Massachusetts—assembled his teachings and experiences as well as his discoveries in Japan and produced one comprehensive presentation—*The Macrobiotic Way of Zen Shiatsu.*

All of the above-mentioned people have practiced the macrobiotic way of life as their daily lifestyle and diet. David Sergel and his family also utilize the macrobiotic diet and principles of nutrition in their daily lives. In fact, most of the leading teachers and practitioners of the art of shiatsu and related arts share the view that proper dietary practice (i.e., whole grains, vegetables, beans, bean products, sea vegetables, and occasional consumption of fruits, fish, nuts, seeds, and natural snacks) is essential to adjust both physical and mental energy in a healthful and peaceful way. Dietary adjustment, in fact, is the fundamental and primary method of energy adjustment.

The art of shiatsu as described in the book of *The Yellow Emperor's Classic of Internal Medicine* published 3,000 years ago in China, has a unique and important position in health maintenance and care, equal to acupuncture, and moxibustion, herbology and other healing arts. Beyond the maintenance of physical health, the art of shiatsu is also related to spiritual development. Like other arts dealing with the body-energy adjustment, it can help us achieve a peaceful state of mind and more spiritual states of consciousness in which we can envision the oneness between the individual and the universal. This is the underlying philosophical background for the art of shiatsu.

So while these body energy adjustment arts are very helpful to improve unhealthy symptoms, both physical and mental, they also contribute to the development of a deeper understanding of humanity within the universe. Accordingly, the spirit of Zen, as well as the spirit of religious traditions, are very closely associated with the spirit of these traditional healing arts. Consequently, the title of this book carries the word of *Zen*. But this word does not indicate a certain sect of Buddhism such as so-called Zen Buddhism, but rather represents the spirit of Zen meditation which is essential in the performance of shiatsu and related healing arts.

David Sergel, after studying macrobiotics in Australia, went to Japan where he studied the art of shiatsu for several years while continuing to practice the macrobiotic way of life. Through these experiences he developed his unique comprehensive understanding of the art of shiatsu. He then taught this art in Boston at the Kushi Institute, and later throughout America, Europe, and Australia, as one of the chief teachers of shiatsu and related arts. Because of this broad understanding not only shiatsu massage but also macrobiotic dietary practice and the meridian system have been very well introduced in this book.

David and other teachers of shiatsu and related arts will be recognized in the future as contributors to human health and development, especially in the unification of traditional Eastern and modern Western health approaches. Together with my friends and associates who are dedicating their efforts to macrobiotic education, the natural food movement, or ecological concerns for the benefit of humanity on this planet, I highly recommend to every individual and family and community this book—*The Macrobiotic Way of Zen Shiatsu*—with the hope that everyone begins to help each other through these simple, practical, and wonderful healing arts.

Michio Kushi
February 2, 1989

Preface

My interest in natural healing began with macrobiotics which I had been practicing for a number of years before beginning the study of shiatsu. My attraction to Zen Shiatsu was in large part due to the way I saw it blend, in both practice and philosophy, with macrobiotics.

Since macrobiotics focuses on diet, this daily ritual must inevitably have an overall larger effect on our health than a shiatsu treatment which one rarely receives more than once a week. By placing Zen Shiatsu within the larger context of macrobiotics we can reinforce and make more effective the benefits of Zen Shiatsu. This integration is the primary goal of this book.

Some people may question how Masunaga would feel about this approach. Masunaga's approach to healing was spiritual with a deep faith in the natural healing power. He was empathetic with macrobiotics and the natural foods movement. Indeed, not only was there a large selection of natural foods for sale in the waiting room of his clinic, but our small classroom was lined with crates of tamari soy sauce and crocks of umeboshi plums. Further, lunches served to the staff were in the main macrobiotic. Masunaga often spoke in terms of yin and yang, and although his approach was based more on the traditional Chinese view of light and shade, the outcome was much the same as that presented by macrobiotics.

Besides integrating macrobiotics and Zen Shiatsu there were other aspects that I wanted to cover. The first was to disseminate as much practical information from my time of study at Masunaga's school as was possible. The second was to compile a body of knowledge I felt was necessary to understand in order to provide a worthy service to those who receive shiatsu. The third was to pass on information from my own personal experiences.

In closing I should emphasize that this book is based on the teachings of Shizuto Masunaga and Michio Kushi. While I have endeavored to remain faithful to their teachings, I have interpreted them in my own way, leading to the possibility of errors or misunderstandings. For those who find this to be the case I apologize. However, at the possible expense of this occurrence I feel it important that Westerners share their experiences of shiatsu. To date very little has been written on shiatsu by Westerners, yet it is here in the West that shiatsu is now receiving wide interest. I hope the thoughts expressed in this book stimulate and encourage others to write on this subject with the larger intention of spreading shiatsu, by providing greater understanding and training quality shiatsu practitioners.

Acknowledgment

My deepest thanks to my parents for their continued love and encouragement.·

My deepest thanks to Shizuto Masunaga and Michio Kushi.

Mr. Masunaga, along with a very supportive staff, made every effort to help non-Japanese students understand Zen Shiatsu. I would also like to thank at Masunaga's school, the Iokai Shiatsu Center, Mrs. Masunaga for her encouragement with this project, and Hirai Hidemasa, upon whose approach to Zen Shiatsu, my own practice is based. In addition I would also like to thank Suzuki sensei, Kono sensei, and the staff at Iokai.

I have much to thank Michio Kushi for. It was Michio who gave me the opportunity to teach in Boston and it was he who arranged for the publication of this book. Apart from the opportunity to learn from him, Michio always remains in my mind as an inspiration—for his ceaseless efforts toward the betterment of life on this planet and world peace.

In Australia I would like to thank a long time family friend David Rich for his support and inspiration, especially in my youth, and Daniel and Marcea Weber who with great spirit and enthusiasm established Sydney's first macrobiotic center.

In Boston there have been a number of people who through their love, encouragement, support, and friendship have enriched my life in numerous ways. In the approximate order that I met them I would like to thank Norman Cohen, Aveline Kushi, Solveig Eskedahl, Karin Stephan, Jeffrey Denner, Estee Rappaport, Donna Cowan, Steve Goldin, Daniel Do Amaral, David Woodman, and Maya Tewari. In addition I would like to thank the various teachers I studied with and the staff of the Kushi Institute, as well as the Boston and indeed the world macrobiotic community.

In the preparation of this book, without any exaggeration, a greater team of helpers one could not have wished for. Special thanks to Steve Goldin who edited the entire project with the love and care of a personal possession. In addition I would like to thank the following: Lynne Paterson, macrobiotic cooking teacher and Iyengar yoga instructor from Miami, who modelled for the photographs; Daniel Do Amaral for his fine photography; Millicent Harvey who arranged the photo session and took care of the lighting; Tom Boode-Petersen whose superb illustrations far exceeded my vision of them, and Tom Atwood of Page Magic for a beautifully typed manuscript. In addition I would also like to thank Evelyn Harboun for a substantial contribution to the chapter on the macrobiotic diet, and Norman Cohen for numerous suggestions on various parts of the text. Deepest appreciation also to Alex Jack for his editing and suggestions, Marc Van Cauwenberghe who edited the chapter on meridians, and David Woodman who helped with the editing of the practical material. My thanks also to Nancy Aronson, Wayne Yee Mon, Odile Corbel, Austin Lyons, and Andy Harrop for their editorial assistance, and to Allejandro Gonzalez whose illustrations for class were an inspiration to proceed with this project.

I would also like to express my thanks to the publishers and authors of the various books I referred to in preparing this text. I would especially like to thank Rudolph Ballentine, Ted Kaptchuk, and Felix Mann.

Finally my deepest appreciation to three very patient people, Mr. Iwao Yoshizaki, Mr. Yoshiro Fujiwara, and Ms. Yotsuko Watanabe of Japan Publications, Inc., for their continued support on a project that was way overdue, and to Toyoko my wife and Takeshi my son—yes it's finished!

Contents

Chapter *1*

The Philosophy of Shiatsu

"... touch is, I suppose, the most primitive sense, but this gives rise to the purest feeling of identity ... Sight is the most intellectual sense and hearing is next but there is a great distance between them and their object; whereas with touch there is an immediate coming together. We must experience that. It is the same as intuition, not just relative intuition but collective or total intuition. When this takes place there is real understanding of reality and the experience of Enlightenment."

Daisetsu T. Suzuki[1]

Were we to ask a friend to massage our shoulders, most likely he or she would employ rubbing, pinching or kneading motions, forward, backward or in circles across the muscles. However, if we were to receive shiatsu, we would simply feel stationary pressure at some particular point, then at another and so on. In the first massage there is movement; both giver and receiver are conscious of the giver actually "doing" something. In contrast, the latter massage seems relatively motionless: it might remind us of Rodin's sculpture of "The Thinker," where he giving elbow shiatsu to his own knee. At first glance it may seem strange that the latter "non-doing" massage can actually be effective. The philosophy and mind behind this approach differ distinctly from our Western world view. Since that philosophy and mind are very practical in nature, we first need to gain greater understanding of this outlook in order to enhance our ability to give effective shiatsu.

Shiatsu or "finger pressure" evolved in Japan in this century from Anma, a style of massage imported from China centuries earlier. While its deepest roots lie in an instinctive application of pressure to relieve areas of bodily pain, the theoretical base of shiatsu is classical Chinese medicine. The style of shiatsu on which this book is based also reflects the cultural background of Japan, permeated by the philosophy of Zen Buddhism. Shizuto Masunaga created and developed this style throughout a thirty year career until his death in 1981. It is known as Zen Shiatsu.

Macrobiotics, or life embracing the "largest view," is a practical philosophy based on the ways common to traditional peoples. As it is popularly known, macrobiotics was first introduced from Japan by George Ohsawa, a teacher, poet, philosopher, and world traveler, who began teaching in Europe during the 1930s. Macrobiotics, according to Ohsawa, applies to all, of whatever religion, culture or geographic location. The ultimate goal of macrobiotic practice is the attainment of absolute freedom. The compass to reach this goal is an intimate understanding of the forces of yin and yang; a comprehension of an order common to all aspects of the infinite universe. The foundation of this freedom lies in our daily diet.

Since the same cultural soil gave form to both shiatsu and macrobiotics, we might expect to see strong possibilities of a harmonious integration between the two. In fact as we delve deeper, we see evidence that shiatsu arose from a macrobiotic mind and is thus according to this view, from its foundation, a macrobiotic practice.

This chapter is devoted to showing the connection between macrobiotics and Zen Shiatsu. It is divided into three sections. The first section deals with aspects of Oriental philosophy pertinent to the practice of shiatsu. These aspects are presented in a macrobiotic model: the spiral of materialization—a form which illustrates the process of spirit becoming matter. We will see how various stages along this spiral apply to Zen Shiatsu. The second section utilizes information presented to show how the traditional cultures of Japan and China, and modern industrialized nations developed along different "axes" as a result of their diet. Since we are dealing with Oriental massage this section will focus more on Oriental culture. The final section draws on preceding information to show how Zen Shiatsu is a product of a natural philosophy; of a macrobiotic diet and view of life. Zen Shiatsu will be contrasted with Western massage. The importance of the way we touch, implications of the macrobiotic connection, and the Zen of Zen Shiatsu will also be addressed.

1. The Spiral of Materialization

One Infinity

Oriental philosophy speaks of an infinite universe without beginning or end, expanding in all directions at infinite speed. Lao Tsu describes it thus in the *Tao Teh Ching*:

> "There is something formless and perfect,
> Ever-existing, even before the birth of Heaven and Earth.
> How still it is! How quiet!
> Abiding alone and unchanging,
> It pervades everywhere without fail.
> Well may it be the mother of the world.
> I do not know its name,
> But label it Tao."[2]

Tao, meaning the Way, or Path, was a term of convenience used by Lao Tsu to describe what essentially cannot be expressed in words. In Confucianism, Tao is Tai Chi, the Supreme Ultimate. Buddhists call it Sunyata (Sanskrit), Taikyoku (Japanese), the Absolute, the Void, Emptiness, or Nothingness. Macrobiotic philosophy often refers to Tao as One Infinity. The Tao is both manifest and non-manifest. It produces heaven and earth, man and woman, yet transcends all dualities; it is beyond time, space, and causation. The Tao is empty, hollow, a void. However it eternally produces, permeates and nourishes all.

D.T. Suzuki, the eminent Buddhist scholar who first presented Zen to Western audiences, describes the relationship of the individual to One Infinity in this way:

> "According to the Zen point of view, the universe is a circle without a circumference, and everyone of us is the centre of the universe. To put it more concretely: I am the

centre, I am the universe, I am the creator. I raise the hand and lo! there is space, there is time, there is causation. Every logical law and every metaphysical principle rushes in to confirm the reality of my hand."[3]

In this passage, Suzuki contrasts the Absolute with relative existence, pure sensation with self-awareness. Since Suzuki's image of the universe has no circumference, there can be an infinite number of centers. Each human being is a center of the universe, a microcosm of the macrocosm. Each contains all that preceded his or her creation. Every individual is One Infinity in themselves. All objects or beings, animate or inanimate have or are "Buddha nature." This level of consciousness constitutes Enlightenment: it describes the essential goal of Buddhist practice.

The Absolute can neither be grasped from the outside nor understood by logical or conceptual thought. "Stop up the aperture of the vessel, and shut the doors (of the senses)," says Lao Tsu. The Absolute lies within. Like a mirror which reflects and takes on the image of whatever appears in front, the unchanging Absolute exists only to be revealed in its pure state when the reflected object departs. The reflected object represents the individual's impression of the outside world and his conceptual thought, that only exists because of this external stimuli.

The way to the Absolute lies in an intuitive mode of understanding. This true awareness arises from what Lao Tsu refers to as "Wu-Wei," literally non-doing. More specifically, Wu-Wei denotes non-interference, the absence of human willful effort. The Tao always strives toward balance and harmony. To awaken to the Tao, the individual endeavors to unify the mind and body through an attunement with nature. When living inherently in such a state one abides by and consequently expresses the Tao, one lives by Wu-Wei. Zen Shiatsu is an expression of Wu-Wei.

Buddhist paintings commonly depict the Absolute as a circle known as "Ensō," an image of purity and emptiness. Carried over into our daily lives this circle reminds us of the all-inclusive nature of the infinite universe and the wholeness of each individual. This holistic view extends to shiatsu massage. The giver views each receiver as possessing within his or her own healing power. The shiatsu practitioner's role is to nurture this innate life-force.

Yin and Yang

Within the ocean of Infinity endless streams of motion flow in all directions. When and wherever such streams intersect, One Infinity differentiates into two opposite forces: contraction and expansion. The contracting force we call yang, the expanding force, yin. Yin and yang constitute the two poles of One Infinity.

From the interaction of these two forces in various proportions all relative phenomena arise. Between these two poles all relative phenomena exist and by these two forces all relative phenomena are governed. Everything constantly changes; the life of any phenomenon consists of the continuous movement from the extreme of one pole to that of the other in endless cycles.

We can sense this rhythm in our daily life experiences. The oneness of breathing involves continuous repetitions of inhalation followed by exhalation. Endless cycles that move from the extreme light of day to the extreme dark of night compose the oneness of each day. Likewise the seasons of the year move from the extreme heat of summer to the extreme cold of winter. Like waves, movement is always followed by rest, conversation alternates with silence. Likes change into dislikes, war into peace, hate into love. Success follows failure, sadness changes into happiness, poverty into wealth, sickness into health, and so on in never-ending cycles.

Thus the oneness of any entity or process is comprised of two antagonistic yet complementary forces. One cannot exist without its opposite, each is defined by its opposite, each seeks its opposite for completion.

George Ohsawa called the phenomenon of differentiation from One Infinity a "dualistic monism," and interpreted it with seven universal principles and twelve laws of change. This cosmic constitution is the Order of the Universe, which Ohsawa described as the Unique Principle. According to Ohsawa, the Unique Principle applies to every phenomenon in the relative world and forms the basis of all macrobiotic studies and practices.

The seven principles are the following:

1. Everything is a differentiation of One Infinity.
2. Everything changes.
3. All antagonisms are complementary.
4. There is nothing identical.
5. What has a front has a back.
6. The bigger the front, the bigger the back.
7. What has a beginning has an end.

The twelve laws of change are as follows:

1. One Infinity manifests itself into complementary and antagonistic tendencies, yin and yang, in its endless change.
2. Yin and yang are manifested continuously from the eternal movement of One Infinite Universe.
3. Yin represents centrifugality. Yang represents centripetality. Yin and Yang together produce energy and all phenomena.
4. Yin attracts yang, yang attracts yin.
5. Yin repels yin, yang repels yang.
6. Yin and yang combined in various proportions produce different phenomena. The attraction and repulsion among phenomena is proportional to the difference of the yin and yang forces.
7. All phenomena are ephemeral, constantly changing their constitution of yin and yang forces; yin changes into yang, yang changes into yin.
8. Nothing is solely yin or solely yang. Everything is composed of both tendencies in varing degrees.
9. There is nothing neuter. Either yin or yang is in excess in every occurrence.
10. Large yin attracts small yin. Large yang attracts small yang.
11. Extreme yin produces yang, and extreme yang produces yin.
12. All physical manifestations are yang at the center and yin at the surface.

To apply this philosophy practically we must first know how to identify something as yin or yang. Identification can be made more clearly by viewing ourselves as between Heaven and Earth. From a metaphysical point of view, Heaven—the creative principle—is yang, symbolized by man. Earth—the receptive principle—is yin, symbolized by woman. From our physical point of view, Heaven connotes the heavens above, an infinite yin expanse, while yang, finite matter, composes Earth. In both man and woman, Heaven symbolizes the invisible world of consciousness or mind. Earth represents the physical, practical world: the body with its senses and emotions.

We can depict yin and yang (Fig. 1):

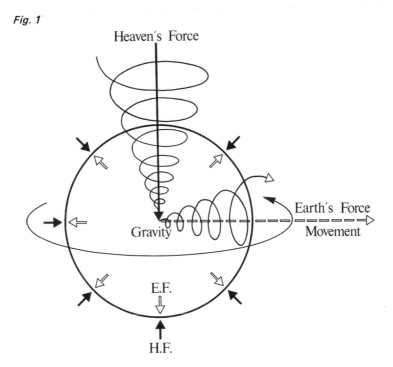

Fig. 1

The earth revolves on its axis in a counterclockwise motion, receiving the force of heaven in counterclockwise spirals from all directions toward its center. The strongest influence of this heaven's force comes from the north pole. Conversely, this same counterclockwise rotation causes earth's force to move away from the planet from all points in clockwise spirals. Earth's force is strongest coming from the equator. Heaven's force is centripetal: it moves from periphery to center, downward and inward, contracting, gathering, condensing, and materializing. Thus heaven's force is yang; it creates yang objects and tendencies. Earth's force is centrifugal motion: from center to periphery, upward and outward, expanding and ascending, dispersing, separating, differentiating, and decomposing. Earth's force is yin, creating yin objects and tendencies. Basically we experience heaven's force by what is known as gravity, while earth's force predominates in horizontal movement such as walking. When still we draw in more of heaven's force, while when in motion we draw more on earth's force.

We can classify the different qualities of any object according to yin and yang. From the above diagram (Fig. 1) and explanation, we can see that top is yin, bottom yang; periphery yin, center yang; outside yin, inside yang. A horizontal shape is more yang than a vertical one, since the horizontal surface is more open to the stronger influence of heaven's force.

Following similar reasoning, an object with broader shape toward the top would be yin in comparison with the broader shape toward the bottom, since the former shows the predominance of earth's force rising, while the latter, the predominance of heaven's force descending. For this reason we often see the symbols ▽ and △ used for yin and yang respectively. As well, vibrations of a shorter wavelength and higher frequency would be yin by comparison with vibrations of longer wavelength and lower frequency. Since the vibration of the color purple has a shorter wavelength and higher frequency than the color red, we would say purple is more yin and red more yang. Since water tends to make things expand, the higher the liquid content of an object the more yin, the drier the more yang.

The following list contains a fuller explication of such polar relationships (Table 1):

We classify into yin and yang by comparison. Since, as we have observed, everything changes, some points need to be emphasized about making comparisons. To begin with, there are no absolutes. Categorization into either yin or yang implies an overall tendency, or the stronger force of the two. "More yin" or "more yang" would be more appropriate designations. Therefore, when we make this type of comparison we should consider the following relationships:

(1) Comparison of a particular aspect of a phenomenon at different points in time
For example, in terms of atmospheric influence daytime is considered yin since energy is rising, while nighttime is yang as energy is descending. Further, midday is more yin than early morning since energy reaches its zenith toward midday. In the same way, the middle of the night when energy reaches its nadir is more yang than mid-afternoon.

Considering human life span, infancy is physically more yang than full maturity when we take on a more upright posture. Old age, when we begin to contract, is more yang than full maturity also. Overall though, physically speaking, the infant being smaller, is more yang than the old person.

In the life of a vegetable, one at full maturity is more yin than the same vegetable before it is ripe, since earth's force has become stronger. An overly ripe vegetable, however, is even more yin since it is beginning to decay: earth's force is now overly dominant.

(2) Comparison of two or more different aspects of a particular phenomenon
For example, while daytime is yin in terms of atmospheric influence, its effect on the individual is yang since it induces physical activity. Conversely, while nighttime is yang in terms of atmospheric influence, its effect on the individual is yin since it induces relaxation.

Regarding an individual person, physical activity expresses a more yang quality, while shyness a more yin quality. In the same way, mental activity expresses a more yin quality, while a gregarious nature may express a more yang quality.

When examining vegetables the red color of a tomato expresses a more yang quality. Conversely, the high liquid content, short life span, and relatively short growing period in a warm environment all express more yin qualities. Taking a carrot, for

Table 1

	YIN∇*	YANG△*
Attribute	Centrifugal force	Centripetal force
Tendency	Expansion	Contraction
Function	Diffusion	Fusion
	Dispersion	Assimilation
	Separation	Gathering
	Decomposition	Organization
Movement	More inactive, slower	More active, faster
Vibration	Shorter wave and higher frequency	Longer wave and lower frequency
Direction	Ascent and vertical	Descent and horizontal
Position	More outward and peripheral	More inward and central
Weight	Lighter	Heavier
Temperature	Colder	Hotter
Light	Darker	Brighter
Humidity	Wetter	Drier
Density	Thinner	Thicker
Size	Larger	Smaller
Shape	More expansive and fragile	More contractive and harder
Form	Longer	Shorter
Texture	Softer	Harder
Atomic particle	Electron	Proton
Elements	N, O, P, Ca, etc.	H, C, Na, As, Mg, etc.
Environment	Vibration ... Air ... Water ... Earth	
Climatic effects	Tropical climate	Colder climate
Biological	More vegetable quality	More animal quality
Sex	Female	Male
Organ structure	More hollow and expansive	More compacted and condensed
Nerves	More peripheral, orthosympathetic	More central, parasympathetic
Attitude, emotion	More gentle, negative, defensive	More active, positive, aggressive
Work	More psychological and mental	More physical and social
Consciousness	More universal	More specific
Mental function	Dealing more with the future	Dealing more with the past
Culture	More spiritually oriented	More materially oriented
Dimension	Space	Time

* For convenience, the symbols ∇ for Yin, and △ for Yang are used.
Reprinted with permission, *Macrobiotic Diet*, Kushi, Michio and Aveline, with Alex Jack, 1985, Japan Publications, Inc. p. 37

example, we see the downward growing single condensed orange root as more yang by comparison with the upward growing, multitudinous green leaves.

(3) Comparison of a particular object with a different object of the same group
Between two people alike in many respects, the one who is shorter we would consider more yang.

Between two root vegetables, a carrot and a daikon for example—the carrot is orange, the daikon white; the carrot usually smaller with less liquid content; the carrot is sweet, the daikon pungent. In all respects the carrot is more yang.

If we compare two root vegetables of the same species, that which is smaller, all other things being equal, is the one which is more yang.

Thus to classify any phenomenon, we need to consider a number of different variables. The overall predominating quality determines the category into which we classify that phenomenon.

The principle of a dualistic monism is symbolized in Chinese philosophy by the Tai Chi Tu (Fig. 2). The circle represents One Infinity, while each half represents yin and yang. In one version of the Tai Chi Tu the left half is clear, rising upward. It shows earth's rising force, which peaks during the daytime. In contrast, the dark right half moves downward. It in turn symbolizes heaven's downward force, which is strongest at night. The two smaller circles show us that nothing is wholly yin or wholly yang. There is always yin within yang and vice versa. The middle line is visualized in constant motion as yin changes into yang and vice versa.

Fig. 2

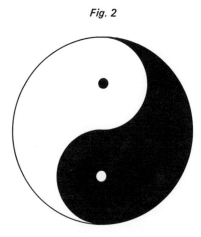

Zen Shiatsu is in all respects a practical application of yin and yang. This can be seen in the following qualities:

1. The giver and receiver are viewed two-as-one.
2. The giver harmonizes yin and yang within to apply what we call "natural leaning pressure."
3. We always place both hands on the receiver's body yet they perform different functions. One hand always remains stationary, which is yang, supporting or stabilizing the yin moving hand which gives shiatsu.
4. The application of pressure to a point draws the receiver's mind into his or her physical self thus helping to unify the mind and body.
5. In diagnosis we perceive the receiver's energy as one unit. The appearance of excess energy in certain areas of the body indicates a proportionate deficiency of energy in other areas. Whenever and wherever there is excess, elsewhere there must be deficiency.
6. The changes that come about as a result of shiatsu can benefit the receiver both physically and mentally.

The Logarithmic Spiral

The Tai Chi Tu further depicts two logarithmic spirals (Fig. 3). The spiral with the unbroken line describes the evolutionary process culminating in the appearance of human beings. The other spiral describes the return journey of the spirit to One Infinity upon physical decomposition. We refer to the former figure as the spiral of materialization, the latter as the spiral of spiritualization. These two spirals can be depicted together (Fig. 4): the direction of the former moving inward in the direction of the center, the latter outward toward infinity.

Fig. 3

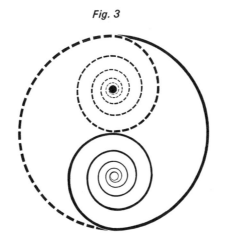

Fig. 4

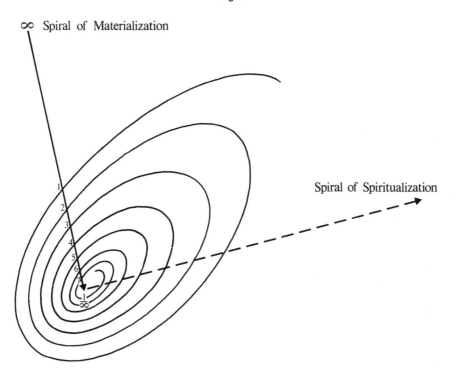

The logarithmic spiral is the macrobiotic mandala: it represents the evolution of the relative world. All relative phenomena are the outcome of process along the spiral of materialization.

A logarithm multiplies by the second number with each following number in a series. For example, a logarithm with a ratio of 1: 2 would be 1, 2, 4, 8, 16; of 1: 3: 1, 3, 9, 27, 81, and so on. The spiral is two dimensional. One can visualize its three dimensional counterpart, the helix, by viewing the peripheral spiral as close by and the center in the distance or vice versa. The thread of a screw depicts a helical shape. The logarithmic spiral in macrobiotic philosophy is a line connecting One Infinity with a final physical state. Each coil of the spiral depicts a new stage in the process of evolution toward the material. With each half turn of the spiral polarity changes to its opposite. Thus, the spiral shows the interconnectedness of yin and yang, two poles of one continuum. Since the distance between extremes shortens with each new stage, we can see that the process speeds up and causes greater density and heat as it approaches the center. The space between the coils of the spiral going toward the center can be seen as another spiral going in the opposite direction (see Fig. 4).

In the macrobiotic model the spiral of materialization leading to the creation of humanity occurs in seven stages:

1. One Infinity
2. The world of polarization: the bifurcation of One Infinity into two antagonistic yet complementary forces, yin and yang
3. The world of energy or vibration—*ki*
4. The world of preatomic particles
5. The world of elements or nature: soil, water, air
6. The vegetable kingdom
7. The animal kingdom, culminating in humanity

In other words, humankind is the terminus of the spiral of materialization. We begin our return journey to One Infinity from the time of conception. For example, during pregnancy the fetus takes on a more yang, curled up shape, similar to that of half the Tai Chi Tu. Soon after birth the baby is still contracted in shape. Later on it begins to expand, first crawling on all fours (a reflection of our evolutionary connection with apes). It then stands vertically and the child's consciousness begins to develop more rapidly.

The evolution of consciousness is depicted in seven stages that lead back to One Infinity. Macrobiotic philosophy views these stages as levels of judgment. In order, these levels of judgment are—mechanical, sensorial, emotional and aesthetic, intellectual, social, ideological and, ultimately, supreme judgment, or the capacity to transcend all dualities. No stage can be skipped: each one evolves into the next.

Spirals occur throughout nature. They are found within the shapes of galaxies, whirlwinds, tidal waves, and seashells. Branches of a tree grow from a trunk spirally as does the hair from the crown of our head.

The spiral applies to any and all situations. When applied to history, it tells us that our present civilization is fast approaching the end of a spiral of materialization. This process will ultimately develop into a spiral of spiritualization. It will lead to a new, more spiritually directed civilization.

With reference to learning shiatsu, the spiral illustrates why progress may be slow in the beginning, yet accelerates with practice and experience. Since speed implies streamlining, spirallic development involves eliminating the unnecessary. Advanced shiatsu then, does not necessarily mean the addition of new techniques but rather, refinement and simplification. As we learn more precisely where and how to apply pressure, our shiatsu becomes more effective. This principle can be seen in the martial arts. While a technique may be structurally simple, the power of execution comes from hours of training in positioning and timing. In other words, there is depth within simplicity.

A Zen Shiatsu massage expresses the spiral. We begin in the sitting position with the receiver facing away from us. This position facilitates the receiver's concentration on our shiatsu. We progress through three more positions—on the side, stomach, and back, and finish with shiatsu to the *hara*. The hara is the body's center of energy and the massage throughout has been to effect change in the hara. The approach has been from periphery to center.

Ki

The interaction of yin and yang gives rise to the world of vibration or electromagnetic energy. This energy is called *ki* (Chinese: chi). Together, One Infinity, yin and yang, and ki constitute the invisible worlds in the spiral of materialization. Ki is the universal life-force. The terms consciousness, spirit or simply energy all convey the notion of ki. The fact that the ideogram for ki, 氣 is so commonly used in their language demonstrates that traditionally Japanese people have seen life in terms of ki energy. In both Macrobiotics and Zen Shiatsu, ki is an integral concept.

We can distinguish between two basic types of ki:

1. Universal or primal ki—Universal Consciousness
2. The manifestations of primal ki—all phenomena in the relative world

The Japanese often defined relative phenomena by attaching some prefix to the term "ki." For example, in Japanese, weather or "tenki" is comprised of the characters of heaven and ki, while the characters of thunder and ki make up "denki," meaning electricity. Likewise, in classical Chinese medicine that aspect of our body which protects us from external sources of illness is known as Wei Chi or protective chi. The Chinese refer to hereditary factors in one's makeup as "Hsien-Tien-Chi" or inherited ancestral chi.

We can further classify relative phenomena into two basic groups: those possessing more yin ki and those possessing more yang ki. Yin ki represents ki in its more invisible state that we know as spirit or energy. Yang ki represents the more condensed or materialized forms of ki that we call matter. Applying the spiral we can see that they are in essence one and the same. Yin ki could be considered as spiritualized matter and yang ki as physicalized spirit or energy.

In traditional Japan all objects of nature, both animate and inanimate were worshipped as spirit. In the West we often ascribe a gender to or personify animate or even inanimate objects. We might for example refer to our car or boat as "she" and even give it a personal name. In light of the above, one might consider this practice at times as an attempt to define that object's spirit. The more empathy we have for any object, the more likely we are to discern its true spirit or ki nature.

It is a basic principle of Oriental healing that each individual possesses his or her own innate healing power—a power that arises from the balanced flow of the body's ki energy in harmony with the movement of universal ki. Conversely, disease arises when this flow of ki energy becomes distorted. For example, ki can accelerate, slow down, weaken or stagnate.

According to the macrobiotic view, our being consists of two bodies as one: our invisible bioplasmic body or ki constitution which connects us with the world of spirit, and our protoplasmic or physical self, evolving from and nourished by our bioplasmic body.

One's principal connection with universal ki is a spiritual channel that runs vertically through the center of the body. Along this channel are seven major energy centers where ki energy accumulates and is transformed. These transformers are known as *chakras*. From the chakras, channels commonly called meridians carry ki energy to the various internal organs. Meridians of ki energy connect each internal organ with the periphery of the body, passing through the superficial layers of the skin. The meridians of each internal organ link in these outer layers to form two circuits, one for each side of the body. Ki flows along these circuits in endless cycles, ideally, in harmony with the flow of universal ki.

Along each meridian minute holes known as *tsubo* allow ki to enter or exit from the body. From each main meridian a multitude of branches feed ki to each and every cell of the body. The flow of energy along the meridians consists primarily of universal ki. The food we eat, the air we breathe, our emotional state and environmental influences also carry their own varieties of energy which can influence meridian ki flow. Residues of excess and improper food can collect under the superficial layers of the skin as hardened fat that blocks the exchange of ki through the tsubos.

Since we live in a dynamic relative world, ki flow never maintains a balance that is static. Yin is always greater than yang or vice versa. When we observe nature we notice that extreme movement in one direction always generates movement to an equal and opposite extreme. Nature always strives for balance and harmony. Taken as an expression of the order of the universe, one can apply this principle to attain optimum health by reducing extremes found in ki flow along the meridians.

In normal health we experience our being as oneness, the kind of oneness we do not necessarily realize until we lose it. We notice that when we eat something disagreeable we feel uncomfortable in the stomach region. When we have a toothache our attention becomes focused on that tooth until the pain is cleared up. When we lose love we "feel" it in the heart. In each of the above examples, ki energy became focused in a certain area and our mind was drawn to and held on that place until we reestablished a state of harmony.

Mind is infinitely greater than body. However, the mind cannot move with optimum freedom until the mind and body work in harmony. Since, according to classical Chinese medicine, the functioning of the internal organs affects us both physically and psychologically, difficult situations such as those previously mentioned cause distortions in the functioning of the internal organs. These disturbances will in turn be reflected in the flow of ki along the meridians.

There are various ways to restore equilibrium. Adjustment in diet is one of the most fundamental approaches. Basic changes in lifestyle including the environment in which one works or lives may be required. Psychological assistance or emotional support may be needed. In shiatsu we deal directly with the meridians. Knowing where and how to apply pressure, we endeavor to draw the ki flow back into a state of balance.

Aikido master Koichi Tohei refers to ki as "the infinite gathering of infinitely small particles."[5] In macrobiotic terminology, what Tohei speaks of describes a yangizing process. Consequently, in comparing two similar objects, we could say that the one observed to be overall more yang would possess stronger ki.

Let us consider from this viewpoint how diet can affect our outlook. In macrobiotics, classifying all foods according to yin and yang gives us the basic idea of their quality of ki energy. Comparing the two most fundamental food groups, animal and vegetable, the first is the more yang and therefore carries more yang ki. Animals are active, dense and heavy, and nourished by red blood. Their ki energy moves overall in a downward and then outward direction. Conversely, the vegetable kingdom is stationary, grows upward and is nourished by green chlorophyll. However, the consumption of animal food which is extreme yang, requires making a balance with extreme yin such as sugar. By comparison, a diet based on grains and vegetables is more centered.

From another perspective this grain and vegetable regimen is yang compared with the wide diet embracing animal food and sugar, since center is yang and periphery yin. Furthermore, from the spiral of materialization we observe that humanity evolved from the vegetable kingdom. Moreover the ki energy of animal food spirals downward in contrast with that of the vegetable kingdom, which moves upward. Since we are evolving toward the greatest expanse of One Infinity, consumption from the vegetable kingdom is in harmony with our evolution (Fig. 5).

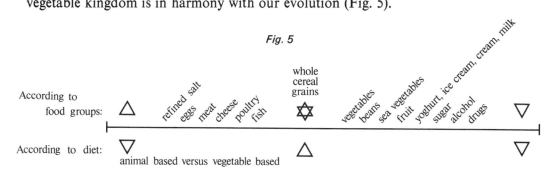

Fig. 5

Thus a grain and vegetable based diet is gathering or yangizing. It possesses stronger ki than an animal food based diet. Although the food groups are more yin, the simplicity of the diet is more yang. One further emphasizes the yang quality by choosing the more yang varieties in each food group, by cooking, and by using salt.

Within human beings, universal ki manifests primarily as mind (yin ki) and body (yang ki). Since we know that yin and yang combined produce energy, we can say that the human entity has its greatest strength when mind and body are unified. However, since mind has infinite potential while body is finite we can see that mind ultimately rules body. We know that the condition of our body reflects in our thinking and that the condition of our mind is reflected in our body condition; but ultimately, mind rules body.

The eating of a macrobiotic diet makes our body strong, which in turn strengthens our mind. Further, eating macrobiotically is eating according to a principle. Principle is a function of the mind, while action a function of the body. By choosing our food consciously, observing its effects and adjusting what we eat accordingly, a macrobiotic approach strengthens our mind. It harmonizes mind and body by drawing the mind into the body.

Ideally, physical expression is a spontaneous manifestation of our mind's intentions. The more refined the integration of mind and body, the closer is the connection with universal ki, and, consequently, the stronger our own ki. Mind and body achieve greatest unification in a state of relaxation, which, as we shall see, means that heaven's force predominates. Mind, or yin ki, too, is more an expression of heaven's than earth's force.

Referring back to Tohei's dictum then, when we exercise we do not need to develop muscular strength to attain physical power. Our most important consideration is to simply concentrate on what we are doing. For example, by putting our mind into a stretch while performing a yoga *asana* we draw the mind into the physical self— uniting mind with body. In like manner, when we give shiatsu we unite mind and body. We bring consciousness into our hands at the point of pressure, as we feel for a living response from the receiver.

In shiatsu we diagnose by touch. We can perceive the quality of ki by the quality of the physical body.

Man and Soil Are Not Two

> "Man patterns after Earth;
> Earth patterns after Heaven;
> Heaven patterns after Tao;
> Tao patterns after Innate Freedom."
>
> Lao Tsu[6]

Open any book dealing with Oriental culture and one soon becomes aware of a constant reference to nature. Expressed either directly or indirectly, nature is revered and the way of nature seen as a guiding force for life. A famous saying in Japanese expresses their relationship with nature: "Shin Do Fuji"—man and soil are not two. The macrobiotic diet is based on this principle. The individual's relationship with nature constitutes his or her fundamental connection with One Infinity.

In macrobiotic philosophy the parallel evolutionary development of nature's plant and animal life is considered significant. Particular animal and vegetable species evolved together as illustrated in Fig. 6.

The most advanced and evolved food is seen to be whole cereal grains. Grains are botanically unique in that they are fruit and seed as one, the center of the food spiral. Ohsawa described grains as the most balanced food. He supported this idea with scientific evidence (e.g., the potassium-sodium ratio of grains closely approximates that found within and surrounding a human cell). The Chinese ideogram for rice 米 is an image of balance in itself. Grains, though rooted to the soil, tend to grow vertically. While earth's nourishment reaches the plant through the roots, heaven's nourishment penetrates it through "antennae," small seed hairs that surround each grain. From this viewpoint we could say that in terms of physical food grains are for hu-

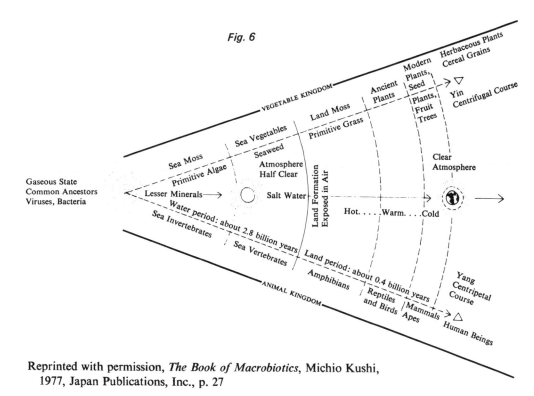

Fig. 6

Reprinted with permission, *The Book of Macrobiotics*, Michio Kushi, 1977, Japan Publications, Inc., p. 27

manity the most direct connection between heaven and earth. For this reason macrobiotic people who wish to develop spiritual clarity will for short periods of time of 3 to 7 days eat a diet consisting primarily of whole cereal grains (supplemented by miso soup, greens, condiments, and tea).

From a macrobiotic perspective grains have helped humankind to develop. When man discovered fire he learned how to cook, making grains suitable for digestion. The vertical growth pattern of grains, transmitted into the human frame, helped posture become more erect. By standing upright, human beings received the forces of heaven and earth more directly. Further, just as grains grow at the top of a stalk, consuming them not only strengthened the spine but also nourished the brain: through the consumption of grains consciousness evolved. Grains have a long storage life, and are the most widely available food on this planet. Another indication that grains constitute the principle food for humanity is found in our tooth structure. We have eight teeth designed for cutting, four for tearing and twenty for crushing. Cutting is suitable for vegetables, approximating 25 percent of a macrobiotic diet. Teeth designed for tearing reflect the consumption of animal food which is approximately 12.5 percent of the diet. Over 60 percent of our teeth are designed for crushing —ideal for whole cereal grains.

Thus, in eating macrobiotically we consume a diet of whole natural foods centered on grains and vegetables. Ideally all food is grown in our local region, within a maximum distance of 500 miles of our home. When eating animal food, fish is chosen over meat, chicken, eggs or dairy. Viewing Fig. 6, we see that the biological distance between fish and humans is much greater than that between other mammals and humans. When humans eat fish, fish becomes human. When humans eat meat, humans become more animal: one's development is hindered since the polarity lessens. Since humanity is the terminus of a spiral of materialization, eating animal food in excess goes against the flow or will of the universe. This way of life ultimately leads to an unnatural or untimely death. Moreover, since the evolution of animals is moving downward toward the spiral's material center, overconsumption of animal food leads to attachment and possessiveness. It leads to a life of attachment to material acquisition, and blocks the individual's progress toward humanity's ultimate destiny of absolute freedom.

2. Yin and Yang and Life's Axes

In this section I will endeavor to show how the traditional cultures of Japan and China developed along a different "axis" than modern industrialized nations as a result of their different diets. Let us again compare heaven's force and earth's force for a better understanding (Table 2):

Table 2

	Heaven's Force unifies integrates	Earth's Force differentiates causes decomposition
Moves Toward:	inside, a point, bottom, back, center	outside, front, periphery, away from a point
Predominates:	when stationary in colder months in mountainous regions in overcast, wet weather at new moon from late afternoon until night in confined or enclosed spaces	when moving in warmer months in valleys, on plains in sunny, bright weather at full moon from early morning until early afternoon in open spaces
Creates:	precision simplicity refinement warmth punctuality	 complexity multiplicity coolness tardiness
Promotes:	relaxation/thought when sitting relaxation/sleep when lying down	desire to move when stationary desire to arise when lying down inability to sleep
Nourishes or Creates in the Human Being:	mind bioplasmic body (invisible) the inner life principle character, formality, discipline structure skeletal, nervous systems	body protoplasmic or physical body the senses action personality, informality shape digestive system

The predominant movements of heaven's force and earth's force in relation to the Earth (see Fig. 1) can be depicted as two axes along which we live our lives:

1. A vertical axis descending from top to bottom—uniting heaven and earth, and dominated by heaven's force
2. A horizontal axis moving across the planet, dominated by earth's force

A vertical axis is the axis of unification. It is primary, yang, and positive. Since earth is derived from heaven, a horizontal axis is secondary. It is the axis of differentiation—yin and negative. We understand this perspective intuitively when we describe the directions of a compass, always first from north to south, then east to west. A vertical axis could be considered the spiritual axis, since intuition, the invisible energy of heaven, predominates. A horizontal axis could be described as the material axis: it carries the energy of the physical earth. A vertical axis implies superior-inferior relationships and suggests an axis of quality. Conversely, a horizontal axis conveys the idea of expansion; it suggests an axis of quantity, and deals with equality and inequality.

Let us imagine a group of people on each axis. Since the vertical axis implies integration of the forces of heaven and earth, we can see that those on the primary, vertical axis would be unified within. The situation would be akin to listeners tuning in their receivers to the same radio station, and picking up the same signal of empathy, cooperation, and common sense. On the secondary, horizontal axis, earth's dominating force would emphasize the expansive tendencies of each individual. They are therefore likely to first separate from each other but ultimately to intersect or come together. We can illustrate this principle with the example of new settlers in a land, who move out, stake a land claim, and establish boundaries. Once these individual boundaries are established, any traveler is then viewed, depending upon the circumstances and inclination as either guest or intruder. Horizontal movement then suggests competition, conflict or greed on the one hand, or sympathy or pity on the other. Refinement along a vertical axis, that is, of heaven's and earth's forces within each individual, ultimately leads back to Nothingness—oneness with the Absolute. This proc s is represented in each human being as degrees of spiritual power, according to the level of refinement of these forces. As there is no direct connection with heaven and earth, movement along a horizontal axis depends upon self-power. Since earth's force causes decomposition, self-powered movement away from the vertical axis ultimately ends in spiritual decay.

Life on the two axes can be seen as waves. We could take for example a high and narrow wave (high amplitude and frequency), and a low and wide wave (low amplitude and frequency). The higher one rises on a vertical axis, the less one expands horizontally and vice versa. It is difficult to move in both vertical and horizontal directions at once. At different times of the day, at different times of our lives, we tend to live on one axis more than the other. Comparing the lifestyles of various individuals, we can identify innate tendencies to emphasize one axis over the other. When we compare cultures we can see the same qualities. Let us examine modern industrialized nations, and the traditional, agricultural, vegetarian-based cultures of the Far East, with special reference to Japan and China.

From a macrobiotic point of view the core difference between the two aforemen-

tioned cultures is diet—the heavy consumption of animal food by the modern industrialized nations versus the vegetable based diet of the traditional Far East. As we have
seen, the energy of animal food is yang, moving downward toward the earth. Within
the individual this movement leads to attachment, possessiveness, and stagnation. As
a consequence this person seeks for release, or yin. Such release would be movement
along a horizontal axis, the axis dominated by earth's expanding force. Since the
consumption of animal food leads to desire for extreme yin, a simpler diet of grains
and vegetables can be seen in contrast as centered, or yang. Thus, being predominantly vegetarian, the initial movement of traditional Oriental people was toward the
center. However, while remaining rooted to the soil, the overall energy of the vegetable kingdom is directed upward.

Thus we have two basic movements, which can be graphically depicted (Fig. 7):

Fig. 7

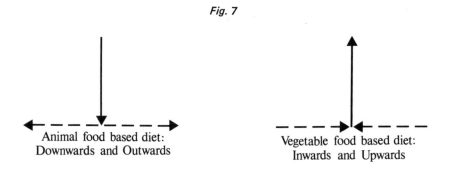

Animal food based diet:
Downwards and Outwards

Vegetable food based diet:
Inwards and Upwards

Through their dietary habits, cultures demonstrate an organic tendency to favor one
axis over the other. The consumption of animal food led to a horizontal axis culture,
while a vegetable food based diet led to a vertical axis civilization.

Let us compare these cultures diagramatically (Fig. 8):

Fig. 8

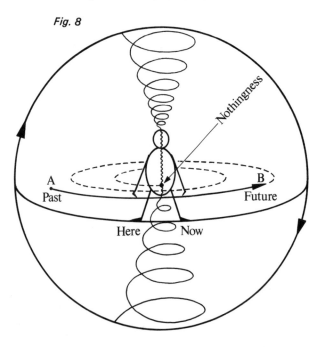

Movement along a horizontal differentiating axis from A to B has given rise to analytic and linear thinking; it manifests in such concepts as past, future, and progress. God is seen as existing outside the individual in another world above. Horizontal axis people see the earth as something below or inferior to the human being, something to be conquered, exploited, possessed. The downward energy of animal food has influenced these people to seek within the earth for energy and resources. Subconsciously they reach toward heaven in a material way by using these resources to build telescopes and space ships. While they express an interest in both heaven and earth, overall they see little or no connection with or between either world. Each person is on his own. This axis is visualized in the extreme by the automobile: its horizontal thrust emphasizes self-power, individuality, and speed.

Nourished largely by grains and vegetables, ancient Orientals looked upward. Earth's force discovered heaven's downward force. Heaven's force is infinitely greater than earth's force; earth's force is attracted to heaven's force. Paradoxically, heaven's force directs the individual back down to a point. Growth in consciousness depends upon concentration on whatever one is doing. There is a harmonizing of heaven's and earth's forces, of the invisible with the visible, of the spiritual with the material. God lives within. The harmony of the two worlds appears in the unification of mind with body, of thoughts with behavior. Daily life becomes spiritual practice. Heaven can be realized on earth.

Further, unification of mind and body requires that one live in harmony with the surrounding environment. Rooted to the soil, these people became sensitive to the movements of the universe around them. Adapting to nature's rhythms through subtle adjustments in their diet and manner of life ensured harmony with the Tao, a life in the here and now. Integrating yin and yang, they were able to internalize the unique principle and apply it to all facets of their lives. The vertical axis is realized in the extreme by sitting in deep meditation.

We symbolize negative by a straight horizontal line —. Yet positive is indicated by a cross +, not by a vertical line only | . In other words true positivism embraces the negative. It needs to be emphasized that we move on both axes and that movement along both axes ensures a fulfilling life. What is important is the order in which we implement them into our lives. Since earth evolved from heaven our first step is to harmonize along a vertical axis. Again in the words of D.T. Suzuki:

> The intellect looks outwardly, takes an "objective" view of things. It is unable to look inwardly so as to grasp the thing in its inwardness. It attempts to achieve a unitive view of the world by what is known as the objective method. This objective method may work well, but only when the inside view has first been taken hold of. For the unifying principle lies inside and not outside. It is not something we arrive at; it is where we start. It is not the outcome of postulation; it is what makes postulation possible.[7]

Earth's force horizontal axis qualities should be carried out within the context of heaven's force vertical axis qualities. Analytic, conceptual thinking has its role within the context of an intuitive mode of understanding. Materialism has a place within the context of a spiritual view.

To fully understand the two axes, there is another aspect that needs to be considered. While the ground at our feet appears flat, we know the earth to be actually round. In the same way, we can see that movement from A to B is also a spiral, as movement from B is ultimately a circle returning to A. Moreover, from the spiral of spiritualization we can see that all people are ultimately moving in the same direction. However, the wider the diet, the slower is movement toward the center and direct connection with the forces of heaven and earth, and ultimately with One Infinity.

When we change from a typical modern to a macrobiotic diet we are likely to soon notice feeling lighter, more optimistic, and less attached. Moreover, we become aware of the effects of our daily diet on body and mind. We can see a relationship between physical well-being and our emotions and frame of mind. This self-observation may be regarded as the first stage on a spiral moving toward the center, of change from a horizontal to a vertical axis way of life.

Religious people often speak of the "inner life," "God-given inner strength," "an inner light"—all images of the spiral's center. By meditation and other spiritual practices one can move even closer to this center. As the Buddhist masters tell us, in advanced states of meditation "body/mind drops off." That is, body sensation and linear thought disappear. Such body/mind is more a product of earth's force. Only the spirit body nourished by heaven's force remains. Another passage from Lao Tsu illustrates this process:

> To learn, one increases day by day;
> To cultivate Tao, one reduces day by day.
> Reduce and reduce and keep on reducing,
> Till the state of non-action is reached.
> With non-action there is nothing that cannot be done.[8]

Ultimately the individual returns to Nothingness, oneness with the Absolute.

Observations of traditional Japanese culture offer interesting insights that further demonstrate this process. We first note that Japan is an island country. Historically, until this century Japan was never conquered and foreign influences were absorbed by choice. Islands are yang compared with continents not only because of smaller size but also because of the surrounding salty seas. Also, islands approximate Suzuki's image of the universe as a circle without a circumference: while the perimeter cannot be seen, its all inclusive influence can be felt.

In addition we note the following:

1. Japan is a small predominantly mountainous country, supporting a very large population on a limited area of inhabitable space. It is subject to periodic natural disasters from earthquakes and typhoons.
2. Japan is one race of people with a long history.
3. People traditionally ate mild variations of the same diet. It was quite simple, based on grains and vegetables, and comparatively salty.
4. Japan has had a scarcity of natural resources and domestically grown food.
5. Until this century the people were small in height and centered in their hara. Western people by comparison have tended to be centered in their chest.
6. Japan experiences a four season climate.

All of these factors either are or create yang. One aspect of yang is the ability to absorb yin while still maintaining the original yang core. Japan dramatically demonstrates this quality. No other country in the history of civilization has ever so thoroughly absorbed the greatest of two opposite cultures, namely China and the West. However, they have preserved the essence of their original culture, while blending these outside influences to become distinctly their own.

Further, since the Japanese environment is so yang, we can expect whatever has been imported to undergo a further yangizing process. This process is reflected in the simplification, precision, refinement, and miniaturization we see in the Japanese products flooding Western shores. Modern Japan is very much a horizontal axis culture, with its economic and industrial power reaching to every corner of the globe. Still the spiritual legacy handed down from generation to generation has been a guiding force in the way Western culture has been adapted. While modern Japanese culture appears very Western, the way of practice is distinctly Japanese. Even though much of its meaning has been forgotten, traditional culture remains pervasive, and still highly respected. It exists both alongside and integrated with Western ways.

Through various customs and practices still carried on today, we can gain a glimpse of the traditional Japanese mind. We may begin with communication.

When Japanese people greet each other they bow. This practice shows the predominating influence of heaven's force—a contracting movement from north to south. The communication is vertical: it emphasizes mental vibration from one to the other. In the West one looks the other straight in the eye and firmly shakes hands. We could call this greeting horizontal communication. In the same way a Westerner "takes a person for their word," while the Japanese place more emphasis on the *feeling behind* the words. The former once again could be seen as horizontal communication versus vertical or intuitive communication in the latter. We notice that they refer to themselves as part of a collective "We Japanese" which shows a large view in comparison with "I." Japanese people will have little trouble agreeing with you, nodding their head from north to south as they answer "yes, yes." However, it is rare to see a horizontal movement implying "no," and further we find most Japanese people indeed have difficulty in actually saying "no." In this case "yes" reflects the positive vertical axis while "no" the negative horizontal axis. At some point in a conversation one will be asked when they are leaving Japan, rarely if ever when one arrived. The former is yang as it implies definition in time, while the latter is yin since the length of the visit is open-ended. When a Japanese signals someone from a distance to come to them, the arm will be extended horizontally, palm down, and bent downward at the wrist; the movement of the arm would be downward. Exactly the opposite would be the case in the West. Once again the former is yang, latter yin. Finally, the Japanese tend to appear quite shy and reticent. This manner is yang compared with the more open and expressive ways of the West. It suggests that the force coming in is greater than the force going out.

In writing the Chinese and Japanese begin, on what is to the West the last page. The writing is vertical, down the page; it begins in the top right hand corner, with the next line to the left of the first. In this form we see both vertical and counterclockwise movements, exactly the opposite to those of the West. Further, when a letter is addressed, Japanese begin by writing the name of the country first, then state, town, street, street number, family name, first name. In this order we clearly see movement from periphery to center, the direction of heaven's force. The case in the West is again exactly the opposite.

In traditional paintings, especially the Zen Buddhist works in black ink, we notice the paintings are most often vertical and comparatively small. The subject matter occupies a small space, often toward the bottom, leaving the remainder of the painting relatively empty. Generally the paintings are a landscape or scene of nature. This subject strongly contrasts with Western religious works. Paintings found in the Vatican for example, a central expression of Western religious images, are not only huge in size by comparison, but most often horizontal in shape. The subjects are nearly always people, with figures filling the whole canvas. Moreover, the paintings are in color and many portray bloody battle scenes in the name of God. The Orient once again demonstrates more the influence of heaven's force while the West that of earth.

Various art forms are practices of training in the "Way," or Dō (Japanese for Tao). They include Shodō, the way of writing; Sadō, the way of tea; and Kadō, the way of flower arrangement. In these practices we are likely to find much ritual, precision, refinement, and attention to detail. They focus on the most subtle of movements. In ritual there is a slowing down of earth's force and consequently a maximization of heaven's force. Precision, refinement, and attention to detail are all the outcome of this yangizing process, drawing the mind into the action. Often the practitioner is stationary, sitting in seiza. Also most practices in the "Way" are carried on indoors within confined spaces.

The Japanese home emphasizes the internal. Houses are often surrounded by high fences that seal off the outside world. Windows have been traditionally made only of a translucent white rice paper. This kind of window shields out the external: one's attention is directed inward. An effort is made to draw nature into the home in the form of miniaturized plants and rock gardens.

The extreme yang environment of Japan has even produced a distinct form of violence. The Japanese, for a long period, by choice continued to use swords in combat while the West employed rifles.[9] In Japanese swordsmanship, the blade is raised above the head and the strike is made vertically and downward. Conversely, the trajectory of a bullet is horizontal. Even in Western fencing the strike is more horizontal than vertical. Japanese culture in general appears to have produced a high incidence of self-inflicted violence. Even today reports in the daily press of suicides are almost as common as accounts of murder in the West. Often suicide involves whole families and in some cases extended families. A common form of suicide, jumping from tall buildings, clearly shows a subconscious surrender to heaven's force.

Finally, Zazen, sitting in meditation, clearly shows the emphasis of heaven's force. First, the posture of Zazen is more yang than kneeling in prayer, since sitting is more contracted than kneeling. Second, the movement of the hands in Zazen is downward resting in the lap, while in kneeling in prayer the hands are pointed upward. Third, basic instruction in Zazen emphasizes concentration on the breath: the mind follows the breath to one point in the lower abdomen, known as the *tanden*. Fourth, the practitioner of Zazen sits to discover "Who am I?" By comparison, Western philosophy has traditionally begun with the question "What is Man?" In the former, study is directed toward the person practicing, while in the latter there is separation between Man and the person studying Man. The Eastern represents an inwardly directed unifying force—heaven's force. The Western represents a differentiating force moving away from the individual. This is earth's force.

Overall then, we see two interrelated movements in Japanese culture. We see movement from periphery to center or from bigger to smaller. We see movement going toward the inside or toward the self. These movements suggest heaven's force predominates in traditional Japanese culture.

Understanding this approach to Oriental culture is extremely relevant to the practice of shiatsu. Heaven's force directs the mind to a point. In shiatsu, that point is literally a point. It is a tsubo or pressure point. We know that the origins of classical Chinese medicine go back at least several thousand years. We may speculate that the people of those early times, influenced by a grain and vegetable based diet, readily tuned into heaven's force. They were inspired to develop a system of medicine that (1) dealt with heaven's invisible energy, and (2) involved points on the surface of the body (tsubos), points that were an integral part of this invisible energy system. For a therapeutic treatment this system employed acupuncture and massage working on the tsubos. Since Japan is a more yang environment than China, the kind of massage that became Japanese was more simplified or yang than the Chinese counterpart. Chinese massage used pressure points, often employing movement over these points. It also employed kneading, tapping and rubbing techniques. By contrast, shiatsu, the Japanese style of massage, focused largely on stationary pressure to these points.

3. How Does Zen Shiatsu Work?

The commonly held view considers shiatsu as "acupuncture without needles," with pressure performing the same function as needles. It suggests that invisible currents of electromagnetic energy emanate from the giver's fingertips. By knowing where and how to apply shiatsu, according to this view, we can inject or withdraw ki from the receiver's body. For example, by applying pressure to an area of stiffness, the giver's ki would melt away this condition. Or by applying pressure to an area that feels empty, that area would be filled with ki emanating from the giver. In this approach effectiveness is sometimes equated with strong pressure.

While ki may indeed emanate from the giver's fingertips it may not be in this way or only in this way that shiatsu works. Masunaga's approach to emphasize another side, that the healing ki of shiatsu *lies within the quality or spirit of the touch in itself*, as compared with the idea of some invisible current that emanates from the touch. That is, his approach focuses on how the receiver responds to touch.

As we have seen, shiatsu is stationary pressure to a point. More precisely, in Zen Shiatsu we apply "natural leaning pressure." Natural pressure is the vertical application in a relaxed state of the giver's hands to the receiver's body. It is the pressure of heaven's force which is yang. Leaning pressure is the horizontal movement of the body from one hand to the other to apply deep pressure. This movement contains the influence of earth's force. In other words, the giver harmonizes yin and yang, heaven's and earth's force within, at the point of pressure. However, body movement follows the application of the hands. Further, in Zen Shiatsu we *always* apply both hands to the receiver's body. Yet one hand, when possible the left, always remains stationary, supporting the other hand, which moves. Again, movement follows the application of the stationary hand. Moreover, this moving hand simply moves from one point to the next. At each point, the moving hand stops, and by the leaning movement of the body stationary pressure is applied. Upon the release of pressure, the moving hand maintains body contact, sliding to the next point where it once again stops, and the same procedure of applying pressure is repeated. Thus we see that the dominating force in Zen Shiatsu is heaven's force, and that movement, the influence of earth's force, takes place within the context of heaven's force. We see in Zen Shiatsu, in two ways, body movement and arm movement, vertical and horizontal axes; yet the horizontal axis role is within the context of a vertical axis one. In addition, since heaven's force is far greater than earth's force, we can see the importance of the "non-doing" stationary hand.

Heaven's force predominates at night or when we are still. At these times, we open up to the influence of heaven's force, which induces relaxation. In a vertical sitting posture this force activates the mind. In a horizontal lying down position it causes us to sleep. In the latter state we are consuming heaven's force. It recharges our batteries; it revitalizes us. Zen Shiatsu is in itself, by the technique of application, this heaven's force. It causes the muscles and flesh to relax. Tension drops away and this yang pressure connects with the yin invisible ki constitution from which the physical body arises. By connecting with the ki constitution we connect with the receiver's spirit. Further, in a state of relaxation, shiatsu becomes for the receiver a kind of meditation. Yang attracts yin. The yang pressure of shiatsu draws the receiver's mind, by comparison yin, into the body at the point of pressure. The receiver's mind is attracted to a point, and it follows the pressure from one point to the next throughout the entire body. Point by point the receiver's mind once more unites with body. Sometimes this pressure may even cause the receiver to almost fall asleep. In this state, shiatsu becomes even more effective and the giver opens the receiver to even deeper, more yin states of consciousness.

We can now compare shiatsu with Western massage. Modern Western culture lives predominantly on a horizontal axis. Since this axis is dominated by earth's force it emphasizes movement, and that movement is toward the periphery. In terms of the human entity it means emphasis on the outer physical as opposed to the inner spiritual body. Exercise regimens, emphasizing the muscles and cardiovascular system are followed to develop this physical body. Oriental exercise regimens by comparison are internal. They focus on developing ki. In like manner, the kind of massage that has arisen in the West employs manipulation to this physical self, with such motions across the body as rubbing, pinching, and kneading to effect changes in the muscles and blood flow. The massage is peripheral (Fig. 9).

Fig. 9

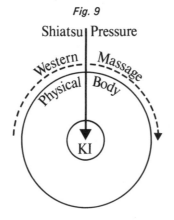

In the same manner Western medicine treats symptoms that appear on the surface. However, this peripheral body evolved from invisible ki. Neither Western massage nor Western medicine deal directly with the origins of the problems appearing in the physical body, which according to traditional Oriental medicine are caused by distortions in the flow of ki energy. Moreover, whereas Western massage, often called "bodywork," deals solely with the physical body, shiatsu, by connecting with the receiver's ki, not only treats the physical body, but through the physical connects with the receiver's mind. The origin of disease is in the mind.

The spiral of materialization tells us that the spiritual and the material lie on one continuum. In Masunaga's theory, the body condition is seen to reflect the individual's psychological state. Masunaga observed two opposite extremes in the distortion of ki flow. These conditions are called *kyo* and *jitsu*. Kyo refers to an underactive state, a condition of deficiency or emptiness, while jitsu refers to an overactive state, a condition of excess or fullness. Mentally, kyo reflects what we have chosen to conceal or ignore. Others are not likely to discern this condition from a person's appearance. Likewise, in the physical body, one cannot easily detect a kyo condition by simple observation of the body surface. Only upon the application of pressure can we clearly see that the muscles in that area are flaccid, or lacking in tone and resilience. Conversely, a jitsu condition reflects a psychological state where energy is concentrated, what we focus much thought on, what we are most interested in and probably what we are most keen to share with others. Likewise, in the physical body a jitsu condition projects from the normal body surface, easy to recognize. It is full of energy. The muscles are full and round in a appearance. They may be either resilient or tight and stiff.

In Zen Shiatsu we literally point out these conditions to the receiver. Along a kyo meridian for example, we hold stationary pressure on a point for a prolonged period. We could liken conventional shiatsu theory on this technique to a car at a gas pump filling up an empty tank. That is, from the giver's hands or fingers, ki emanates to fill an emptiness. The Zen Shiatsu view is quite different. Nothing is added from the outside. The meridian is empty because psychologically the receiver has chosen to ignore some aspect of his or her life and it is this attitude that manifests in this physical condition. The giver holds on the point to simply draw attention in the receiver's mind to the "depth" of the problem. The giver is trying to draw the receiver's mind back. The greater the weakness, the longer and deeper is pressure held on the point, since the receiver is slow to acknowledge this condition. The receiver's mind wants to be somewhere else. Through touch the giver is trying to say something like, "Please be aware of this!" With a jitsu condition energy is moving outward, but the giver's pressure is going against it. Force confronts force. Yang repels yang. Such pressure elicits a quick response. Jitsu represents the abiding mind, the mind that has become attached to something. The giver's pressure in this situation is saying something like "You're stuck, please move on!" What we are doing through the touch of Zen Shiatsu is sending a message, we might even say, giving advice.

The challenge of Zen Shiatsu is three-fold. Through touch, how can we apply pressure so that the receiver will (1) "hear" our message, (2) accept it, and (3) act upon it? Our pressure must be strong enough for the receiver to concentrate on what we are doing. We do not want his or her mind to wander elsewhere. Conversely, it must not be too strong, in which case the muscles will tense up, preventing the penetration of our pressure. The strength relates to the hearing, the gentleness to the acceptance. However, acting upon our advice automatically follows acceptance. For where the mind moves, ki moves. In a kyo state, the way pressure is applied causes ki to move to the point, in a jitsu state away from the point. In Zen Shiatsu, the energy that moves to the kyo area comes from the jitsu area; in this way a balanced state is reestablished. Nothing is added on or withdrawn by external pressure.

Technical virtuosity and theoretical knowledge are important aspects of shiatsu. However, they are only stages along the spiral, secondary to, and necessary for, enhancing the quality of touch. Above all, Zen Shiatsu is the spirit or language of touch.

Zen Shiatsu — The Language of Touch

Touch is symbolic. Intuitively, we all know how to convey a message through touch. When we wish to issue a warning to someone, one hand is sufficient. Fingers prod the receiver. The inference is heightened awareness and possibly separation. If a person is asleep and we wish to wake them, again one hand only is enough. With a clasping motion, perhaps to an arm, we may shake them. Movement causes the receiver to awaken from their reverie.

Love and caring are different. To display affection we embrace with both hands. If that affection is deep love, then the hands tend to remain stationary. We draw or are drawn closer to the loved one and we hold for a period of time. If the affection is sensual, then quite probably the hands will move.

Consider some different forms of displaying affection. We could take for example a situation where our partner, or someone else we really care about, is doing something, we clearly see to be harmful to them, and we wish to bring it to their attention. In this predicament, we face the other person. Both hands may grasp the receiver's upper arms, and along with an expression such as "Can't you understand what I am trying to say?," the receiver is shaken forward and backward. In a more hypothetical example, the one we love has just passed on yet we do not want them to die. Perhaps we would lightly clasp the upper arms and with very gentle shaking motions utter something like "Don't go, please don't go!"

From these examples we can see that we intuitively use prodding, shaking, and motion to stimulate action. Two hands applied to another convey love, caring, or affection. Holding for a period of time conveys depth of such affection.

In light of the above, we can see in Zen Shiatsu, how the way we touch conveys a message to the receiver. In Zen Shiatsu we always apply both hands to the receiver's body. Straight away we imply unity and that we are giving of our all. Holding pressure, the prolonged application of shiatsu to a point, suggests involvement and the depth of caring. One hand always remains stationary supporting the moving one. The stationary hand conveys the message of support. However, the way that hand is held also implies a message. If the hand is applied firmly it implies firm support, loosely —wishy-washy support. The supporting hand can be applied close to or at a distance from the moving hand. Closely applied support can indicate that support is actually "close at hand." At a distance it can imply that we support the receiver but he or she has his or her own freedom. It may also imply a lack of real support. If our shiatsu is precise in application it indicates clarity of expression, figuratively and literally, getting to the point. If the pressure is sharp it may imply overly direct communication. If it is too strong the receiver's reaction of bodily tension may indicate that the "message" is more than he or she can handle. If throughout the massage we always apply just the right pressure, enough to keep the receiver's mind on the point, yet not so strong that he or she tenses up (implying that he or she does not wish to hear what we have to say), in this state there is real rapport between giver and receiver.

We could continue these illustrations on and on. Communication through touch can be subtle. All the nuances of touch add up to our message. The effectiveness of this message depends not only upon what is said but also the quality, condition, and spirit of the person saying it. Our message and the way we convey it must be just right for each receiver.

The Relationship of Macrobiotics and Zen Shiatsu

Traditionally both the Japanese and Chinese people consumed a diet that was largely macrobiotic: a diet of locally grown natural foods, centered around whole cereal grains and vegetables. Through their philosophy, literature and traditional practices, we can see that their view of life and consequently their way of life was macrobiotic. They began with the largest view and came down to the smallest. They tuned into heaven's force, and endeavored to harmonize their life on earth with the way of heaven. From this mind, kinds of massage evolved that were suitable for these people. Shiatsu was one outcome. From this perspective let us now focus on the giver and receiver in a Western context.

With regard to the receiver we can clearly see a different kind of body that develops on a Westerner who consumed a standard modern diet and that same person after following a macrobiotic regimen for a period of time. More than likely the former body would be less flexible, and the flesh, ligaments, and muscles more dense, hard, stiff and heavy. The Western diet develops the physical body at the expense of the spiritual body. The tsubos become blocked, preventing the interchange through these holes of the body's ki with universal ki. Consequently, stagnation arises. Sometimes when such people receive shiatsu for the first time the experience may be uncomfortable. Shiatsu is yang and their overall body condition is too yang. Yang repels yang. Thus pain or discomfort may arise. It may take a number of massages before they are used to and respond positively to shiatsu. In addition, it is not uncommon for these people to find difficulty relaxing. They may anticipate the giver's next move and adjust their body accordingly, independent of the giver's actions. For example, if an arm is raised, it is quite possible that if the giver lets go, the arm will remain suspended in midair, when it should naturally fall to the side. This kind of unconscious tension inhibits the possibility of effective shiatsu.

By comparison, better results can be obtained from shiatsu with a person who lives and eats macrobiotically. Their flesh, though strong and resilient, is less dense or hard. When giving shiatsu, ki moves more easily in the macrobiotic than the non-macrobiotic person and consequently the individual responds more positively to such a massage.

By following a macrobiotic diet and way of life, the receiver can reinforce the benefits gained through shiatsu. Whether the receiver is eating macrobiotically or not, the practitioner can in all confidence make individual recommendations based on macrobiotic principles. The macrobiotic approach is universal, appropriate for all people. The macrobiotic practitioner's prescription pad is dietary and way of life education based on the natural order. It is an education for sound physical, mental, and spiritual well-being.

For the giver of shiatsu, a macrobiotic diet and way of life will better enable him or her to grasp the principles of shiatsu technique. Too often, those who eat an excess of animal food feel the need to use strength, to push or pull, to apply abnormally strong pressure and to apply pressure before applying proper support. There may be a lack of empathy for the receiver. In the giver's mind it is the giver who is healing the receiver. This mind arises out of a horizontal axis life, one that sees no intimate connection between the individual, and heaven and earth, one that emphasizes self-power. Such a view gradually disappears as one's diet changes. The effectiveness of the easy way, of natural leaning pressure in a relaxed state, becomes more obvious.

For the giver of shiatsu, the macrobiotic diet and way of life can have even further meaning. To understand this meaning we need to discuss the Zen of Zen Shiatsu.

The Zen of Zen Shiatsu

Whether we express it as identity, two-as-one, or two phenomena or beings as not-two, Zen relates to the experience of oneness. It is a realization of oneness between the individual and the Absolute, a true awareness of the oneness of all. By calling his style of massage Zen Shiatsu, Masunaga implied that the experience of Zen can be realized through the practice of Zen Shiatsu. We shall focus on this state purely in terms of the giver.

Zen Shiatsu is a meridian systems technique: that is, the practitioner applies pressure to a number of points along a line. Some of these points may be tsubos, some not. While stationary pressure is applied to each point, the overall treatment is very dynamic; pressure is applied to numerous points over the body's surface. It is a style with a distinct form or procedure, where one movement naturally flows into the next. It is a comprehensive approach and it is yin and yang in motion. No matter what the person's condition, the same basic pattern or form is followed for each receiver. Within that overall form, specific adjustments are made for each person's condition.

In this chapter we have seen in various ways how Zen Shiatsu expresses the principle of Wu-Wei; non-doing or non-interference. There is no pushing or pulling, only leaning and pressing. Moreover, in the transfer from giver to receiver we do not consider it our primary goal to add to or withdraw from the receiver's ki. The receiver is a holistic entity with his or her own innate healing power. When the giver applies pressure the goal is to stimulate the receiver's ki to move and to show the receiver to where that ki can be redirected. The deficiency in one area is restored to a state of balance by drawing the receiver's own ki from an area of excess to that of deficiency. Balance, harmony, oneness and wholeness are reestablished. Thus, the crux of Zen Shiatsu is touch, to apply pressure in such a way that the receiver responds to our touch, to change within at a subconscious level.

In Zen Shiatsu, the giver's mind moves into the hands to feel for a response from the receiver, at the point of pressure, and the receiver's mind is drawn to that point. In other words, if one's shiatsu is effective, the minds of giver and receiver become one at the point of pressure. If this state continues throughout the massage then a rapport will arise between giver and receiver. In this state Zen can be experienced. However, from a Zen point of view when this experience does not take place, the giver needs to self reflect. The giver must consider the changes to be made within to bring about a better outcome.

The receiver then, is a mirror of the giver's condition and inspires the giver to further develop his or herself. To the macrobiotic person, one's condition depends upon one's whole way of life including diet; it is based on an understanding of yin and yang, of the order of the universe. By improving one's way of life, one's shiatsu becomes more refined and effective.

From this view shiatsu can be seen as a Dō, as a training in the Way. The goal of such training is to become one with the Tao and to consequently express the Tao. The giver as an entity within his or herself becomes a channel of Universal spirit; the will of heaven takes over and one's shiatsu becomes Universal massage.

For the practitioner who chooses this path, the macrobiotic way of Zen Shiatsu leads, through touch, in the words of D.T. Suzuki, to a "real understanding of reality and the experience of Enlightenment."

Chapter 2

Macrobiotic Cosmology

The Five Phases of Energy Transformation

Fig. 10

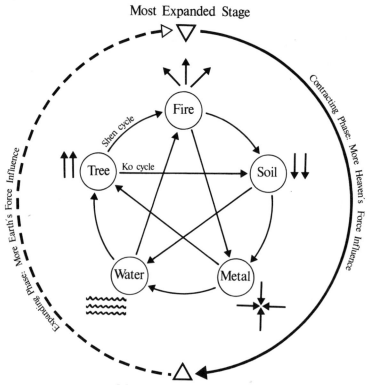

While yin and yang represent the two poles of One Infinity, stages of change are recognized between both extremes. In Japanese this theory is known as "Yin-Yang-Go-Gyō." Though commonly translated as the Five Elements, the Five Transformations or Five Phases of change would be more appropriate since, as we can see from the literal translation "yin yang five to go," movement is implied. The ancient Chinese called these five transformations Tree, Fire, Soil, Metal, and Water. These naturally occurring phenomena are used to represent universal qualities of energy. This earthly symbolism demonstrates Oriental qualities in our model of life's axes described in the previous chapter.

The Eastern psyche, contrasted with that of the West, can be observed when one considers the symbolism of their respective astrological systems. These systems are compared by Lama Govinda, a renowned Buddhist adept and scholar:

When the Greeks identified the planets with certain gods [Mars the god of war, Venus the goddess of love] they projected into the sky qualities of their own psychic experience symbolized in the images of their gods. This was a genuine procedure derived from an inner reality . . . In ancient China, however these equally experienced tendencies (of human emotions) [Year of the Tiger, Boar, Sheep] were not projected into the starry sky, but were retained in our earthly surroundings.[1]

According to our model of life's axes (pp. 28–35), the Greeks displayed an expanding horizontal axis culture by projecting a personal quality into a world outside of their own. The Chinese conversely, living more on a heaven's force-dominated vertical axis, could see the universe in the ground at their feet.

This direct connection of heaven and earth can also be seen in their political system. John Blofeld, a noted authority on Taoism and Chinese culture, writes on this outlook:

The Chinese people have been called a materialistic people on the grounds that the popular conception of the heavenly regions is of an astonishingly close replica of the structure of the Chinese Empire in the world below. However, this judgment ought to be reversed, the traditional Chinese view being that the entire universe is composed of spirit and that the Chinese Empire was a replica of heaven, not the other way around.[2]

Again according to Lao Tsu, "Man patterns after Earth" and "Earth patterns after Heaven."[3]

In Five Transformation Theory, this pattern has all phenomena classified into one of five phases.

There are four aspects of the theory that we need to consider: the symbolic nature of each quality of energy; the correspondences of each symbol; the relationship between the different phases of energy; and finally, the application of this system to healing.

The Five Transformation Theory can be represented on an axis model. The correspondences of each phase of change can be viewed as lying along five vertical axes, occupying according to their nature, different planes of existence on each axis. In essence, all correspondences on each axis would intrinsically carry the same quality of energy. Conversely, relationships of each quality of energy to another, since they lie on a cyclical plane of movement, can be considered horizontally: one quality of energy supports or controls another.

The Symbolic Nature of Each Quality of Energy

One can theorize that the Five Transformation system arose from the penetrating observation of ancient sages who discerned this pattern throughout nature and ultimately within themselves—a microcosm of the macrocosm.

We can emulate the ancients. We can look at each symbol in its natural state. We can take a tree for example, observe its character, and see how its qualities appear within a person. These observations of nature will help us to understand the traditional correspondences (p. 46) as well as further behavioral correspondences suggested in Chapter 4.

Tree Nature Energy

Tree nature is symbolic of vegetation. It has an overall tendency to grow upward and outward. Thus, ascension and expansion are basic qualities of this energy.

To gain a more complete picture we can observe other qualities of trees in their natural state. Beginning underground as a seed, trees grow from darkness into light and grow toward the light. Trees have roots, a trunk, joints, branches, leaves, fruit and seeds, rings which tell of its age, and a skin of bark. Trees can be seen as symbols of life's cycles, passing through stages of birth, development, maturity, old age, and death. Throughout the year they undergo stages of change—new leaves of a light green in the spring; flourishing growth and darker leaves by summer; leaves changing color and falling in autumn; and leaves lost by winter. Trees are a symbol of growth— they grow upward, branch out and blossom. Although trees and vegetation grow rapidly in the beginning and in spring, overall they suggest steady, even and controlled growth. Generally speaking, trees only adapt well to new environments of similar nature. Though firmly rooted to the soil they are resilient and responsive, bending this way and that with the wind: they are strong yet flexible. Branches do not break easily—they snap when they break, usually when they are dry or taking too much pressure. The gentle quality of trees makes us feel peaceful and tranquil in their presence. When they die, trees become rigid, then they rot and decay—a process of fermentation. Fermented vegetation has a sour taste. Trees are independent of each other, but in a natural setting different species live in harmony. Trees depend upon soil for a base and nourishment, and water for nourishment as well. Trees can be destroyed by fire, especially if they become too dry.

Fire Nature Energy

Fire nature energy is rapidly ascending and spreading. It is energy in its most dynamic, expanded, and free state. Fire gives light—it is bright and clearly stands out. Fire can be warming, drying, or weakening. It radiates and we feel its presence. Fire needs to be fueled. It attaches or clings to a thing, absorbing and exhausing all of that object's energy. Fire envelops, spreads rapidly, and can rage out of control. Fire is ephemeral— it needs to be fueled constantly and lasts only as long as there is something it can absorb energy from. It is a penetrating, very concentrated energy. Fire needs wood to burn. Water puts it out or traps it, preventing it from spreading. Fire warms the earth, drawing things to life, or parches it, destroying life. Fire melts metal.

Soil Nature Energy

Soil nature energy is downward energy—gathering, condensing, solidifying, and stabilizing energy. Soil is solid: it provides a foundation and stability, a base. Mother earth nourishes and nurtures: it gives life. Soil can be fertile or arid and barren. Fertile soil is moist or damp. Arid soil is dry and crumbles or turns to dust, which is easily blown away by the wind. Soil is frugal: it provides the basics, the necessities, the fundamentals. Soil serves others: it gives impartially. Good quality soil does not move much—it is stable. Trees bind soil keeping it together, or can exhaust it. Metal provides nutrients. Fire gives soil life through warmth, or parches it. When soil dries, it cracks. Water softens and nourishes soil: in excess, water causes soil to become soggy or muddy or washes it away. When the cold freezes, soil remains dormant.

Metal Nature Energy

Metal nature energy is energy in its most yang state: the most condensed, solid, materialized and inwardly directed.

Metal brings to mind man-made objects and industry. Metal objects are distinct and separate entities—they have a clearly defined shape and often, sharp edges. Metal objects tend to be heavy and hard and may be difficult to move. Metal is solid and it is difficult to change this quality—it is generally impenetrable except by heat, other metal objects, or over a long time by water. The surface of unfinished metal may be rough, but with refinement and polish it can become smooth, shiny and reflective. Metal objects are useful and dependable—they are images of structure, strength and endurance. However, metal objects themselves break down or break apart. Metal in the form of man-made objects can destroy trees. Metal is melted by fire. Metal in the form of man-made objects can remove soil. Metal repels water.

Water Nature Energy

Water in its natural state can be described as floating or dissolving energy. Water is fluid and flows. Water seeks the lowest level. At rest water is level. Water can manifest in different states—it can be soft, hard, brittle or wet. Water is a medium: things dissolve in, sink in, and float on water. Water takes on the shape of whatever it flows into. It may appear dark from a distance, but clear upon closer inspection. Water connects things. While it may appear quite motionless, water can actually be moving quite swiftly. Water can be shallow or deep, and deceptive in either way. Water permeates—it goes where other phenomena cannot reach: it is very adaptable. It is difficult to swim against its current—water can be powerful and dangerous. Water tends toward coldness in its natural state. Water stagnates or "dies" when separated from the main source or when not flowing for too long a time. Water provides nourishment for trees and puts out fire. Soil disrupts water's path. Water goes around metal objects or rusts or wears them away.

We can gain further insight into the nature of water energy by exploring the qualities of a river. Rivers flow: a river begins high up in the hills or mountains as rivulets, which are small, narrow and shallow. They follow the easiest course of nature, meandering here and there—they do not really know where they are heading. As the river progresses and takes form, it gets into a groove, penetrates deeper, and carves out a path for itself. As the river becomes bigger, its path becomes straighter and generally it gets even deeper. It usually empties into a larger bulk of water such as the sea or a lake. Rivers can dry up.

The Correspondences

Table 3 presents the most common correspondences. It is an adaptation of a table compiled by Michio Kushi. Sections marked with an asterisk come from the book *Tao* by Taoist Master Ni Hua Ching. Other references are listed in the bibliography.[4]

By observing the correspondences in Table 3 relating to development, seasons, and time of day, we can clearly see how each manifests the corresponding intrinsic energy. Taking time of day as an example, morning mirrors a period of expansion and often of rush. One gets up and prepares to leave the home for the day's activities. The middle part of the day is often the busiest, while things tend to quiet down and become more settled in the afternoon. Toward evening one returns home, often to

Table 3 The Correspondences of the Five Transformations of Energy

	Tree	Fire	Soil	Metal	Water
Energy	Upward	Very active	Downward	Solidified	Floating
Organ Energy:	Liver	Heart	Spleen-Pancreas	Lungs	Kidneys
	Gallbladder	Small intestine	Stomach	Large intestine	Bladder
Development*	Birth	Growth	Maturity	Harvest	Storage
Direction	East	South	Center	West	North
Season	Spring	Summer	Late summer	Autumn	Winter
Color	Green	Red	Yellow	White	Black
Adverse Environment	Windy	Hot	Humid	Dry	Cold
Time of Month	Increasing half-moon	Full moon	Obscured moon	Decreasing half-moon	New moon
Time of Day	Morning	Noon	Afternoon	Evening	Night
Animal	Chicken	Sheep-Lamb	Ox, cow, bull	Horse	Pig
Grain	Wheat, barley	Corn	Millet	Rice	Beans
Vegetables	Upward growing	Enlarged leafy	Round	Contracted, small	Root plants
Fruits	Plum	Apricot	Date	Peach	Chestnut
Physical Roots	Eyes	Tongue	Lips (mouth)	Nose	Ears
Sense	Sight	Talking	Taste-touch	Smell	Hearing
Physical Systems	Tissue, muscles, tendons	Blood vessels	Muscles, flesh	Skin, body hair	Bones
Physical Branches	Nails	Facial color	Breast, lips	Breath	Head hair
Skin Color	Blue, gray	Red	Yellow, milky	Pale	Black, dark
Odors	Rancid, oily	Burning	Fragrant	Fishy, rotting	Putrefying
Tastes	Sour	Bitter, hot	Sweet	Pungent, spicy	Salty
Emotions	Anger	Joy, laughter	Wonder, worry, sympathy	Grief	Fear
Spirits	Soul	Spirit, inspiration	Intelligence	Astral ghost	Will, aspiration
Physical Liquids	Tear	Sweat	Slaver	Mucus, snivel	Saliva
Physical Changes	Gripping	Anxiety	Sobbing	Coughing	Shivering
Roles	Color	Odor	Taste	Voice	Liquids
Voices	Shouting	Talking	Singing	Crying	Groaning
Mode of Action*	Twitching	Itching	Hiccuping	Coughing	Shivering
Moral*	Benevolence	Humility	Trustfulness	Rectitude	Wisdom

gather together with family members for dinner. At night one lies down in a horizontal position to sleep, to replenish and store up energy and perhaps enter the floating world of dreams.

The Energetic Relationships

These five qualities of energy connect with each other in fixed patterns of unending cyclical change. Two main cycles are traditionally recognized: a supporting, nourishing, or creative one known as the Shen cycle; and a controlling or destructive one known as the Ko cycle (see Fig. 10). Symbolically we can begin each cycle with tree nature energy.

In the Shen cycle, tree energy engenders fire energy, which in turn engenders soil energy, which in turn engenders metal energy, which in turn engenders water energy, which in turn engenders tree energy, and so on and on. This process is mirrored in the procession of the seasons, the changes of energy throughout the day, and the cycle of life from birth to old age and death. It can also describe emotional states which may change within seconds, or changes within the galactic cycle which may take millions of years.

Water, tree, and fire, all represent energy in various stages of expansion, while soil and metal represent energy in stages of contraction. In this cyclical progression, when rising energy predominates descending energy wanes and vice versa. We can be more specific and see how one type of energy, when dominant, affects its opposite. This relationship is known as the Ko cycle.

In the Ko cycle one quality of energy controls that which follows it by two. Thus tree controls soil, soil water, water fire, fire metal, and metal controls tree energy. For example, if tree energy becomes dominant, soil energy wanes or becomes weaker.

A third cycle, of less importance, is also recognized. It is the rebellious or competitive cycle, which is the Ko cycle in reverse. For example tree energy rebels against metal energy, metal rebels against fire, and so on.

In his book *Chinese Geomancy*, Stephen Feuchtwang interprets tree nature energy in the following way:

> Wood is understood to be all vegetation, which is fed by Water, and swallows, covers, binds earth, is cut down by metal implements and ignites.[5]

In his book *The Inner Structure of the I Ching*, Lama Govinda writes about *Sun*, the Chinese name for one of the trigrams associated with tree nature energy:

> . . . Sun, in the image of wood, is that which penetrates everywhere with its roots, takes everything nourishing into itself and leads it upward into the realm of light. It does so imperceptibly, and yet it is so strong that it can split rocks.[6]

If we take the image of tree nature energy in relation to soil to be binding and penetrating with its roots, then perhaps we can see how the Ko cycle is the catalyst of change within the Shen cycle (see Fig. 10). That is, while tree energy is perceived in nature to be upward energy, its relationship to soil is through its roots, which have a binding or contracting effect on soil. In the extreme we can see that contracted soil becomes rock or even metal. Following this analogy, fire melts metal to become water, soil combines with water to become nourishment for trees, metal's contracting effect on trees dries them out, making them burn more easily, and water controls the movement of fire, leaving ashes to become soil. In this way we can see the integrity of the system. As such it has an unlimited number of applications in understanding natural phenomena.

Applying the Five Transformations to Healing

In macrobiotic healing the basic approach evaluates energetic distortions within an individual, which parallel the condition of the various internal organs. In Zen Shiatsu we are looking for examples of the most extreme excess and the most extreme deficiency. Once these distortions have been identified the next step is to restore health in the individual by directing their energy back into a state of balance and harmony. In Zen Shiatsu this state is achieved by drawing energy away from the meridian of excess and directing it to the meridian of deficiency.

In evaluating a person's health, there are four kinds of diagnosis, carried out in the following order:

1. *Bō-shin—Observation.*   Bō-shin includes evaluation of posture, mannerisms, and general behavior. It also includes evaluation of the face, hands, and feet, diagnosing discolorations, texture, and markings on the skin.
2. *Bun-shin—Listening.*   Bun-shin not only includes listening to the complaint, but also the manner in which it is expressed. The tempo and pitch of the voice, as well as the emotion behind the words can all correspond with one of the Five phases.
3. *Mon-shin—Questioning.*   The information gathered from observation and listening will guide the practitioner to this next step: asking the type of questions that will help to confirm the diagnosis.
4. *Setsu-shin—Touch.*   Final confirmation comes through touch. What we are looking for through touch will be explained later on in this chapter.

In the first three modes of health evaluation Table 3 can be very helpful. First, when we look at the correspondences relating to season, environment, and time of day, atmospheric energy is focused in the corresponding organs. Consequently, deficiencies or excesses are likely to become more apparent at these times and places. For example, from practical experience we know that liver and gallbladder problems arise more often in the early morning or in spring; heart problems in summer; and lung problems such as colds and runny noses in autumn; kidney and bladder problems appear more often at night or in winter.

Second, the words in the table should be taken metaphorically as well as literally. For example, soil energy relates to the sense of taste. The individual may reveal a poor ability to discern the different tastes of food. This may indicate problems with the stomach and spleen-pancreas. However the way they express themselves through appearance may imply a "lack of taste," and the way they expressed a thought or emotion may have been "in very poor taste." These examples may also indicate soil energy imbalances.

We could take as another illustration a combination of correspondences, for example, emotions and environment. We may consider an angry environment (tree), or a frenetic, excitable, hot environment (fire). These environments may have two effects, one affecting the corresponding organ, the other the organ controlled by this energy. We may find the person with a heart problem (fire) spends a good deal of time in the company of excitable or hysterical people (fire). The chronic worrier (soil) may live with a spouse who is always angry (tree).

Third, the principle of moderation can be considered by taking the five tastes and foods as examples. On the one hand a particular taste or food may be the one to recommend for nourishing a particular organ if we find that such a taste or food is not being consumed. Considered from another perspective, if we find that the same taste or food is consumed very often, this excess may turn out to be the very cause of the problem and what we would recommend to avoid or restrict.

Fourth, various parts of the body not only reflect the condition of a corresponding physical organ by their state of functional health, but can also, through their appearance, tell us of the condition of the corresponding organ. For example the ears correspond to the kidneys. Therefore if an individual complains of an earache, ringing in the ears or poor hearing ability, it may indicate problems with the kidneys. In addition, the color, texture and markings of the skin at the ear, can also tell us of the condition of the kidneys.

The Invisible Body — The Ki Constitution

Fig. 11

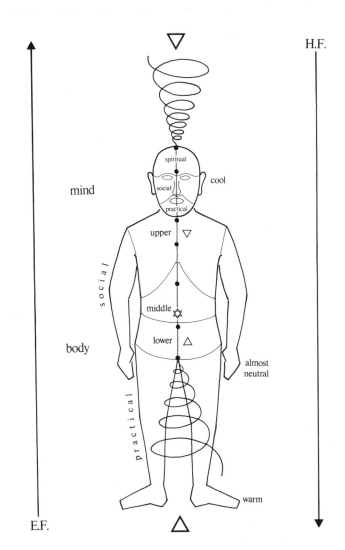

To Taoists the human entity has its roots in both heaven and earth. Earth's energy nourishes more the peripheral physical "tree" (the torso corresponding with the trunk, the limbs with the branches) through the physical food we consume. Whereas this body branches outward, they believe that there is a spiritual body with roots in heaven that enters the physical body from the head and branches downward and inward. The trunk of this spiritual body is described by Michio Kushi as a spiritual channel running vertically through the center of the body. Along this channel of the body, the energies of earth's force and heaven's force directly interact. At seven major "joints" these energies collide. In Indian spiritual philosophy these joints are known as chakras.

The collision of these energies causes branches to form: streams of ki energy or meridians around which the physical body develops. These meridians in turn branch and further branch, feeding ki energy to each and every cell (the leaves of this spiritual tree).

Again demonstrating the Oriental view of correspondences, Michio Kushi further teaches that this human entity is a microcosm corresponding with a giant spirit body that exists in space.[7] It is from this cosmological perspective that he develops his view of the body. This subject is worthy of an entire book in itself, but this chapter will concentrate on those aspects pertinent to the practice of shiatsu.

Mr. Kushi likes to illustrate the energetic foundations of the human body with the following demonstration. Take a metal object such as a ring or pair of nail clippers (we shall call it a pendulum) and connect it to a piece of cotton thread a few inches long. Without moving your hand, hold it a few inches above the heads of both a male and a female. Soon the pendulum will begin to spin, counterclockwise over the head of a male, clockwise over the head of a female. If they hold hands, the object will cease to move. Since we know that heaven's force spirals counterclockwise and earth's force clockwise we can see that males carry or are dominated more by heaven's force, while females by earth's force. In the same manner, when we hold the pendulum over the open palms of either a male or a female, it will spin clockwise over the right palm and counterclockwise over the left. This movement suggests that the right side of the body is dominated and nourished more by earth's force, while the left, heaven's force. The function and structure of the body supports this view, for in females the left breast and ovary tend to be located a little lower than the right and the right breast and ovary a little larger. The same can be said for a male's testicles. Moreover, the digestion of food takes place more on the left side while nutrients are carried away from the small intestine upward to the liver via the portal vein on the right side. We see that movement through the colon ascends on the right side and descends on the left. We also see that the majority of people are right-handed; the moving side of the body tends to be the right.

Looking at the body from top to bottom, we see that the head, which is closer to heaven carries out more yin invisible functions associated with coolness; while the feet attached to the earth carry out more yang physically active functions associated with warmth. The hands should be in-between, almost neutral. In terms of energetic nourishment, the lower part of the body (the lower abdomen on down) is nourished by more downward moving energy while the upper body (from the diaphragm on up) is nourished more by upward moving energy. The middle part of the torso is nourished by a balance of both forces.

We need to remember the following: top is yin, bottom yang; inside yang, outside yin; center yang, periphery yin; front yin, back yang. (See Fig. 11.)

The Physical Body

The physical body arises from the ki constitution. However, while the mind is nourished more directly through this ki constitution, the physical body is nourished to a large degree by the quality and quantity of physical food we consume. Of course, both mind and body are also affected by our emotional and environmental influences.

1. THE ENERGY OF FOOD

"You are what you eat" is an expression popularized by the natural foods movement many years ago. The English language is replete with idioms expressing human behavior in terms of animals, plants and their products: to charge like a bull; to chicken out; to pig out; to be as gentle as a lamb; a silly cow; an egghead; a turkey; a nut; fruity; addressing a person as "sugar" or "honey." Yet rarely if ever is any connection made between the consumption of these things and our behavior—an outcome of the horizontal axis culture's tendency to separate subject and object.

Conversely, since the traditional Chinese culture was vertical axis, they were accustomed to thinking in terms of correspondence and drawing that correspondence back to their own selves. That which resembled some human quality in nature was seen to be possibly beneficial to the human entity. Da Liu, a practitioner and teacher of Taoism for over fifty years illustrates this outlook in the Taoist search for immortality:

> Obviously, the natural substances that compose the human body—flesh, bones, blood and so on—are not sufficiently durable to last indefinitely. Even with special care, the tissues of the body are likely to deteriorate and die after little more than a century. Perhaps then, it was concluded by Han Wu Ti and others that one must transform the tissues into more long lasting substances in order to prolong life. According to such reasoning, the secret of longevity for buildings is that stone and metal survive longer than clay or wood. Thus, Han Wu Ti reasoned, he would transform his tissues by consuming [powdered] jade mixed with the moisture of the heavens.[8]

From centuries of observation and testing, a highly sophisticated system of herbal remedies based on the Five Transformations has been developed to help treat a multitude of ailments.

The macrobiotic choice of food too is based on this system of correspondences, supported by centuries of practical experience by traditional cultures. These correspondences then have resulted from humanity's intuitive understanding of the yin-yang quality of a food. By taking into account various factors including the shape of a food, its taste, color, origin, growing season, water content, and life expectancy we can see how a food will affect our health, mentally, physically and spiritually, positively or negatively. Thus we can change ourselves and help control our lives by what we eat. Let us then consider the effects of various foods in the macrobiotic diet.

Whole cereal grains have already been discussed with this approach. The image of a stalk of rice corresponds with our head and spine, our brain and nervous system. While firmly rooted to the soil whole cereal grains grow vertically toward heaven, nourished by heaven's force absorbed through the tiny antennaelike projectiles on the outer coating of each grain. This vertical quality transmutes into the human entity in the form of a naturally upright spine. The grains growing at the top of the stalk correspond with mental nourishment. Whole cereal grains thus open us up to the influence of heaven's force: they are a practical way to develop our consciousness.

Three types of vegetables also illustrate the principle of correspondences; root, leafy greens, and round-shaped. Root vegetables are hardy and grow downward. These factors suggest yang—that they carry a strong quality of energy toward the lower part of the body—the lower abdomen, the reproductive organs, and the legs. The consumption of root vegetables in balanced proportions will nourish and strengthen these areas and provide a sense of groundedness and stability. In addition, if we take into consideration the different types of root vegetables and their energetic correspondences, we can then more clearly determine which organ will be most affected.

Let us, for example, compare *daikon* and burdock. We see that burdock grows longer and narrower. These qualities suggest that its energy is directed more inward and downward, and that it nourishes more the small intestine. Its bitter taste, correlating with fire energy, also supports this view. We can further assume that it would strengthen the function of the reproductive organs. On the other hand, daikon is pungent and white in color, both qualities corresponding with metal nature energy, which corresponds with the large intestine. Metal produces water. We note that daikon not only nourishes the large intestine but may also help to induce urination in an overly contracted kidney condition.

The tops of root vegetables grow upward suggesting a yin energy that nourishes more the chest region, the lungs especially. Their peaceful energy is said to contribute to a like state of mind. Leafy greens such as kale, mustard, and collard also grow upward. Direct growth from the soil as well as their green color would suggest that these vegetables nourish more the liver and gallbladder functions all tree energy correspondences. Round-shaped vegetables such as squash, onions, and cabbage grow close to the ground and therefore receive more a balance of upward with downward forces. This balance corresponds with nourishment of the middle section of the abdomen, the kidneys, liver and gallbladder, and stomach and spleen-pancreas. In addition, since these vegetables grow so close to the surface of the earth and their flavor, the predominantly sweet taste associated with soil energy, we can see that they would tend to nourish more the stomach and spleen-pancreas. Soil controls water. Thus they may also affect the kidneys.

Beans are clearly similar in shape to the ears and kidneys, all three corresponding to the water phase. Thus it is not surprising to see that azuki beans are renowned for their beneficial effects on the kidneys. Black soybeans can be used to improve reproductive functioning, also a water phase correspondence.

Sea vegetables are soft and flexible, yet they must be strong and durable to withstand life in the ocean. Sea vegetables thus promote the functioning of the blood (the body's sea) and its vessels. They alkalize the blood, have blood anticoagulant properties and can have a beneficial effect on arteriosclerosis. They can also contribute to softening tumors. *Kombu* is believed to improve sexual vitality (water phase). *Hijiki* has long been renowned for promoting strong and lustrous hair. To ancient Orientals, hijiki's long black strands, waving to-and-fro in the sea, must have reminded them of their own hair.

Tree fruit if consumed in excess can lead to a cold condition in the intestines, loss of sexual vitality, an expanded heart condition, more rapid and shallow breathing, talkativeness, scattered thinking, and more active movement of the arms. If we were to superimpose an image of a fruit tree over our torso and upper body, we could visualize how the roots of the tree sap energy away from the reproductive organs and intestines, displacing it upward and outward as a dispersed kind of energy in the upper body, much like the movement of the branches of a tree growing upward and outward.

All foods can be classified according to the Five phases (see Table 4). Such categorization can be useful in a number of ways. In the case of vegetables such classification most often corresponds with the season in which they mature, the time that we are most likely to consume them. However, vegetable foods which can be stored, can be used out of season to create balance if necessary. In this way we can help maintain our health. This table can also tell us what foods, if consumed in excess, may be the cause of a problem. In this situation we need to consider both the nourishing and control cycles. For example salt in balanced quantities promotes the functioning of the kidneys. In excess it creates hardness in the same organs. Through the control cycle it would also affect the heart such as in its involvement with high blood pressure. The sour taste promotes the functioning of the liver and gallbladder. In excess though, its astringent effect creates a tightening of the muscles. Through the control cycle it could also be the cause of worry. In the same way, the sweet taste can be beneficial to the stomach and spleen-pancreas. It can nourish and relax these organs. In excess it weakens them, leading to worry, and through the control cycle, fear.

While there is bound to be some disagreement on such classification, Table 4 provides a guide to the categorization of foods. Some foods have been classified under more than one phase. It may be because a food grows in more than one season, or it may be that a food contains qualities of both phases. Some types of foods, for example sea vegetables, are listed as a general category while varieties of that food group are listed under particular phases. Every food group contains elements of the other five phases within it.

Table 4 Classification of Foods According to the Five Transformations

Tree	Fire	Soil	Metal	Water
Quality of Energy: Upward	Very active	Centering Downward Relaxing	Solidified	Floating
Five Colors: Green	Red	Yellow	White	Black
Five Tastes: Sour	Bitter, hot	Sweet	Pungent, spicy	Salty
Effects of Five Tastes: Astringent Gathering Contracting	Drying Eliminating Dispersing	Nourishing Relaxing	Dispersing	Softening Hardening
Cooking Styles: Steaming Tempura Deep-fry	Boiling Grilling Stir-fry Quick sauté Roasting Toasting	Pressure-cooking *Nishime*	Baking *Kinpira* Long-time sauté	Stewing Simmering

Tree	Fire	Soil	Metal	Water

Whole Cereal Grains:

Tree	Fire	Soil	Metal	Water
Barley	Corn	Millet	Brown rice—	Beans as a
Hato mugi	Long grain		short, medium	general category
(Job's tears)	brown rice	Sweet brown	Wild rice	Buckwheat
Wheat berries		rice	Rye	
Oats				
Wild rice				

Grain Products:

Tree	Fire	Soil	Metal	Water
Cracked wheat		Mochi	Seitan	*Soba* noodles
Bulgur				
Couscous				
Amazaké				
Fu				
Sourdough bread				
Sprouted bread				
Udon				

Vegetables:

Tree	Fire	Soil	Metal	Water
Broccoli	Bok choy	Brussels	Broccoli	Cabbages
Celery	Burdock	sprouts	Brussels sprouts	Kale
Chinese	Carrot tops	Cabbages	Carrots	*Kuzu*
cabbage	Chicory	Carrots	Carrots tops	Rutabega
Chives	Collard greens	Fresh green	Cauliflower	Dried daikon
Dandelion	Cucumbers	beans	Daikon	Dried
Greens	*Daikon* tops	Green peas	Daikon tops	mushrooms
Fresh	Dandelion	Onions	Ginger	Dried
mushrooms	greens	Parsnips	Horseradish	vegetables as
Green peas	Endive	Pumpkin	*Jinenjo*	a general
Leeks	Escarole	Rutabaga	Lotus root	category
Mugwort	Lettuce	Squash—	Lotus seeds	
Scallions	Mustard greens	fall, winter	Mustard	
Shiso leaves	Rappini	String beans	Mustard greens	
Sprouts	Snow peas	Sweet daikon	Parsley	
Ume	String beans	Sweet turnips	Red radish	
Wild	Summer squash		Turnips	
vegetables as	Turnip greens		*Wasabi*	
a general category	Watercress		Watercress	
	Zucchini			

Beans/and Fermented Bean Products:

Tree	Fire	Soil	Metal	Water
Miso	Black-eyed	Chick-peas	Black soybeans	Beans as
Natto	peas	Kidney beans	Miso	a general
Tempeh	Red lentils	Pinto beans		category
Green lentils	*Tofu*	Whole dried peas		*Azuki beans*
Mung beans		Yellow soybeans		Great northern
				beans
				Dried tofu

Sea Vegetables:

Tree	Fire	Soil	Metal	Water
Wakame	*Aonori*	*Arame*		
Sea palm				

Tree	Fire	Soil	Metal	Water
	Dulse	*Mekabu*	Hijiki	Sea vegetables as
	Nori			a general
				category
				Agar-agar
				Kombu
Fish:				
Shellfish:	Very Active	Smaller	Very Compact	Freshwater
Littleneck clams	Ocean Fish:	Ocean Fish:	Ocean Fish:	Fish:
Mussels	Eel	Cod	*Chirimen-iriko*	Perch
	Octopus	Halibut	(Tiny dried	Trout
	Squid		fish)	Flounder
			Salmon	
			Sardine	
			Smelt	
			Tuna	
Seeds:				
Flaxseeds	Apricot seeds	Pumpkin seeds		Dark sesame
Poppy seeds	Sesame seeds			seeds
	Sunflower seeds			
Nuts:				
Cashews	Brazil nuts		Almonds	Chestnuts
Peanuts	Cashews		Pine nuts	
Walnuts	Macadamia nuts			
	Pistachios			
Fruit:				
Lemons	Apricots	Sweet apples	Grapes	Black berries
Limes	Cherries	Cantaloupes		Dried fruit as
Persimmons	Oranges	Currants		a general
Plums	Strawberries	Melons		category
Raspberries		Peaches		Watermelon
Sour apples		Pears		
Tangerines		Raisins		
Tree fruit as a general				
category				
Seasoning:				
Miso		Sweet brown	Brown rice	Sea salt
Sauerkraut		rice venegar	vinegar	
Ume vinegar		*Mirin* (Sweet	Horseradish	
Vinegar as a general		cooking wine)	*Tamari* soy sauce	
category				
Umeboshi plum				
Oil:				
Peanut	Corn	Light sesame	Soybean	
Oil as a general	Dark sesame	oil		
category	Sunflower			
Safflower				

	Tree	Fire	Soil	Metal	Water
Pickles:					
Ume pickles					Long-term pickles
Sweeteners:					
Barley malt			Grain syrups over all	Rice syrup	
Condiments:					
Chives with miso			*Gomashio*	*Tekka*	*Shio* Kombu
Dandelion miso					Shio nori
Scallions with miso					
shiso leaves					
Wakame powder					
Umeboshi					
Beverages:					
Barley tea		*Bancha* tea	Amazaké	Roasted brown rice tea	Kombu tea
Beer		Dandelion tea			*Mu* tea
Green magma		Grain coffee			Spring water
Saké		Nachi green tea			Well water
Soy milk					
Ume tea					
Foods That Are Generally Avoided:					
Carob		Alcohol	Beef	Cheese	Pork
Chicken		Black tea	Butter	Eggs	
Ghee		Coffee	Sweet wine		
Maple syrup		Chemicalized food			
Sour cream		Chocolate			
Milk		Cream			
Wine		Dry wine			
Yogurt		Eggplant			
		Honey			
		Irradiated foods			
		Lamb			
		Microwaved foods			
		Red pepper			
		Soft drinks			
		Sugar			

Even though a food may relate to one of the above correspondences, we should keep in mind that the way of preparation can substantially alter the energy of that food. Daikon, a popular vegetable in the macrobiotic diet, is a good example. Daikon has the ability to dissolve excess fats and eliminate mucus. However, the manner of preparation influences the location in the body it will affect most.

- Grated daikon with a dash of tamari soy sauce to taste, a more yin preparation, is often recommended in small amounts to dissolve more peripheral fats.
- Daikon cooked in miso soup may be a more appropriate way of taking daikon to dissolve hardened fat in the arteries, since miso as a blood cleanser will draw the energy of daikon to this location.

- Raw daikon with *bancha* tea, since it involves a liquid, directs the pungent quality of daikon to the kidneys, aiding to relieve problems of urinary retention for example.
- Cooking daikon *nishime* style (p. 84), a more yang preparation, draws out a sweeter taste. Since soil controls water it could be effective in softening hardened fats within the kidneys.

Table 4 shows us the energetic correspondences of various foods and consequently the internal organs such foods will nourish if consumed in a balanced way. However the effect is subtle, more noticeable by the balanced state of health that arises, which we so often take for granted. Conversely, the long time consumption of more extreme foods, or the excess or unbalanced consumption of more healthful foods will have more noticeable effects, most often of a negative nature. The following descriptions can aid the practitioner in understanding the condition of those people who come to receive shiatsu.

1. *Salt (including sea salt and salt products)*

   The overall body is tight, hard and inflexible, especially in the legs and back. The flesh is hard, there is loss of weight; they may appear skinny. The skin is dry, withered, contracted, grayish in color, showing signs of premature aging. Other indications include the following: dark colored skin, especially around the eyes; dryness in the extremities; poor circulation in the extremities and thus coldness, especially in the feet; premature graying of hair; short, cryptic expression; inflexible, rigid personality, short temper; tremendous appetite; overly sleepy; lack of energy (in extreme cases); water retention and kidney related problems.

2. *Eggs*

   Flesh, ligaments, and muscles are tight and hard, yet the body is still fleshy. The skin may be yellowish in color, smooth, with little body hair and shiny. The head of a male may be bald and pointed. Very deep hardness in yang organs and in yang locations—liver and pancreatic problems especially; creation of cysts, tumors, pus and boils; yellow fat accumulations in the whites of the eyes; yellowish vaginal discharge; strong body odor especially through breath or flatulence; withheld quality to the personality, as though there is a shell around them; hard on the outside but emotionally gentle; difficulty in self-expression; prone to fits of anger; very rigid personality, may appear cold, possibly cruel; strong sexual stimulation—promotes many short-term relationships; sense of loss and anguish.

3. *Meat (particularly beef)*

   The more yang quality of meat gathers deep inside and downward. The more yin quality, excess fat, gathers toward the periphery. Body overall very hard, tight, stiff, dense and heavy; leathery thick skin, often sweaty; thick set, heavy build; shoulders on a male well-developed; forward stoop (often tends to look down toward the ground); overall heavy feeling, focused in expression between eyebrows and over brow; tightness in the lower back region; loss of hair on males toward the crown; forceful in expression, overbearing, aggressive, impulsive, pushy, insensitive to others, thoughtless, rough, loud, violent; discharges the energy of meat through very active physical behavior; likes to be surrounded by open space; enjoys the natural environment and outdoor activity.

4. *Chicken*

   Overall body tightness and hardness; tight ligaments, muscles and flesh; scrawny appearance; feisty; rounded upper back; tightness and hardness around the shoulder blades; rough quality to the skin; a gathering of fatty accumulations just below the skin surface; the skin may become slightly yellow; fatty accumulations around the throat, possibly causing thyroid and parathyroid problems; increased stiffness of hands and feet, fingers, and toes; swollen and painful joints; extreme itchiness in the joints; wobbly thin legs; lack of strength in legs; hands and feet beginning to take on the shape of a chicken's feet; protruding heels; deep hardness in the pancreas and associated region; excessive blinking; glassy eyes, often requiring glasses; pointed nose and features; pecking, jerking gestures; difficulty in relaxing; tight, thin lips; very sharp senses; impulsive; picky with their food, scavenger mentality; henpecking; cowardice; likes to make a comfortable home (building a nest).

5. *Dairy Food*

   Pronounced bone structure; large bones and frame; thick skin which is insensitive to pressure; white milky complexion, white patches under the skin; fine, light-colored body hair of a fine texture; slow, dull reactions; yin insensitivity—insensitive to subtle nuance; very mucous forming; mucous accumulation in the sinuses and lungs; white-colored vaginal discharge; strong body odor; tends not to sweat so much; soft quality to the eyes, which may bulge very slightly in shape; gentle, kind character; overly agreeable; tendency to be followers; sentimental, childish, mentally immature; frigid; does not make a home.
   Cheese: Heavy, dense body; fat accumulation in hips and legs, and under the skin, creating dry skin; whitish, yellowish complexion, callouses on the feet, pancreatic problems
   Milk: External softness from a coating of excess fat; milk excess gathering more around breasts and arms; fine white hairs on face
   Ice cream: Pinkish color to the skin; creating kidney stones and hearing problems
   Butter: Oily, smooth, yellowish skin

6. *Fish*

   Muscles, ligaments and flesh tending to be softer than with the overconsumption of other kinds of animal food; sharp senses; narrow view—tunnel vision; smooth, soft flowing expression; constantly moving around; group identity, orderly, nonconfrontational; cool, more mental personality; devour or be devoured mentality; possible cause of crossed-eyes; shellfish can create intestinal and shoulder cramps.

7. *Bread and Baked Food*

   Bread is a dry contracted food that expands with liquid. Thus: puffy skin, bloated cheeks; *white bread*—white, puffy, pasty skin; *white flour combined with sugar*—white, puffy, pasty skin with pink or reddish overtones or pimples; dry skin; an excess of bread and/or baked flour products discharges through mucus and crusty formations; crusts and sometimes callouses on the feet; white crust—white milk bread; crust formation on the inside corners of the eyes—gallbladder problems; most affected organs—lungs and large intestine, pancreas, liver, and gallbladder; dense, hard, inflexible body; intestinal problems; causes flatulence especially when combined with sugars.

8. *Fruit*
    Not so fleshy or well-covered; skin overly red, bluish or purplish, especially in the fingers or toes; opened pores of skin, allowing oils to escape, creating thick, dry, puffy skin; fragile skin, easily bruises; itchy skin resulting from excess fats from fruit sugar; darkish, reddish complexion; coldness in body; cold hands and feet; loss of sexual vitality; ascending, outwardly dispersing energy—thus much nervous, frenetic, unfocused energy, "up in the clouds," "spaced out," chatterbox, tendency to often look upward toward the sky; skeptical, analytical, sentimental, emotional; heart problems—irregular heartbeat (arrhythmia), expanded heart; runny nose, colds; watery eyes, cataracts, excessive blinking; "wide eyed"; hair thinning; dandruff; in males loss of frontal head hair; high pitched voice—irregular tempo of voice indicating irregular heartbeat (often signified by a cleft in the tip of the nose); weak lungs, rounded shoulders, stooped spine; very long, thin nose.

9. *Sugar*
    Loose skin and flesh and possibly overweight; brown or dark complexion; brown patches on the skin; freckles; expanded features; astigmatism; cataracts; expanded, open skin pores; moody; depressed; dispersed thinking; loss of direction, scattered, confused; schizophrenic; crying easily; lacking endurance

10. *Recreational Drugs*
    Expanded pupils, sluggishness, slow, scattered; insecure and fearful; lack of vitality; bluish color in the extremities, under eyes and on hands

11. *Water*
    Flabby, full skin, muscles and flesh; swollen, puffy general appearance; swollen ankles; swollen, distended abdomen; puffiness or swelling under the eyes; wet hands; watery, unclear, deep voice; frequent urination

2. CONSTITUTION AND CONDITION

In giving shiatsu and advice we need to consider both the receiver's constitution and condition. The constitution of individuals refers to their characteristics formed before birth. The constitution is determined by the health and vitality of the parents and ancestors, as well as the diet, environment and lifestyle of the mother during pregnancy—embracing her mental, physical, and spiritual quality. The condition of an individual refers to his or her present state of health influenced by diet, emotional and environmental factors. While one's constitution is largely determined at birth one's condition is subject to change, even from day to day.

Constitution
Basically we can divide people's constitutions into more yang or more yin types.

1. A More Yang Constitution
Such people tend to have a strong frame or bone structure. The face has a more round or angular shape with the lower half more prominent than the upper and facial features gathered more toward the center. The eyes may be narrow, the eyebrows thicker and slanted downward toward the nose. The nose may be wide and flat, and

the mouth small—about as wide as the nose. The ears may be large, with substantial lobes. The body is comparatively smaller, compact, and integrated. The shoulders tend to be square in shape, the area of the palms larger than that of the fingers. In good health the body tends to be fleshy and there is an aura of strength, sturdiness and vitality. There is a tendency to be aggressive and dynamic, more physically than mentally active. In thought and action they tend to be quick, precise, and creative.

Center is yang. In life such people tend to move in two basic directions. First they may move further toward the center, intensifying the center—excelling at what they do, becoming leaders in their field. Negatively this movement may be expressed as self-absorption or egocentricity. On the other hand, they may also move toward the periphery. Vertically, this movement manifests as spiritual development. Horizontally it manifests positively as an embrace of space or negatively as a wasting away of their inherent yang energy.

2. A More Yin Constitution

These people tend to have a more fragile or delicate frame, bone structure and appearance. The face tends to be either more vertical, or the upper half more pronounced than the lower. Facial features tend to be more spread out, and more rounded than angular. For example, the eyes tend to be more round in shape, larger and further away from the nose. The eyebrows may be thinner and slant downward on the outside. The nose may be longer and narrower, or the mouth may be quite large. Such people tend to be taller and thinner. The shoulders tend to slope and the fingers may be longer than the palm and the hands overall not so fleshy. Such people tend more toward mental or artistic interests, more quiet, introspective and less sociable. They tend to be less physically strong or dynamic and perhaps more sensitive.

Periphery is yin. Those with more yin constitutions will tend to move in life in two basic directions. They may move toward the center, looking for a center or grounding, they tend to be followers. Or they may move even further toward the periphery becoming less practical, more cerebral and eccentric.

Condition

Basically we can divide into more yin or more yang conditions.

1. An Overly Yang Condition

The operative words are tightness, dryness, and hardness, which can be used both literally and metaphorically. Muscles and flesh tend to be tight and stiff, and movement and gesturing tends to be sharp, angular or mechanical. The lips may be tight, the skin dry and drawn. There may be a tendency to clench the fists, to grind the teeth during sleep, and locked jaw. The skin may be yellowish or dark, especially around the eyes. The nose may be congested. They may suffer from constipation. There may be a tendency to feel hot and they rarely blink. There is a tendency to lean forward when sitting or walking and a sense of impatience, aggressiveness or insensitivity to the feelings and rhythms of others. Communication tends to be short and to the point. There may be a tendency to talk loudly and the possibility of a heavy appearance or feeling. They may be antisocial with a desire to exclude or be critical of others for not living up to their expectations.

2. An Overly Yin Condition

The operative words are looseness, wetness, and softness, which can be used both literally and figuratively. There is a tendency toward a lack of integration or coordination in movement; slouching when sitting, and walking more on the heels. The mouth tends to be open, with more salivation, and the body tends toward being cold. It may even appear slightly bluish in color in more extremes. The palms may be wet. The complexion may be white or pale. Such people may be long-winded, never getting to the point. They may be scattered in their thoughts, daydreamers, and procrastinators. They may be overly dependent on others and there is a tendency to exclude themselves from the company of others, often preferring solitude.

Those people with a more yang constitution may have either an overly yin or overly yang condition. The same principle applies to those with a more yin constitution. Moreover, a yang condition can be caused by either an excess of yang, or a deficiency of yin. A yin condition can be caused by either an excess of yin or a deficiency of yang. These conditions may be more clearly understood when illustrated diagrammatically (Fig. 12):

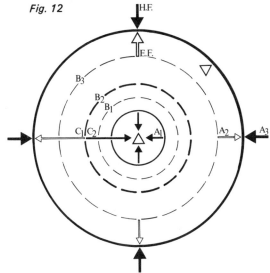

Fig. 12

The outside circle represents the human entity. This entity arises from the interaction of yin and yang forces. Yang represents gathering or stored energy; yin represents releasing energy. Yang energy (A_1) moves toward the center, while yin energy (A_2) moves toward the periphery. The entire entity is externally under the yang influence of heaven's force (A_3). Imagine the center of this outside circle to be another hollow circle. The consumption of yang energy moves toward the center, filling up this circle. If yang is consumed in excess, it spills over into the next concentric zone, defined by B_1, and so on until the entire entity becomes filled with yang. Conversely, yin energy consumed, moves first to the periphery, filling up the outer zone defined by B_3. Yin in excess spills over B_3 into the next concentric zone, then over B_2 and so on until the entire entity becomes filled with yin.

Let us assume B_2 to be a dividing point between an equal balance of yin C_1 and yang C_2 energy. If yin moves over B_2 toward the center then it begins to affect stored yang by releasing it to the periphery. Conversely, if yang moves over B_2 toward the periphery it will absorb or dry out yin, or force yin to the surface.

From this description we can discern the following processes:

1. *Yang contracts.*   Excess yang causes the overall entity to contract.
2. *Yin expands.*   Yin causes the overall entity to expand.
3. *Yang expands in the extreme.*   As each zone fills up with yang, the overall effect is one of expansion. However since this expansion results from the backing up of yang contracting energy, we can expect this entity to be hard, dense, tight, and probably heavy. This we call a yang excess condition.
4. *Yin contracts in the extreme.*   If yin backs up all the way to the center then all stored yang energy is released and the entity collapses under the external influence of heaven's yang force. However this kind of contraction will contain softness and weakness. It describes a yang deficient condition.
5. *Yang remains constant, but excess yin is consumed.*   In this condition the overall entity expands. The surface of the body appears round and full. It is called a yin excess condition. Since yin releases yang, this condition, if it becomes chronic, leads to a yang deficient condition.
6. *Yang remains constant but insufficient yin is consumed.*   In this condition the entity first overall contracts. The person may lose weight, the flesh becomes thinner and either tighter or loose, since there is a lack of energy moving outward. While there is inner strength the body surface appears flat and the skin lacks muscle tone, or resilience. It describes a yin deficient condition.

When we understand these processes we can more clearly comprehend Masunaga's approach to diagnosis through touch, known as Kyo Jitsu-Ho Sha.

Kyo and Jitsu

Kyo and Jitsu are terms used to describe conditions of energy distortion within the physical body. Kyo refers to a condition of deficiency or emptiness: the dispersion or absence of energy. Jitsu refers to a condition of excess or fullness: the localization or buildup of energy. A kyo condition can be caused by a deficiency of either yin or yang factors. A jitsu condition can be caused by an excess of either yin or yang factors. Thus four basic conditions can be observed: Yin kyo, meaning yin energy is deficient; yang kyo, meaning yang energy is deficient; yang jitsu, meaning yang energy is in excess; yin jitsu, meaning yin energy is in excess. Yin kyo and yang jitsu are both more yang conditions. Yang kyo and yin jitsu are more yin conditions. Jitsu is dynamic. Kyo is flat, dull or listless. The terms kyo and jitsu can refer to a person's overall condition or to the condition of a particular meridian and its associated internal organ.

To aid in our understanding of Masanaga's theory of energy distortion we can visualize the human body as a circle, the circumference divided into twelve interconnected parts. Each part represents a meridian of ki energy related to a particular internal organ. The twelve meridians connect to form a circuit along which ki moves in unbroken cycles. If the movement of energy from one meridian to the next is balanced then we can expect a state of good health. However, since we live in a relative world, distortion always exists, because yin is always greater than yang or vice versa. The object of shiatsu is to minimize these distortions. In this theory, the energy quotient of the human entity is always seen as one. If there is more energy focused in one particular meridian there must be proportionately less available for all other meridians. One cannot add to or take away from one meridian without this effect permeating through all other meridians.

Masunaga viewed the body as physically reflecting a psychological state. We can illustrate his approach by taking as an example a conversation among a group of people. When a subject arises, the one who is interested will likely respond by contributing. The more interesting the subject to that person, the more quickly will he or she likely contribute and quite possibly, ultimately dominate the conversation. This situation represents a jitsu condition. A jitsu condition reflects something that a person is interested in, something that they like to display, or wish to express and share with others, the way they would like the outside world to see them. Consequently, the bodily manifestation of a meridian in this condition appears as protruding from the normal body surface, localized and easy to be seen. The muscles in such an area are likely to be more pronounced, the surface of the skin exhibiting a full or round appearance.

Referring back to the conversation, if someone openly criticizes this person's interest or point of view, the person being criticized will most likely take it personally, perhaps even feel hurt since their heart is obviously involved in this subject. However, simultaneous with this hurt there will be a reaction or counter to the criticism. Since so much energy is focused on this interest, it will be difficult for criticism to "get through" since this person has a good deal of energy to lodge a response. In the physical body, sharp direct shiatsu to a jitsu meridian resembles criticism and it will elicit a similar response. The receiver will react quickly with pain or discomfort: and in addition, a sharp angle of pressure will have difficulty staying on the muscle. It will tend to slip off. The operative words for a jitsu condition are visibility and reaction.

If in this same conversation a subject arises that an individual does not wish to discuss, more than likely the group will be unaware of the sensitive nature of the topic until the conversation turns directly to the person in question. However, with a question, the group will most likely encounter resistance from the individual to respond. If the group is not sensitive to the subtle nuance of body language and voice tone, and continues to probe, it is quite probable that he or she will close up, refusing to answer the question. The situation represents a kyo condition, reflecting an area of our being that we choose to conceal or ignore, and in this theory, the motivating force behind the external appearances.

In giving shiatsu to a meridian in this condition we will from visual observation be unlikely to discern any difference in the flesh through which the kyo meridian passes and the normal flesh condition. The surface will appear flat. However with shiatsu, which is akin to a question in the conversation, we will immediately see that the flesh is soft and flaccid or lacking in resilience. If pressure is applied too sharply or quickly, akin to a lack of sensitivity to the sensitive nature of the subject of converation, there will be either muscular resistance or tension in the surrounding area to protect the meridian; or there will be overall body contraction as a response to pressure, akin to refusing to answer the question. The stronger, sharper or quicker the application of pressure, akin to a forceful and direct question, the more likely will the muscles contract, making shiatsu pointless.

In our conversation, to elicit a response from the person in question, we would need to show empathy, that we cared about them. We would need to display warmth, show that we supported them, and were considerate of their feelings. In shiatsu the same is true. We need to apply a supporting hand close to the area receiving shiatsu, akin to emotional support. We need to apply pressure slowly and gently, akin to a slow and gentle approach in questioning, and we have to wait for the muscles to relax, opening up to our pressure (responding to our question) before we apply even deeper pressure. We may have to stop and hold our pressure two or three times before we actually connect with the kyo meridian. Holding, then applying deeper pressure corresponds with further probing in the conversation. Deep pressure corresponds with becoming deeply involved with the person's problem. The operative words for a kyo condition are thus concealment and resistance.

In summary, jitsu is located by asking oneself "What stands out about this person that they are they keen to show?" "What would they have us believe?" Kyo may be located by asking oneself, "What's missing?" or "What's lacking?," in their nature. What is their motivation to present themselves to the world in this way? We can illustrate kyo and jitsu conditions diagrammatically (Fig. 13):

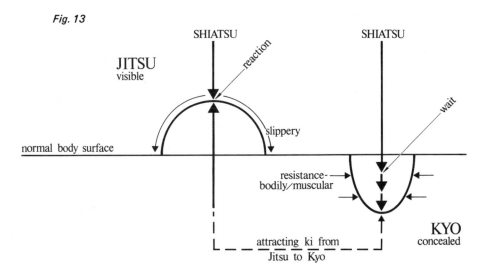

Fig. 13

In this diagram we see a line with the words "attracting ki from jitsu to kyo." This aspect of Zen Shiatsu is quite unique. Referring back to our circle we see that all meridians are interconnected. Therefore a kyo meridian and a jitsu meridian are interconnected. These conditions tell us that since the individual has focused more attention on one aspect of his or her life, proportionately less is available for other aspects. There is a tendency to maximize our strengths and ignore our weaknesses. However, as we see from our circle of twelve interconnected parts, strengths and weaknesses are interconnected. Thus such a way of life ultimately leads to the downfall of the entire organism, in much the same way that a chain is only as strong as its weakest link. In the Zen Shiatsu approach, rather than expending energy to maximize a strength, more should be devoted to building up a weakness, restoring the entire organism to a state of balance. This condition is the optimum state of health the individual can enjoy at that time. Since kyo and jitsu are interrelated, the energy needed to build up the weakness should come from the area of strength. Thus, the first tenet of Zen Shiatsu is to "TREAT KYO FIRST." By certain techniques in the application of pressure we redirect or draw energy away from the jitsu to the kyo area. In this way the jitsu area naturally subsides and the kyo area fills up: balance is once more established. Nothing is added, or withdrawn by external pressure.

Before describing the various conditions we are likely to encounter there are a number of things we need to be aware of. First, in the Zen Shiatsu approach meridians are considered in pairs: lung and large intestine; stomach and spleen-pancreas; heart and small intestine; bladder and kidneys; heart constrictor and triple heater; gallbladder and liver. One yang "solid" organ is paired with one yin "hollow" organ. If one partner of a pair is kyo then both are kyo in comparison with the other five pairs of meridians. However, one meridian of the pair will be slightly more kyo or jitsu than the other. Second, to restore the entity to a state of balance we focus our treatment on the pairs of meridians of greatest opposite distortion.

Another important factor is the general difference we will find in the flesh conditions of those who eat a more vegetable quality or macrobiotic diet and in those whose diet is centered around animal food. Generally speaking, those people who consume large quantities of animal food will have bodies that tend to be harder, more dense, tighter, stiffer, and generally heavier than those who eat macrobiotically. The vegetable quality of the macrobiotic diet creates a flesh which is soft yet strong, which in a healthy state is firm and quite resilient to touch, and quite fleshy. However, those people who have eaten an overly salty macrobiotic diet will be thinner and their bodies harder and tighter. Various conditions of the body can now be described in some detail.

Feeling for Ki

In shiatsu we diagnose by touch. We can perceive the quality of ki by the quality of the physical body. Those with more yang constitutions have the capacity, at least, to possess strong ki. Those with strong ki are overall quite fleshy but not fat. However such people tend to gain weight quite easily since they have a slower metabolism. Further, the overall shape of their body tends to be plastic rather than muscular, devoid of the appearance of the skeletal structure. The flesh is soft yet strong, firm yet supple and there is good muscle tone. With shiatsu, upon the release of pressure, the flesh quickly resumes its original shape.

In comparing a body overall, areas that are less fleshy reflect a more chronic deficiency of ki flow along the meridians in that area. Areas that are overly muscular or tight reflect a more chronic excess of ki energy. Deficiency of ki flow along any meridian is reflected in flaccid or stringy muscles or those with little resilience to touch. Excess of ki is reflected in overly tight muscles that are painful and slippery to the touch.

We can further describe different body conditions:

Hardness.   Hardness is yang. Hardness represents stagnation and a chronic condition. It represents a way of life that a person has become accustomed to, stubbornness and resistance to change. The harder the body the more stubborn and the greater the resistance.

Softness.   Softness is yin and represents sensitivity.

Fleshiness.   The quantity of ki in reserve. The more fleshy (but not fat), the more active is the person likely to be.

Thinness.   Less reserves of ki. Overall a deficiency of ki, especially if the flesh is loose or soft.

Firmness.   The individual's ki is integrated.

Tightness.   Stagnation of ki. Ki is withheld.

Stiffness.   Stagnation of ki. Ki is dormant.

Flaccid muscles/looseness/lack of muscle tone.   Ki is deficient or dispersed.

Resilience of the muscles to touch.   Ki is active.

Slippery feeling.   There is an abundance or excess of ki.

Sometimes seemingly opposite tendencies arise:

Tight but thin.   Ki is integrated but there is a limited supply, which the individual is reluctant to expend.

Thin but slippery.   Overall there is a deficiency of ki, but at this point in time the individual needs to focus their energy in one particular area. This condition applies more than likely to a particular meridian.

Fleshy but loose.   The individual is constitutionally strong but presently not so active.

When describing the four basic conditions into which we classify an overall condition, we should keep in mind, that each condition suggests a tendency. Each classification is not mutually exclusive. For example a person may have both a yin and yang excess condition or both yin and yang deficiencies. However in each case, either yin or yang will be prevalent. Further, we can note that a yin excess condition in the extreme turns into a yang deficient condition as can a yang excess condition, but the latter is more unlikely. A yin deficient condition may in the extreme turn into a yang excess condition. The following descriptions are to an extent generalizations, and possibly more extreme than what one is likely to encounter. However, within each depiction there are the main descriptions which we can see in a variety of gradations.

An Overly Yang Condition

1.   YANG JITSU—YANG IS IN EXCESS

In this condition (Fig. 14a), yin releasing energy is about normal. However yang gathering energy has backed up to such an extent that the skin surface appears expanded, the flesh exhibiting a full and round appearance. This condition represents an excess of stored energy, abundant reserves in the extreme. It is most often caused

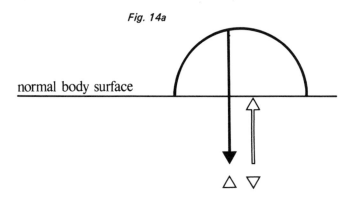

Fig. 14a

normal body surface

by a diet of excess animal food, and salt, along with much physical activity. Since yang predominates, it most likely suggests a focus of energy on the physical, practical, social or material realms. Since yin is normal it suggests that such energy can be expressed and that such expression will generally be positive, cheerful, optimistic, warm, and perhaps even passionate. If yin is less than normal or yang is much in extreme then release will not be so easy. We could liken such a condition to a large group of people all trying to hurriedly exit through a narrow door. There may be pent-up emotions with periodic outbursts, stagnation and inability to change.

Mentally this condition is reflected in thinking quickly, clearly, creatively, simply, precisely, and dynamically. Thoughts will tend to focus mostly on one particular interest, which is usually of a more practical nature. In some cases these people may be too attached to, or live in the past. Or they may be short-sighted, satisfied with short term at the expense of long term gain. They may be rigid, stubborn, and display resistance to new ways of understanding. Physically they tend to be dynamic and expressive, precise, punctual, quick, and alert, with the ability to follow through and complete whatever they set out to do.

More Yang Constitution

These people have a strong physical base oriented toward the practical, social, and material domains of life. They are often very dynamic and ambitious: workaholics, overachievers and those with a strong sex drive. They have the ability to think on a practical but grand scale and realize that dream. However, they may become too focused on one thing, narrow or rigid in their outlook. There may be difficulty in relaxing and little time given over to peace, quiet or self-reflection. There may be a tendency toward self-centeredness, impatience, thoughtlessness, and lack of consideration for others. In more extreme cases an agressive spirit may turn into occasional outbursts of anger or even violence, especially when strong yin such as alcohol is consumed in excess, releasing energy upward, causing the individual to become "hotheaded."

More Yin Constitution

These people have a stronger mental or artistic base directed toward putting into practice an idea or concept. While the idea may come quite easily, the practice may be more difficult. The idea may be far greater than is for them possible or practical. They are directed toward the physical, using their yang energy to focus on one thought or idea which they explore deeply. However a successful outcome may take longer to realize than they had planned.

Body Condition

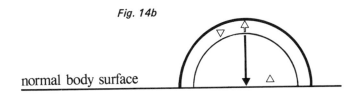

Fig. 14b

normal body surface

The surface is dynamic, appearing to protrude from the normal body surface (Fig. 14b). The outer line is undivided, suggesting firmness or tightness. In this condition yang energy first moves to the center so that the whole entity contracts. The center fills up and yang gradually backs up toward the surface, causing the surface to expand. However this yang expansion causes some degree of density. The muscles will be clearly pronounced, exhibiting a full and round appearance, and be slippery to the touch. Most likely the body will be to some degree hard, stiff, tight or heavy. In more extremes, energy may be very stagnated and difficult to move. We can note that there is figuratively speaking a large fire (yang) below a small amount of water (yin). The effect of this situation may by three-fold: yang consumes or dries out yin, leading to a hot condition; yang forces yin to the surface, leading to a wet or sweaty skin; yang holds yin inside, since the first movement of yang is toward the center—this condition leads to swelling and a taut and tight surface which may be extremely sensitive or tender when touched. We can also note that when we apply pressure, the direction of our pressure is going in the same direction as the predominating yang energy. This condition can be likened to a laundry bag filled with clothes yet with pockets of air within it. Depending upon the quality of yang and the duration of consumption, there may be some degree of softness or slack before we actually connect with the yang center. When we apply pressure, it is to this depth that we first press. In a conversation it would be akin to finally connecting with someone on a topic they are interested in, since at that level the body will react; perhaps it will react with some degree of discomfort, akin to drawing out a response from the person in question on some area of their life they are reluctant to change.

2.   YIN KYO—YIN IS DEFICIENT

Fig. 15a

normal body surface

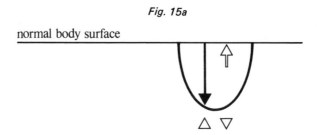

In this condition (Fig. 15a) yang gathering energy is normal while yin releasing energy is deficient. There is plenty of stored energy but an inability to express it. This condition is caused by a lack of dynamic activity or from a diet that is too narrow, lacking in variety, freshness, and lightness. Yin kyo reflects problems of dealing with the physical world, of communicating and sharing with others, of finding satisfaction with one's material accomplishments. Since yang is normal there is ample energy to think and act dynamically and creatively. However, the lack of yin implies the lack of a stimulus to put things into action, to use and express that energy. Without yin, energy cannot be brought to the surface or outward to be shared with others. Yang gradually builds up and the individual appears to others hard or cold, dull, listless, joyless or detached. Yet inside may beat a warm heart and a sense of frustration at not being able to express what they feel. There may be a tendency to become self-centered, spending too much time thinking about oneself.

Mentally this condition reflects in the person who has the yang energy potential to think creatively and dynamically. But they lack the yin nourishment which would stimulate their imagination, inspiration or idealism, causing them to settle for the mundane, routine, and tried and tested. Instead they could be searching for new ways to replace the old or, exploring new ideas. There will be a tendency to think seriously and materialistically, usually focusing on one train of thought, which they may have difficulty in expressing clearly. In their physical behavior such people may appear cold, hard, or "uptight." There may be a lack of interest in their appearance, wearing the same style or color of clothes day in and day out. For relaxation, they may be set in their ways, preferring routine forms of amusement when they could be exploring new kinds of experiences.

More Yang Constitution

These people have a strong physical base with ample energy to become successful in the material world, to which they are directed. However there may be trouble finding enjoyment in whatever they do. This double yang situation with a lack of yin may create a deep frustration that they cannot express what they feel inside. Since this condition implies excess energy moving toward the self, they may become quite self-centered. They may have trouble getting along with people, creating a space between themselves and others by being overly critical or harsh.

More Yin Constitution

These people have a stronger mental or artistic base but their energy condition limits them to the physical. They are inherently more comfortable with mental activity but lack the uplifting yin energy to ignite the mind's processes. They have difficulties dealing with the realities of everyday life. This situation arises because the physical energy they possess is limited by their innate yin constitution, a situation amplified by the lack of yin in their present condition. It prevents them from seeing the enjoyment that can possibly be gained from such activity. Consequently there may be a tendency to become too serious and pessimistic.

Body Condition

Fig. 15b

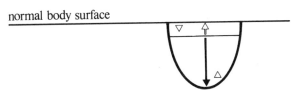

normal body surface

The surface of the body is flat (Fig. 15b). The body overall is generally tight but there is a thin veneer of softness covering a flesh which is generally dense, hard, tight, and stiff, but not as extreme as a yang jitsu condition. Likening the condition to a jar of nut butter, if we were to dip a spoon into it and then withdraw it, the movement of the mass would be slow to return to its original shape. Likewise in the body, the flesh is dull and listless, possibly heavy and lacking in resilience or muscle tone. When we release our pressure the body surface returns slowly to its original shape. However if we apply pressure too quickly, there will be localized muscular resistance or tension since the body has ample energy to defend itself. Since a normal fire (yang) is below small reserves of water (yin), we can expect internal heat. The surface may appear dry or hot, or it may appear cold, if the quality of yang is mild and yin is not sufficient to draw this yang to the surface.

An Overly Yin Condition

1. YIN JITSU—YIN IS IN EXCESS

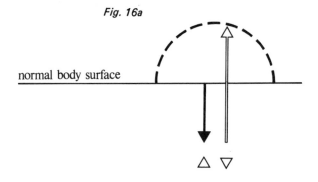

Fig. 16a

normal body surface

For this condition to appear (Fig. 16a), yang gathering energy must be present in approximately normal supplies. However yin releasing energy is in excess causing the body surface to expand. While yang energy lasts there will be a more rapid expression of energy. This energy will tend to move either upward, manifesting as expansion of the mind; or it will move outward manifesting as increased activity in the practical, social or material realms. In each case the individual may be pursuing a variety of interests. This condition is caused by an excess consumption of yin food such as fruit, fruit juice, sugar, alcohol, recreational and some medicinal drugs. Liquids and some lighter forms of dairy food such as milk or butter may also contribute to this condition. Since yang is normal there is ample energy to express and excess yin creates an ease of expression. The problem then becomes one of conserving energy and in using the expressed energy effectively.

Mentally, this condition directs much energy toward intellectual, artistic, aesthetic or religious endeavors. However there may be a tendency to think too broadly, unrealistically or impractically. The individual may be overly idealistic, too cerebral, abstract, future oriented or "up in the clouds." Thus in terms of physical behavior they may appear to be cheerful, optimistic, and outgoing, yet their feet are not firmly planted on the ground. There may be much energy being released but expression may be frenetic or lacking in direction. Verbal expression may be very quick or very slow and "not with it." Such people are open to what is new and probably quite expressive and colorful in their sense of dress.

More Yang Constitution
These people have a strong physical base with ample energy to explore either the mental realms or a variety of practical interests and find success at such ventures. There may be a wide range of interests of artistic or intellectual nature, usually with a practical foundation. If energy is directed more outward then there may be much interest in travel or moving around, with difficulty settling in any one place. Either conceptually or practically such people think expansively. Bodily, they may tend toward overweight. The danger for such people is of not knowing their capacity. In the extreme there is the danger of "burning themselves out," of becoming an empty shell with many psychological and emotional problems.

More Yin Constitution

Such people have a stronger mental base with energy directed toward exploring the mental realm. Consequently there will be an ambivalence toward or difficulty dealing with practical daily affairs, of coming down to earth. Such people may have many fine ideas but there is little energy directed toward putting them into practice. They may tend to be daydreamers or complex thinkers. There may be a broad range of mental interests but difficulty paying attention to any single one for any length of time. They will tend to think and express themselves slowly, with less form or clarity and they may prefer a more alone type of existence.

Body Condition

Fig. 16b

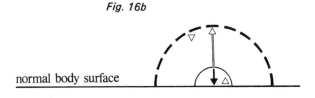

normal body surface

The surface of the body is dynamic appearing as protruding from the normal body surface (Fig. 16b). The outer line is divided, suggesting sensitivity, softness and ease of release. In this condition yin energy first moves to the periphery. Excess yin causes the surface to expand. Further excess then backs up toward the center, releasing yang to the surface. (A pronounced example of this condition in daily life would be the rowdiness that may arise after heavy alcohol consumption.) An image of a yin jitsu condition would be a balloon in various stages of expansion. A balloon is light. When a balloon is only partially blown up it is still soft and the surface comparatively thick. If we press into it, the finger will sink in and when we withdraw it, the balloon will immediately return to its original shape. If we blow the balloon up to its fullest, it is liable to burst; the surface becomes thin and taut. We may not be able to penetrate very deeply pressing into it, for fear of it bursting. These images represent different degrees of this body condition. We can see in this diagram that in this condition the predominating yin force is moving in the opposite direction to our pressure. For this reason, even if the condition is mild, the application of pressure may easily cause discomfort. Overall, yin excess creates a full condition that contains elements of lightness and buoyancy. The muscles will feel slippery and there will be a softness that is absent in a yang jitsu condition. Finally we can note that we have a regular fire (yang) below a large supply of water (yin). Such a situation indicates what we may term a cool condition, though depending upon the proportion of yin and yang factors and the quality of yang being released, it can be a very active condition.

2.   YANG KYO—YANG IS DEFICIENT

Fig. 17a

normal body surface

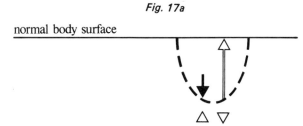

In this condition (Fig. 17a) yin releasing energy is normal. However yang gathering energy is deficient. Energy is released before it has a chance to build up. Such a condition results from the following situations: overexertion without taking care of oneself; stress and tension; not taking adequate rest. With diet it results from the lack of good quality strengthening food. This condition reflects to some degree an inability to deal with the practical realities of daily life. It can be described by such expressions as "running out of energy," "losing one's fire," "burning out." It is the person who tries but cannot meet deadlines, who is never on time, who is always struggling to make ends meet. Expenditures are always greater than savings. Such people may often feel tired and, in the extreme, exhausted or fatigued. Whatever reserves there are never last for long. The flat surface of the body reflects a monotonous and mundane lifestyle. Life is a struggle.

Mentally this condition manifests in the loss of creative thinking or the inability to gather one's thoughts or think quickly or precisely. It therefore leads to a lack of order or clarity in verbal expression, which may sound slow, quiet or tired. In the extreme there is nothing to say or express. In their physical behavior such people are losing their sense of integration. They lack vitality, are perhaps aimless, slow or sluggish in movement and may become sloppy or lose interest in their appearance.

More Yang Constitution
These people have a strong physical base but cannot meet the demands placed on them by their lifestyle. Such a condition often arises from overindulgences or the inability to deal with stress or overwork. What were once challenges have become a struggle. Sometimes this condition results in those who do not know when it is time to slow down and rest, in the case of workaholics for example. In other cases it results from the overconsumption of extreme yin such as recreational drugs. They become an empty shell—burnt out or suffering from psychological problems; they have gone beyond their capacity.

More Yin Constitution
Such people have a strong mental or artistic nature which is forced to deal with physical reality. Besides having difficulty in gathering their thoughts or of thinking creatively, they also have trouble thinking practically or dealing with everyday affairs. There is a tendency to be physically weak or inactive, overly self-conscious, overly dependent on others, or lacking in direction in their lives. They may be thin and pale, overly sensitive to the cold, and tiring easily, require more sleep than is normal. In the extreme, they have no energy left and the life which may have been a struggle becomes a burden.

Body Condition

Fig. 17b

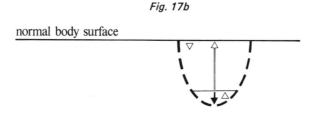

normal body surface

The surface of the body is flat (Fig. 17b). The broken line indicates that the flesh is loose, the muscles stringy or flaccid and there is little ability to withhold energy. The person may not be very fleshy at all through this area, indicating a more chronic condition of the meridian. There is little energy passing through this area, consequently an inability to defend it. However the individual as an entity knows of this condition. When we apply pressure our hand will sink in easily since the muscles in that area do not have the energy to resist. Because the localized area lacks defense, resistance comes from bodily reaction, contraction, and tension that may appear in the most subtle of ways anywhere within the body. This condition can be likened to a jar of liquid with sediment gathered at the bottom. The sediment represents what reserves of yang are left. It will manifest as a deep hardness which is the body's last line of defense to defend this deficiency. In this condition we have a small fire (yang) below a large quantity of water (yin), suggesting that this is a cold condition.

Yin and Yang and The Movement of Ki within the Human Entity

When evaluating a person's health condition the cause is not always clear. Always both yin and yang factors will be present and it is up to the practitioner to determine the factor which is more the cause. Simple overall definitions such as tight, dry, hard for a yang cause; loose, wet, or soft for a more yin cause, are a good beginning.

Let us now go through some of the various movements of ki that we should either consider, or may encounter.

1. *Yang creates, nourishes, and moves toward yang—Yin creates, nourishes, and moves toward yin*

Very simply, we can see this principle in three ways. First, the person whose constitution is yang is so because of yang factors surrounding the mother's pregnancy. She was active and ate a more yang diet for example. Second, if that person has a more yang condition it is because they are consuming an excess of yang. Third, the yin-yang quality of a food gravitates toward an area of the body of like yin-yang quality. For example the effect of sugar, which is more yin, will be experienced in the more yin location of the head. Animal food, which is more yang, will tend to activate the more yang legs and feet. In more subtle ways all food will, according to this principle, nourish or activate different parts of the human entity.

2. *Yang is negatively affected by excess yang and an extreme excess of yin—Yin is negatively affected by excess yin and an extreme excess of yang*

Something that is already yang needs a yin stimulus to release that yang. Excess yang will make yang too tight. Something that is already yin needs yang to keep it integrated. Excess yin will make yin more expanded and weaker. However someone who is already very yang has great capacity to absorb yin. There is a danger of not knowing one's capacity and eventually exhausting the stored supply of yang. Someone who is already very yin needs yang to give strength, but yin changes to yang slowly. If yang is consumed too quickly or in too great an amount, there will be the reaction of a desire to consume extreme yin, to restore a balance that can be more easily coped with. Such people for example become easily exhausted if they are forced to undergo a severe regimen of physical activity.

3. *The greater the yang, the greater the attraction and reaction to yin—The greater the yin, the greater the attraction and reaction to yang*

Focusing on diet, the person who eats too simply or narrowly will more than likely gradually become attracted to yin. Yin may mean a wider diet or it may mean yin quality food. Moreover even a small amount of yin in such a condition will cause a much greater reaction in this person than the one whose diet is already more yin. If they change to a wide diet too quickly they may find that they cannot digest the food. If they consume some stronger quality of yin such as alcohol or a dessert, immediately a strong mental effect will be felt. For the person who has become overly yin, the more yin they become, the more attraction there is for that which will make them strong and moreover, the greater the need there is for such kind of food and the quicker the positive response to its consumption. However if too much yang is taken too quickly, then there will be a negative response. There will be a craving for yin in order to establish a balance with which they feel more comfortable, since yin changes to yang slowly while yang can change to yin quickly.

4. *In excess, yang gravitates toward yin areas—In excess, yin gravitates toward yang areas*

We know that:
1. Yang moves downward and inward. Yin moves upward and outward.
2. Earth's yin force nourishes more the right side of the body. Heaven's yang force nourishes more the left side of the body.

Thus the consumed yang energy will tend to move more toward the lower body, especially the left side, activating more the left side of the abdomen: the stomach, spleen and pancreas, the descending colon, the left kidney, as well as the left leg. Conversely, the consumed yin energy will move upward toward the upper body, especially the right side, nourishing and activating more liver and gallbladder functions, right lung and right arm, the right side of the neck and right brain.

However if yang is consumed in excess, it will first spill over into the lower right side of the body, disturbing the flow of earth's rising energy. This movement will lead to stagnation in the lower right quadrant, leading to tightness in the area of the ileocecal valve, a swollen ascending colon, and a swollen liver and gallbladder. It will also lead to tightness in the right leg, especially along the inside where the liver meridian is located. Conversely, excess yin will spill over into the left upper quadrant, expanding more the left brain, the left side of the chest, and creating a weak feeling in the left shoulder and arm, as well as in the stomach and spleen.

5. *Yang creates warmth, yin creates coolness—But, extreme yang creates peripheral coolness, extreme yin creates peripheral warmth*

Yang energy moves toward the center. However with the consumption of extreme yang, peripheral circulation is retarded, since the energy of extreme yang is directed toward the center. Excess salt consumption will cause this situation. However when the person begins to move, taking in yin energy, circulation and thus warmth should be soon restored to the periphery.

Yin energy moves toward the periphery, releasing stored yang. When an excess of yin such as fruit juice, sugar or alcohol is consumed, the periphery of the body especially the hands and head, will initially become warm, but this condition may be only temporary. Once stored yang is discharged, such foods will create coolness or coldness in the periphery.

6. *Balanced yang creates speed, balanced yin slows down—But, extreme yang slows down, extreme yin speeds up*

Yang is the product of heaven's force, which is a force moving toward a point. Heaven's force creates stillness. When this force is balanced with yin, it can be seen as creating a gathering of energy, which will later be released either by yin or through movement such as physical activity. However if heaven's force is too extreme, far outweighing the yin releasing force, then the individual slows down, becomes or feels heavy, and even sleepy.

Conversely, balanced yin creates deceleration by neutralizing the expressive force of yang. However if much yang is stored, then extreme yin will cause the stored yang to be released, creating more intense activity. However since extreme yin is involved, then such a release of energy may be frenetic or dispersed: there may be a lack of focus or direction in the expression of that energy. Such an action caused by extreme yin lasts only as long as there is stored yang.

7. *Excess yang forces yin to the surface*

In this instance, viewing the body as a sponge can be helpful. Since yang energy moves toward the center, it causes the body to contract. This action in turn forces stored yin to the surface, since the natural movement of yin is toward the periphery. This yang contraction can arise because of either changes in the external environment such as the weather or changes in the internal condition due to diet or physical activity.

We can illustrate the first situation with the effect of the change of seasons from summer to autumn. The cooler weather forces the body to contract. This condition causes any excess yin to rise to the surface. Thus what appears to be a yin condition is actually caused by yang.

Focusing on direct changes to the internal environment, we can take two examples. In the first we can see that after intense activity we begin to sweat. From one perspective such yang activity has made the body tighter, causing excess yin liquid to the surface. In the second, if excess yang food is being consumed this too will force yin to the surface, since excess yang both causes the body to contract and/or it fills the body with yang, leaving little room for yin. For this situation to arise then, the individual's condition is probably already quite yang. A more serious example of this condition may occur when an individual begins the macrobiotic diet but eats too simply or changes too quickly. The yang quality of this diet causes the individual to "shrink," to become too yang. It causes excess the body wants to discharge to come to the surface. Such a result may all be very well unless it causes physical or psychological discomfort greater than the individual is prepared to bear. In this situation the problem is most directly alleviated by widening the diet.

8. *Excess yang holds yin inside*

Sometimes a person's condition may appear yin when the actual cause is yang. As we have seen, yang causes an overall entity to contract, while yin wants to be released. If both forces are fairly balanced then both forces can proceed smoothly. However if yang far exceeds yin, then yin becomes locked inside, often leading to various forms of swelling. Overconsumption of salt can cause this problem. Other examples of how this condition occurs are as follows:

1. *Eating very narrowly after eating very widely.* An example of this situation would be the person who after a long history of drug abuse begins a macrobiotic diet that is too narrow, strict or salty. In such a situation toxins or drugs cannot be discharged.
2. *Consuming yin in a yang form.* The consumption of baked foods containing sweeteners (cookies, cakes) will cause this condition.
3. *Changing a yin condition through excessive physical exercise.* This approach may make the body too tight to allow stored yin to be discharged.

9. *The effect of yin energy consumption will be felt readily—The effect of yang energy consumption takes time*

To someone in good health, the consumption of sugar, for example, will be sensed almost immediately as thoughts become dispersed. Conversely, the energy derived from animal food may not be experienced until hours later, perhaps not until the following day or even longer. We can explain this through an understanding of the digestive process. However, more simply, once we know that yin energy first moves toward the periphery, then already it is close to leaving or being discharged from the body. Conversely, yang energy must first move to the center before it can be disseminated outward and such a process takes longer.

10. *Excess yang creates yin deficiency and vice versa*

When we emphasize consuming yang it will cause an overall yang condition within the body; when we emphasize consuming yin, a yin condition. However this yang (or yin) affects each organ differently, depending upon the type of food consumed. We can take alcohol consumption as an example. Overall, alcohol corresponds with Fire nature energy—it is yin fire. Fire nature energy also corresponds with joy and laughter on the yin side, and the ability to concentrate or become absorbed in something on the yang side. Alcohol consumption (yin fire excess) generally leads to joy and laughter (at least temporarily), but in such a state it may be difficult to concentrate (yang fire deficiency). We can see the effect of alcohol throughout the other transformations.

On the nourishing cycle, yin fire excess leads to yin soil excess. Thus, alcohol which instigates joy and laughter, leads to feelings of sympathy and thoughtfulness. Or one may even burst into song. These qualities all correspond with yin soil.

On the control cycle however, yin fire excess leads to yang metal deficiency. The individual loses the ability to establish order, get their act together, or complete things—all indicative of yang metal deficiency.

Chapter 3

The Standard Macrobiotic Diet

"If one is able to chew the vegetable greens and roots well, he should be able to do all things."—Wang Hsin-min[1]

The Standard Macrobiotic Diet is an approach to eating developed by Michio Kushi. Mr. Kushi has lived in the United States for almost forty years. He has taught and counseled thousands of people both here and abroad. His approach to the macrobiotic diet represents a refinement of the principles set forth by George Ohsawa. It has been most experienced by Western peoples in temperate regions. The dietary guidelines in this chapter (pp. 80–100) are drawn largely from Mr. Kushi's book *Macrobiotic Diet* (Michio and Aveline Kushi with Alex Jack, Japan Publications, Inc., 1985).

In addition to presenting an outline of the macrobiotic diet, the purpose of this chapter is to pinpoint the major ways to adjust the diet according to one's condition, working within each particular food category. This material is employed to show how we can treat the four basic conditions a practitioner will be confronted with in those who receive shiatsu. Since each individual is unique, it can in no way be considered as more than a broad guide. For more information on preparation, macrobiotic cooking books are listed in the bibliography.

The Standard Macrobiotic Diet from an Energetic View

From a macrobiotic point of view all foods can be classified according to yin and yang. Fig. 18 illustrates in a simplified fashion the yin-yang spectrum of the foods that we consume. Refined salt is the most extreme yang food and the vast majority of drugs and medications, the most extreme yin. Whole cereal grains are the most balanced and centered. Human beings, as the highest evolved creatures, have the greatest freedom of dietary choice. The extremes of such dietary freedom have been explored to the fullest by people of the industrialized countries in this century. In the United States over the past seventy-five years those foods comprising the foundation of the standard macrobiotic diet have sharply declined in both quality and consumption. Those foods recommended to be avoided or restricted have sharply increased in consumption and declined in quality.

We can visualize the horizontal line of the diagram as a seesaw, with one end representing extreme yang foods and the other extreme yin. The fulcrum represents whole cereal grains. Thus, in terms of yin and yang, we can see how the consumption of food on one side implies the consumption of food of an opposite kind on the other in order to maintain balance. We can also see that the subtle up-and-down movements created by dietary expansion near the center amplify in ever larger changes the further one moves toward the periphery.

Our life can be seen as movement in four basic directions: inward, manifesting as spiritual development; outward, as social or material development; upward, as mental

78

Fig. 18

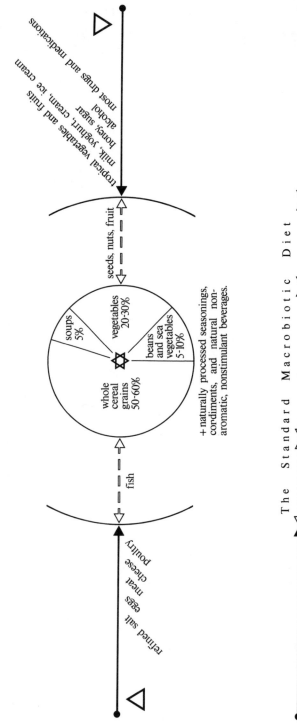

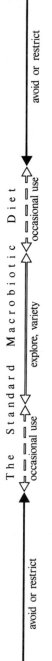

tropical vegetables and fruits
milk, yoghurt, cream, ice cream
honey, sugar
alcohol
most drugs and medications

seeds, nuts, fruit

soups
5%

vegetables
20-30%

beans
and sea
vegetables
5-10%

whole
cereal
grains
50-60%

+ naturally processed seasonings,
condiments, and natural non-
aromatic, nonstimulant beverages.

fish

refined salt
eggs
meat
cheese
poultry

T h e   S t a n d a r d   M a c r o b i o t i c   D i e t

avoid or restrict

occasional use

explore, variety

occasional use

avoid or restrict

development; and downward, manifesting as physical development. Only at the center are all four directions integrated and only there is the individual self united with the spiritual Self of One Infinity. This still point can be achieved by such spiritual practices as meditation, fasting, or semi-fasting on a very simple diet of little more than small quantities of whole cereal grains and liquids. At the extremes, the wide diet consumed by modern people parallels a very dynamic and externally directed lifestyle, with many ups and downs. However in such extremes the individual is likely to lose contact with the spiritual Self. When an excessively yin diet is consumed energy moves upward to the mind and outward in the form of either dispersed thinking or analytical and conceptual thought. The individual loses contact with the body and physical reality and gains only a fragmented spiritual view. When an excessively yang diet is consumed, energy moves downward into the body and outward in the form of attachment to the physical world. The individual loses contact with the spirit and mind. The yin diet person takes a more objective view of life, the yang diet person a more subjective one. At the center though, there is no differentiation between subject and object. As we move away from the center distinction develops and dualism arises. The further we move away from the center, the greater the dualism.

Thus from the dietary changes that have taken place in this century the following conditions can be observed:

1. By ignoring central or principal foods modern persons have lost contact with their spiritual nature, their direct connection through intuition with all other people.
2. The consumption of extreme foods has been associated with extreme forms of lifestyle. No one can deny the enormous advances in travel, communication and material well-being brought about by industrialization and modern technology. However, paralleling these advances, on the negative side there has been a marked degeneration. Individually, there has been a great increase in chronic and terminal illnesses such as cancer and heart disease. Collectively, humankind has destroyed ecosystems globally and faces the possibility of nuclear war. Total extinction of this present civilization is highly possible form within and without.

To reverse this trend the macrobiotic view begins by focusing on the individual. This approach encourages each person to strive to improve his or her own condition. Each will thus be able to live in harmony with the earth and align with the will of heaven. Aligning with the will of heaven we receive divine guidance and the power to carry out heaven's will. World peace begins with each person establishing peace within. This peace is the outcome of sound physical, mental, and spiritual well-being. The individual then radiates this sense of well-being through involvement at other levels: to family, community, society, and the world at large.

Broadly speaking, the macrobiotic dietary approach concentrates on three fundamental steps:

1. Avoid or restrict all kinds of extreme foods.
2. Build up a strong dietary center based on whole cereal grains and vegetables.
3. Explore the center. Within the realms of an appropriate quality diet, choose a wide variety of foods, cooking styles, and food combinations.

By avoiding extremes and building up a strong center we establish a basis for sound physical, mental, and spiritual well-being. By cooking with a large variety of foods, cooking styles and various food combinations, we ensure high level nutrition and dynamic energy.

Within the range of the macrobiotic diet it is easy to adjust one's eating according to the changes in one's life. To develop more spiritually, we eat more simply, more toward the center. To develop more materially and socially we eat more widely, more toward the periphery. To develop more physical power, we eat more from the yang side. To develop mentally, we eat more from the yin side.

The Transition to Macrobiotics

The longer one has been practicing macrobiotics, the easier it is to adjust the diet according to the seasons, age, lifestyle, and other factors. Not all people find the transition to macrobiotics easy and the changes that one will go through do not occur over days or months, but years. However the major changes, the ones that are most difficult to adjust to, are those that occur in the beginning. To make a smooth transition to macrobiotics it is wise to eat very widely for the first few months. (Those with serious health problems are an exception to this approach.) Affirm that you wish to change—that it is your goal. With this outlook, change at the pace your body wishes to change. Those who change too quickly or who eat too narrowly in the beginning are the people who have the most trouble later on, as the body is likely to undergo an extreme reaction.

Begin by slowly eliminating or avoiding extreme foods; move toward the center, toward the standard macrobiotic diet. Simultaneously, begin building up the center. Introduce grains into your diet at a percentage of food intake that your body feels comfortable with. Introduce various soups including miso, plus vegetable, bean and sea vegetable dishes.

To summarize, eat widely in the beginning and slowly increase the variety of macrobiotic foods that you consume.

It will be well worth the time and effort to take a series of cooking classes in this period. For the beginner it would also be wise to consult with someone with many years of macrobiotic experience.

The following dietary guidelines should be considered just that. They provide a framework for you to find a diet that is suitable for you.

Standard Dietary Guidelines*

WHOLE CEREAL GRAINS

Whole cereal grains are the principal food. They constitute approximately 50 percent of the total daily food intake by cooked volume. The percentage may vary plus or minus 10 percent depending upon seasonal adjustments (slightly higher in winter, lower in summer), one's state of health, age, sex, and lifestyle. This category includes cracked grains, whole flour in the form of noodles, and baked, fried, and deep-fried flour in the form of bread, cakes, pancakes, crackers, and the like.

Whole cereal grains and whole cereal grain products include the following:

---

* Regular use=suitable for daily consumption. Occasional use=two to three times per week. Infrequent use=less often. Generally not used=to be avoided or minimized.

Regular use whole grains	Occasional use grains/grain products	Occasional use flour products
Short grain brown rice	Long grain brown rice	Couscous
Medium grain brown rice	Sweet brown rice	Whole wheat noodles
Barley	Mochi	Soba noodles (buckwheat)
Pearl barley*	Bulgur (parboiled	Udon noodles
Millet	cracked wheat)	Somen noodles
Corn	Cracked wheat	Unyeasted whole wheat bread
Whole oats	Steel-cut oats	Unyeasted whole rye bread
Wheat berries	Rolled oats	Fu
Buckwheat	Corn grits	Seitan
Rye	Cornmeal	
	Rye flakes	

Grains

In most macrobiotic households the principal grain is short or medium grain brown rice, usually pressure-cooked, and served once or twice per day.

Other whole principal grains include barley, millet, corn, whole oats, and buckwheat.

For variety and better nutrition, different grains are combined together and with various vegetables, beans or bean products, sea vegetables, seeds, nuts, fish and seafood. When combined, the proportion of brown rice in a dish is usually between 70 and 90 percent, even higher in the case of seeds and nuts.

Brown rice can be prepared in numerous ways besides pressure-cooking. Fried rice creates a richer, boiling a lighter, and baking a stronger taste and energy. By cooking with larger amounts of water, various forms of soft rice can be prepared for those having digestive difficulties.

Different grains have individual properties.

Barley has a lighter, cooling quality, and is recommended for dissolving retained animal food and excess fat. Barley especially nourishes liver and gallbladder functions.

Pearl barley* or "hato mugi" tends to be used for more medicinal purposes. It is useful for dissolving fats, tumors and gathered excess in the lower parts of the body, including the ovarian, prostate, and colon regions.

Millet provides nourishing qualities for the stomach and spleen-pancreas, particularly when served with such sweet vegetables as onions, carrots, and squash. In the form of a soup, millet and sweet vegetables can aid in relaxing a tight pancreas.

Sweet brown rice pounded into the form of mochi is a very energizing food, especially when prepared at home. It can be helpful for gaining weight, creating warmth, creating milk in mothers, and as a snack food.

Oats contain more fat than other grains and are a warming food, making for a hearty winter breakfast. However, since whole oats can be mucous forming, their consumption should be restricted for those with lung and large intestine problems.

Buckwheat is the most yang food in this category and has warming and strengthening properties. It is especially beneficial for kidney and bladder functions and is consumed more often in winter; but since buckwheat has the ability to absorb excess

---

* Jobs Tear, Coix Lachrima, not "pearled" barley (the common species of barley but refined). Also Jobs Tear should be used only in small amounts mixed with other grains 3–5%. It has medicinal value but too large an amount can be toxic.

liquid, it can be appropriately served in an occasional salad in the summer months when we tend to overconsume liquids. For those with serious illnesses, particularly those caused by excess yang, buckwheat is often avoided for a periodoftime.

Grains are usually seasoned during the cooking process: generally one pinch of mineral rich sea salt is added for each cup of dried grain. Grains can also be seasoned with tamari soy sauce and miso, as well as with other condiments.

Noodles

Noodles include partially refined wheat noodles known as "udon," buckwheat noodles called "soba," and wholewheat pasta. Noodles are a popular food since they are easy to digest and can easily satisfy an appetite without being filling. This makes them suitable for luncheons and snacks. Two of the most popular ways of serving noodles are in a tamari broth garnished with scallions, or fried. In the latter form they are usually seasoned with tamari soy sauce and garnished with ginger pickles, scallions or grated daikon. Noodles can be enjoyed a few times per week, but for those with serious illnesses buckwheat or fried noodles are usually restricted.

Baked and deep-fried flour products

When bread is desired, an unyeasted whole wheat or rye sourdough is recommended. Generally, servings are of two or three slices, usually no more than two or three times per week. Bread is best served steamed or with liquids such as soup.

Bread is eaten only occasionally for two main reasons. First, grain once broken begins to lose much of its nutritional and energetic value. While whole grains can be stored for long periods, once broken they deteriorate rapidly. Second, baked or deep-fried flour can be very mucous forming, creating troubles in the lungs and large intestine. It can also cause stagnation, creating problems especially in the large intestine and liver. Overall, such foods possess a hardening and drying energy, creating in the short term a desire for liquids, and in the long term a dense, heavy and stiff body. In addition, baked flour, especially when combined with simple sugars, as is the case with flour-based desserts, can create gas.

Whole cereal grains contain a balance of protein, carbohydrates, fat, and vitamins and minerals ideally suited for human consumption. They also provide more energy and calories than any other food substances. The complex carbohydrates—polysaccharides—in whole cereal grains are gradually and smoothly assimilated through the digestive organs, providing a slow and steady source of energy to the cells and tissues. Whole grains are generally high in B-vitamins and vitamin E.

Many scientific studies have shown that whole cereal grains strengthen the heart and circulatory systems, protecting against high blood pressure, heart attack, stroke, and other cardiovascular disorders. A diet centered on whole grains is also beneficial for the elimination of excessive fats and mucus, reducing body weight, and restoring physical and mental flexibility. Whole grains can also help to detoxify the body from harmful effects arising from the consumption of extreme foods.

Over time, the regular consumption of whole grains and their products as principal food will secure the following benefits to promote physical and psychological health: 1) better digestion and elimination; 2) better blood constituents and circulatory functions; 3) better natural immunity to infection and disease; 4) better nervous system functioning including that of the brain; 5) better hormonal functions; 6) better reproductive functions; 7) improved mental clarity, psychological stability, and peacefulness in human relations; 8) strengthened physical and mental endurance; 9) heightened awareness of the environment and natural world; and 10) deeper spiritual insight and aspiration.[2]

SOUP

One or two bowls of soup constituting 5 to 10 percent of daily food intake by volume is suggested. Since it is highly nutritious, at least one bowl is usually miso soup.

Miso Soup

Miso is a fermented soybean or soybean-grain combination paste, traditionally consumed in Japan in soup form for breakfast. It is yang and alkalizing, providing quick energy for the coming day's activities.

There are numerous kinds but the most commonly used varieties are "mugi" or barley miso, "Hatcho" or plain soybean miso, and "genmai" or brown rice miso. Miso should be processed naturally together with good quality sea salt and usually aged for at least eighteen months. Barley miso is the most popular type and can be used throughout the year. Plain soybean miso is a little stronger in taste and tends to be used more often in the colder months. Brown rice miso, which is sweeter and lighter in taste, tends to be used more often in the warmer months.

The way one prepares miso soup is important. Most often miso soup is prepared with wakame and the miso is not added until the end, after vegetables and other ingredients have been cooked. Miso is diluted in a small amount of soup stock before being added. It is simmered into the soup for a few minutes before serving.

Miso soup can be a deceptive way of consuming excess salt. Indications of this are a salty taste in the mouth, thirstiness, sleepiness, a craving for sweets, or an excessively strong appetite. Thus, the quantity of miso added should be moderate and the taste of miso soup mild. The general recommendation is one level teaspoon of miso or less for each serving of soup.

Besides the quantity of miso, the energy of the soup can be altered by the kinds of vegetables used. For a lighter quality and taste more leafy greens such as kale or Chinese cabbage should be used. More root vegetables such as carrot or burdock could be added for stronger energy. Sweet vegetables such as onions or squash create a richer, sweeter taste. Miso soup should be garnished, usually with grated ginger or chopped scallions, and it should be prepared fresh daily.

Miso is high in vitamins, minerals and good quality fat. Especially in the form of barley or brown rice miso, where grain and bean are combined, it is an excellent source of protein and complex carbohydrate. Since it is a fermented food, miso contains bacteria, lactobacilli which aid in the breakdown of foods and the production of vitamins within the intestines. In addition it strengthens and purifies the blood and lymph systems and may help to prevent radiation sickness.

Other Kinds of Soup

Among the numerous kinds of soup that can be prepared, the following are very popular:

- *Tamari broth.* This soup is a consommé style, seasoned with tamari soy sauce. It is commonly served in place of miso soup or as a broth for noodles.
- *Grain soups.* These soups are often prepared from left-over grains. Grains in this form are warming and strengthening. Prepared with or without vegetables, this is a helpful way for those with digestive problems to take in food. Such soups are also suitable for breakfast and miso can be added for seasoning. Millet soup is an excellent way to soften and nourish an overly tight pancreas. Barley soup helps to relax a tight liver.
- *Vegetable soups.* Sweet vegetable soups, using onions and squash for example, may be beneficial for those attempting to gain weight.
- *Bean soups.* Bean soups are commonly prepared with azuki, chick-peas, and lentils. Azuki bean soup is especially beneficial in relaxing and nourishing tight kidneys.

Soups are taken either before or together with the main meal and should complement it. If the main meal is heavy and contains much variety, then the soup should be light and simple, and vice versa. As well, it is better to use different ingredients in the soup than are part of the main meal. For example a bean soup would complement a main meal without beans, a carrot and burdock soup would balance a main meal lacking root vegetables.

VEGETABLES

Vegetables should constitute 20 to 30 percent of daily food intake. Generally two-thirds should be served cooked and up to one-third in the form of either pickles, pressed or raw salad. Ideally, vegetables should be grown locally, organically, and consumed in season.

Vegetables fall into three basic categories: root, ground, and leafy greens. It is advisable to consume some from each category daily, emphasizing more root vegetables with stronger seasoning and cooking methods in the colder months, and more leafy greens with lighter seasoning and cooking methods in the warmer seasons.

Root vegetables provide strong downward energy; they strengthen the intestines, sexual function, the heart and circulatory system, and the lungs. Leafy greens provide more upward rising energy; they tend to nourish more the lungs and liver-gallbladder functions. Leafy greens tend to be calming yet stimulating to mental processes. Ground and stem vegetables provide more balanced energy and are especially beneficial to stomach and spleen-pancreas functions.

Vegetables are high in complex carbohydrates, fiber, vitamins, and minerals, providing substantial supplies of vitamin A and C, calcium and iron.

The following list shows those varieties commonly used in macrobiotic cooking and those which are generally avoided.

The most popular cooking styles and ways of food preparation in the standard macrobiotic diet include the following methods:

1. *Nishime Style* (also known as waterless cooking). Vegetables are layered in a pot with just enough water to cover the base. The pot is quickly brought to boil, then placed on simmer with the lid on, for twenty to thirty minutes or more. Most often, the main ingredients of this dish are root vegetables and kombu. Since root vegetables are more yang, the time of cooking relatively long, the amount of water

Roots	Ground	Leafy Greens
Regular use:		
Burdock	Broccoli	Bok choy
Carrots	Brussels sprouts	Carrot tops
Daikon	Cabbage	Celery
Dandelion root	Cauliflower	Chinese cabbage
Ginger root	Fall-winter squash	Collard greens
Jinenjo	Onions	Daikon greens
Lotus root	Pumpkins	Dandelion leaves
Parsnips	String beans	Escarole
Red radish		Kale
Rutabaga		Leeks
Turnips		Mustard greens
		Parsley
		Scallions
		Turnip greens
		Watercress
Occasional use:		
Taro potato	Cucumbers	Chives
	Fresh green beans	Endives
	Green peas	Escarole
	Mushrooms	Lettuce
	Shiitake	Sprouts
	Snow peas	
	Summer squash	
	Zucchini	

Generally not used: Among others, artichoke, asparagus, avocado, beets, chili, eggplant, green pepper, paprika, red pepper, rhubarb, sweet potato, Swiss chard, tomato, white potato, yams.

used small and the pot covered, this style of preparation is yang. It gives a centering and grounding effect. This dish is recommended for occasional use, more often in colder seasons, less in spring and summer.

2. *Azuki Kombu Squash.* This dish is comprised of approximately 60 percent squash, 30 percent azuki beans, and 10 percent kombu. It is most often served as a winter dish, since azukis are one of the most nourishing beans for the kidneys, while kombu also corresponds more with the water phase and kidney-bladder energy. Squash, being sweet in taste tends to nourish more the stomach and spleen-pancreas functions. This dish is centering, stabilizing and relaxing. It is especially beneficial to either pancreatic or kidney functions, of either yin or yang condition. This dish is recommended to be served occasionally, less often in summer and more frequently in winter.

3. *Dried Daikon and Kombu.* Drying or roasting a food creates a contracting effect that causes it to absorb more liquid than before, when reconstituted. Daikon is useful in melting away accumulated fats. Also it becomes sweeter through cooking. Both the high water content and sweet taste draw energy to and affect the kidneys, making this dish especially useful for cleansing them of accumulated fats and toxic substances. It is recommended for occasional use in small servings.

4. *Vegetable Tops with Vegetable Roots.* In this dish the vegetables are chopped fine and steamed over a high flame for ten minutes or longer. Vegetables used include

daikon with tops, turnips with tops, carrots with their greens, dandelion roots with their greens. This dish provides a balance between upward and downward energies while activating predominantly lung and large intestine functions. It is recommended for occasional use.

5. *Boiled Salad.* This dish is more yin in nature, from the upward nature of boiling as well as the relatively short cooking time. Boiled salad provides freshness and an overall more outward or peripheral energy. It also helps to balance or neutralize the effects of excess animal protein. It is additionally helpful for people who are too tight or too dry. Boiled salad can be served regularly and should be prepared fresh each time.

6. *Pressed Salad.* A pressed salad involves cutting vegetables very finely, mixing them thoroughly with sea salt, and placing them under pressure, usually either with a pickle press or a heavy weight on a covering plate. Commonly used vegetables include cabbage, carrots, celery, cucumber, mustard greens, onions, and radishes. The vegetables should be kept under pressure for at least thirty to forty-five minutes. However they can be pressed for as long as three or four days, in which case this dish tends to resemble more a light pickle. Pressed salad offers the kind of freshness of raw vegetables. It is helpful in eliminating animal protein, as well as neutralizing acidity and stimulating digestion. It is a good substitute for raw salad. If the taste is too salty, wash off the salt before serving. A pressed salad is usually consumed occasionally and in small quantities.

7. *Raw Salad.* Raw salad tends to be served less often. However it is refreshing in hotter seasons or climates and makes a good balance for animal food. Raw salad can be beneficial for those whose condition is too yang or who crave sweets. When recreational drugs have been consumed over a long period of time, such people are advised to eat widely and raw salad is often suggested. However those with more yin conditions such as skin problems, yeast infections, herpes, candida, as well as people with AIDS should avoid this dish. Generally, raw salad is taken occasionally.

8. *Steamed Greens.* The value of leafy greens cannot be overstressed. Examples such as watercress, kale, collard, turnip, and mustard greens are particularly high sources of vitamin C and calcium, as well as other essential vitamins and minerals. However, the way they are prepared is important. These vegetables should not be overcooked: they should retain a fresh and crispy taste. Fresh steamed or lightly boiled greens can be served everyday.

9. *Sautéed Vegetables.* Vegetables can be sautéed with oil or water. For those with serious illness, oil may need to be restricted. Sauté-style cooking, which uses a high flame for a short period of time, provides more fire nature energy—quick, active, and warming. It is especially beneficial for those with stiff joints and muscles. Sautéed vegetables can be served occasionally.

10. *Kinpira.* Kinpira style of preparation involves cutting vegetables into extremely fine matchsticks. The most commonly used varieties are burdock and carrot. Kinpira is a quite yang dish—only yang vegetables are used, the vegetables are chopped finely, the dish is covered while cooking for a considerable length of time, and if oil is used, stronger heat is diffused into the vegetables. Kinpira is very strengthening for the intestines and digestive functions in general. Small servings are recommended for occasional consumption.

11. *Seitan/Tempeh/Tofu Stew.* This kind of preparation is also known as vitality

stew since it supplies easily digestible protein and quick energy. It is especially beneficial to the circulatory system, warming the periphery of the body by activating blood flow.

12. Sukiyaki. This dish is first prepared in a cast iron skillet, then boiled in a broth and served with a dip. Sukiyaki is made with vegetables, noodles, tofu, tempeh, and sometimes seafood. It provides a quick supply of nutrients, yet it is not heavy since it contains many vegetables. It is especially appropriate for the following situations: in the colder months since it promotes circulation; for those whose energy is stagnated; for those persons who tend to feel tight and/or get cold easily. Sukiyaki can be served occasionally.

13. Tempura. This dish consists of sliced vegetables first dipped in batter and then deep-fried in oil at high temperatures. A large number of foods cook well in a tempura style: seitan, root and some ground vegetables, as well as fish and seafood and some sea vegetables, beans, and grains. Tempura provides light but quick energy and it is appropriate to serve once per week, more often in winter. It is especially helpful for those who have lost weight and for those who are too tight or too dry. It also provides warmth.

14. Pickles. Pickles stimulate the appetite, strengthen the intestines, and aid in digestion. They are especially helpful in the assimilation of whole cereal grains with which they are usually eaten together. Pickles can be broadly divided into light and heavy varieties. Light pickles are quick to prepare and pickled for only a short time— from a few hours to several weeks. Varieties include salt, tamari soy sauce, and to some extent miso pickles if pickled for only a short time, as well as umeboshi or shiso pickles. These kind of pickles provide a lighter quality of energy and are generally recommended in summer, or for those who need to restrict their salt intake. Heavy pickles are stronger in flavor and taste and accordingly provide a stronger energy. They may take from several weeks to several months to prepare and are generally consumed in the cooler months, or by those who lack energy. Examples are miso pickles prepared for a few months or bran pickles. Pickles are usually sliced finely. A few slices each day are generally recommended.

BEANS AND BEAN PRODUCTS

Beans and bean products constitute 5 to 10 percent of daily food intake by cooked volume. The most regularly used beans are those coming from more northerly regions. They are smaller in size and generally lower in oil content. Larger varieties such as lima beans, originating in more southerly areas, are much higher in oil content and used only very occasionally. The other beans in the following list fall in-between these groups:

Regular Use	Occasional Use	Bean Products
Azuki beans	Black-eyed peas, black turtle beans,	Dried tofu
Black soybeans	great northern beans, kidney beans,	Fresh tofu
Chick-peas	mung beans, navy beans, pinto beans,	Natto
Lentils (green)	soybeans, split peas, whole dried peas,	Tempeh
	lima beans	

Essential in most traditional cultures, beans and bean products form an important part of the standard macrobiotic diet. In most traditional cultures grains and beans have been served together. Beans, which are rich in protein and fat, perfectly complement whole cereal grains which are comparatively higher in complex carbohydrates. In addition modern nutritional science has supported the traditional practice: it has shown how the respective amino acids of grains and beans complement each other to form a more complete protein.

For many, a problem with beans is gas. It may be caused by overeating, insufficient chewing, a weak digestive system, or incorrect cooking method or preparation. Usually it is necessary to presoak beans, at least for a few hours and most often overnight, and to discard the soaking water. After the first half hour or so of cooking, the froth on the top of cooking water should be skimmed off. In addition, beans should be cooked with kombu, since the yang minerals in kombu balance the yin protein and fat content of beans. Kombu also tends to draw out the flavor of beans. Presoaking, skimming, the addition of kombu, along with cooking over a low flame for a long period of time will ensure the beans to be thoroughly cooked and easily digested.

Beans can be cooked in various ways, such as boiling, pressure-cooking, baking or roasting. However, the most popular and effective means is known as "shocking." In this method, the beans are cooked over a low flame and as they come to a boil cold water is added to stop the boiling. Repeating this procedure several times during cooking will ensure that the beans are cooked evenly both inside and outside.

Beans are usually seasoned with sea salt or tamari soy sauce and sometimes miso. However, azukis or black soybeans can also be sweetened with a small amount of barley malt or brown rice syrup.

Bean products, namely tofu, dried tofu, tempeh and natto may be taken on a regular basis in place of bean dishes. Of all beans, soybeans are highest in protein and oil. For this reason they are more easily digested following natural processing procedures, such as the making of miso, tamari soy sauce, tofu, natto, and tempeh. Tofu is perhaps the most popular soy food and its bland taste gives it the ability to take on the flavor of whatever food it is prepared with. Tofu is prepared in many different ways in the macrobiotic diet. Since it is quite yin and cooling by nature, it is usually consumed in small amounts. Traditionally tofu has been seasoned with a salty flavor. However in the West tofu has become popular as a base for desserts and dessert fillings, and also as a flavored milk substitute, soy milk. The addition of the sweet taste to tofu makes a yin food very yin and as such is not recommended. However for those on a transitional diet, flavored soy products may prove quite helpful over a short period. Also the textures of tofu and tempeh (a fermented whole soybean product), enable them to be prepared in a variety of ways that often make them an acceptable substitute for those craving animal food.

Overall, beans create a slow, steady source of energy. They tend to be too heavy to be taken as a breakfast food though, and when overconsumed may cause dullness in thinking, slowness in activity, and overweight. In addition to protein and complex carbohydrate, beans are also a valuable source of calcium, phosphorous, iron, thiamine, niacin, and vitamin E. The fat in beans is unsaturated and entirely free of cholesterol.

SEA VEGETABLES[3]

Sea vegetables are recommended for 5 to 10 percent of total daily food intake by cooked volume. All edible sea vegetables are suitable for daily use. However in common practice the most popular varieties are the following:

More frequently	Less frequently	Even less frequently
Kombu	Arame	Dulse
Wakame	Hijiki	Agar-agar
	Nori	Irish moss
		Mekabu
		Sea palm

Kombu and wakame are used almost everyday as a basic ingredient of many dishes. For example, miso soup is nearly always prepared with wakame, and kombu may be used to make soup stocks, or cooked with grain, vegetable, or bean dishes. Since sea vegetables are taken in these forms, it is not necessary to have them in side dishes more than two or three times per week. In such cases hijiki or arame are most often used and a small serving is sufficient. Dulse, agar-agar, Irish moss and *mekabu* all have excellent properties but are generally used less often. Sea palm is a newly available variety with exceptional taste and texture.

Kombu
Kombu is gathered off Hokkaido in Japan, and the east and west coasts of America as well. It is dark green to blackish in color and comes in flat dried strips some 3 to 18 inches long. Kombu needs to be presoaked for a few minutes before use and will expand more than two times its original size. Since it takes a relatively long time to cook, it blends well, in terms of cooking time, with grains, root vegetables, and beans. Kombu is also used in pickling and in some kinds of confectionary. Two popular condiments are made from it. The first, shio kombu or "salt kombu" is very strong. It is useful for vascular diseases and problems with the kidneys and bladder, caused by excess yin. The second, kombu powder is made by baking kombu until it turns black and then grinding it; it can be added in this form to grains and soups. It is used medicinally for some cases of heartburn and in cases of serious diarrhea in children and babies. Kombu tea, made by boiling kombu in water for a few minutes, is helpful for strengthening the blood, calming the nervous system, discharging animal fats and protein, restoring mental clarity, and for kidney-bladder problems caused by excess yang. Overall, kombu is believed to increase sexual vitality, longevity, intelligence, and mental clarity.

Wakame
Wakame comes in dried strips, narrower than kombu and usually 4 to 12 inches long. When dried it is dark green in color, but when soaked turns much lighter. Wakame is harvested from the temperate waters off the coasts of northern Japan, China, Korea and North America. It is usually presoaked, but cooks more quickly than other sea vegetables. Besides being a regular ingredient in miso soup, wakame can be prepared together with many different kinds of land vegetables as a side dish. It is particularly

enjoyable in summer salads. It can be made into a condiment called wakame powder that can be added to grains. Medicinally, wakame is used to reduce high blood pressure and for treating heart disorders in general.

Arame

Arame grows along the coasts of Japan and South America. After drying, arame is shredded. It is black in color and appears threadlike in its dried form. When cooked, it doubles in volume and has a slightly sweet taste. Arame is often sautéed in a small amount of sesame oil, and combines well with root vegetables such as burdock, carrots and lotus root, and dried daikon, as well as with bean products such as tempeh and dried tofu. Arame is also added to soups and salads. Medicinally, arame is used to treat anemia, stomach and spleen-pancreas problems caused by excess yin, as well as many other conditions.

Hijiki

Hijiki grows off the coasts of Japan and China. Hijiki is also black in color and similar in appearance to arame although thicker. It also has a thicker and richer taste and takes longer to cook. When prepared it expands to five times its original volume. Hijiki can be sautéed and combined with root vegetables or bean products in the same way as arame, or used in soups and salads. Hijiki can also be steamed, boiled, deep-fried or baked.

Nori

Nori is cultivated in the temperate waters off the coast of Japan, and also grows on the northeast coast of America. It is prepared in thin sheets that are dark green or purple in color. In Japan it comes in many grades and its quality can be judged by color and flavor. The deeper the color and better the flavor, the higher the vitamin and mineral content. Nori is usually toasted on one side above a low flame before eating to improve its digestability. It is most often used to wrap rice balls or as the outer covering of sushi. However, it can also be cut into thin strips for garnishes in salads, soups, fried noodles or fried rice. A half to one sheet or more can be taken everyday. Nori can also be crushed or ground into a powder. A nori condiment is made by tearing up several sheets, mixing with water and simmering until most of the liquid is boiled away—leaving a thick paste to which tamari soy sauce is added and simmered in. This condiment is beneficial for stomach and spleen-pancreas problems caused by excess yin. It stimulates the appetite and is good for digestion.

Overall, sea vegetables, with the exception of nori, need to be washed beforehand to get rid of grit. Tamari soy sauce is recommended for seasoning more than sea salt and usually added after the beginning of cooking.

Sea vegetables are an important part of the macrobiotic diet since they are excellent sources of vitamins and minerals. They are also high in complex carbohydrates, protein and fiber, and low in fats. There are proportionately more vitamins in sea vegetables as well as minerals, accounting for up to 30 percent of their weight, than in any other food. All vitamins and minerals required by human beings are present in high amounts. Nori is especially high in vitamin A as well as vitamin C and vitamin B_1. Hijiki, wakame, arame, and kombu are all high in calcium and iron content. All sea vegetables, especially kombu and arame, are high in iodine. Sea vegetables are the least processed of natural foods and, with one rare exception found off the coast of the Phillipines, nontoxic. Many varieties of sea vegetables are now being gathered off the coasts of California, Maine, and Nova Scotia.

Since sea vegetables are high in minerals, they help to maintain an alkaline blood condition and are beneficial for improving conditions of high blood pressure, arteriosclerosis, allergies, arthritis, rheumatism and nervous disorders. Sea vegetables can also help to dissolve fat and mucous deposits caused by excessive consumption of animal foods and sugar. Hijiki in particular, which is high in fiber, can strengthen the intestines, create strong shiny hair and purify the blood.

Scientific studies have shown that sea vegetables have strong antibacterial, antifungal, antiviral and antitumoral properties. Sea vegetables reduce cholesterol levels in the blood and reduce fat metabolism. They thereby diminish the risk of high blood pressure and protect against the development of arteriosclerosis. Several varieties of sea vegetables have also been discovered to contain blood anticoagulants and it is theorized that sea vegetables may also protect against radiation.

FISH AND SEAFOOD

For those in good health, fish can be enjoyed in small quantities. Two or three times per week is usually recommended. However this may vary according to the following conditions:

More often	Less often or not at all for
In autumn and winter	Babies and infants
For males	Females
For those living in colder climates	Older people
For those lacking in vitality	Those with serious illness
For those on a transitional diet	Spiritual development

Fish and seafood varieties are recommended as follows:

Occasional Use			Very Occasional Use	
Saltwater	*Freshwater*			
Cod, scrod	Bass	Abalone	Squid	Bluefish
Flounder	Catfish	Clam	*Sashimi*	Herring
Haddock	Pike	Crab	Raw fish	Mackerel
Halibut	Trout	Lobster		Salmon
Mullet	Whitefish	Mussel		Sardines
Perch		Octopus		Swordfish
Red snapper	*Dried:*	Oyster		Tuna
Shad	Chirimen iriko	Prawn		Blue-skin fish
Smelt		Scallop		Red-meat fish
Sole		Shrimp		

Generally, white-meat fish is recommended over other varieties, since it is lower in fats and oils and the texture is softer. Saltwater varieties are generally recommended over fresh, due to the greater dangers of water pollution of inland waters. When purchasing, fish should be checked for indications of freshness: clear eyes; a smooth skin; resiliancy to the touch; good color; intact gills; and lack of a fishy odor. Also the liver, gallbladder, and excretory organs, which filter and store contaminants, should be removed before cooking.

Fish can be served as a soup, as a separate side dish, in stews, with grains, vegetables, and sea vegetables, and in fresh salads. Fish can be prepared in various ways—boiled, steamed, baked, sautéed, pan-fried, deep-fried, tempura style, marinated, pickled, or served raw. Preparations involving oil are used less often, since fish is already comparatively oily; steaming, boiling, and baking are the more common methods. A garnish is usually served alongside to aid digestion. The most common form of garnish is grated daikon served as a small side dish (one or two tablespoons) with a few drops of tamari soy sauce and grated fresh ginger root added. The kind of garnish varies with the type of fish and manner of preparation. Other garnishes include mustard, *wasabi* (grated Japanese horseradish), horseradish, lemon, orange, fresh *shiso*, and chopped scallions. Fish is usually seasoned with sea salt, tamari soy sauce or miso. Other seasonings include brown rice vinegar or umeboshi vinegar, mirin, black or red pepper, and tofu, kuzu or oil sauces. When fish is served as a separate side dish it should be consumed along with a regular serving of whole cereal grain and with two or three times the usual volume of hard leafy greens, such as kale, daikon greens, mustard greens, and collards. These vegetables will help to neutralize toxins and balance the yang contracting effect of fish.

Nutritionally, fish and seafood are high in protein and contain plenty of B-vitamins. Fish is also low in cholesterol, and the type of fat found in fish is unsaturated. A condiment made from *chirimen* or *chirimen iriko* is a good source of vitamin B_{12}. Carp soup, which is recommended for those low in energy, provides fat and protein quickly.

SEEDS AND NUTS

As a supplemental food, seeds and nuts are consumed occasionally, in small volume. While some varieties are consumed raw, normally they are lightly roasted and seasoned with sea salt or tamari soy sauce, or at times with miso, barley malt or rice syrup. They are served primarily as snacks. However, seeds and nuts can also be prepared as condiments, garnishes, or cooked with various foods, for example with whole cereal grains, vegetable dishes, and in breads and desserts. They can also be made into nut and seed butters.

Within the category of supplemental foods, recommendations are made as follows:

Occasional Use	*Less Frequent Use*	*Infrequent Use in Small Quantity*
Seeds:		
Sesame seeds	Poppy seeds	Apricot seeds
Pumpkin seeds	Umeboshi	Sesame butter
Sunflower seeds		
Nuts:		*Nut Butters, e.g.:*
Chestnuts	Brazil nuts	Cashew butter
Almonds	Cashews	Peanut butter
Peanuts	Hazelnuts	Almond butter
	Macadamia nuts	
	Pecans	
	Pine nuts	
	Pistachios	

Seeds and nuts more commonly used are those in each category which originate in temperate zones. They contain less fat and oil and are usually smaller in size. Seeds are used more often than nuts, since they are lower in fat and oil content. Organically grown varieties are preferred since those commercially grown contain chemical contaminants.

Sesame seeds come in both black and brown varieties. In the form of a condiment called *gomashio* (goma means sesame and shio means salt), sesame seeds are an important part of the macrobiotic diet. Like beans, the amino acid content of sesame seeds complements rice to make a better quality protein. Gomashio is also an excellent way to consume oil, and sesame is more easily digested when crushed. The hulled seeds can be ground without the addition of salt to make a butter known as tahini.

Sesame seeds and pumpkin seeds are rich in iron. Chestnuts are low in fat and high in complex carbohydrates. Sunflower seeds may be too oily for those with serious illnesses. Nut butters are more difficult to digest than nuts taken in whole form.

FRUIT

Fruit is consumed primarily for variety and enjoyment. It is preferable that fruit be fresh, locally grown, and eaten in season. Since commercially available fruit is subject to much chemicalization, both during growth and after harvesting, organically grown is recommended. For those in good health, consume in small volume two to three times per week—more often in summer and usually less in winter. With these factors in mind the following choice is suggested:

Occasional Use	To Be Used Sparingly	Better Avoided
Apples	Apple juice	Bananas
Apricots	Apple cider	Breadfruit
Blackberries	Grapefruit	Coconuts
Blueberries	Lemons	Dates
Cantaloupes	Oranges	Figs
Cherries	Limes	Guavas
Peaches	Kumquats	Kiwi fruit
Pears	Tangerines	Mangoes
Plums		Papayas
Raisins		Plantains
Currants		Other fruit juices
Raspberries		Tropical fruits in
Strawberries		a temperate climate
Watermelon		

Fruits recommended for regular use are either low growing (berries and melons), and tree fruits in temperate regions. Apples are commonly used, since they are the most yang: they are small in size, firm, and mild, yet sweet in taste. Citrus (grapefruit, lemons, limes, oranges, tangerines), except for very occasional use in summer, is employed primarily as a garnish or an ingredient for sauces, dressings and dips. Vitamin C, present in high quantities in citrus fruits, is obtained from other sources in the standard macrobiotic diet. Most important are hard leafy green vegetables—

some varieties are higher in vitamin C content than citrus fruits. Fruit juices are consumed less often than fruit since they are more concentrated. Of these, apple juice and apple cider are the most popular. To counter their expansive effects, they may be heated or cooked with kuzu; the binding quality of the kuzu offsetting the expansive effect of the fruit. Tropical fruits are avoided, since both energy and nutrients are too extreme to be balanced by standard macrobiotic foods.

Fruits are served in three ways—fresh, cooked, or dried. Fresh fruit is consumed primarily in season, especially in summer. A pinch of salt is sometimes added, or fresh raw pieces are soaked in lightly salted water before serving, to enhance the sweet taste. However fruit is usually cooked, most often boiled, baked or steamed. A pinch of salt may be added and sometimes kuzu. Dried fruit can be taken as a snack, along with nuts, for example, or cooked. Since dried fruit is more concentrated than fresh one should be careful of the volume consumed. Less fruit is consumed in winter than in other seasons: dried fruit is the most common type of fruit used at this time.

Fruit has a cleansing effect. It helps to eliminate residues from a long time consumption of animal food as well as other accumulated toxins and wastes. Fruit is also a preferable substitute for ice cream or soft drinks and other commercial sweets. However fruit is a cooling food and in excess creates coldness in the body, lowering resistance to colds and flu as well as reducing sexual vitality. Since fruit is high in simple sugars, in excess it creates fat, which can contribute to arthritis, rheumatism, diabetes and heart disease. Generally, too much fruit can lead to dispersed thinking and an ungrounded feeling.

SNACKS AND DESSERTS

In a modern diet, sweets and desserts balance the lack of carbohydrate, or the heavy yang quality of the main meal. In a standard macrobiotic diet, desserts are usually consumed at the end of the evening meal, for variety and enjoyment. For those in good health, desserts are consumed on an average of two or three times per week. If desserts are desired much more than this the cause may be one of the following:
- Eating too yang, especially consuming too much salt
- Not enough whole cereal grain being consumed (or absorbed)
- Food, especially whole cereal grains, not being chewed thoroughly
- A diet too narrow, lacking in variety
- Disease or disorders such as spleen-pancreas imbalances

The first choice of ingredients for desserts is sweet vegetables cooked to bring out the sweet taste—by baking or slow sautéing for example. If a stronger sweet taste is desired, it may be satisfied by a fermented sweet rice product called amazaké. Otherwise grain-based sweeteners such as barley malt or rice syrup are commonly used. Generally a smaller quantity of such products is needed if they are cooked, than if served raw. A great many desserts can be created with these foods, together with a small number of other ingredients (Col. 2). All refined sweeteners, spices and sweeteners from tropical countries, and other extreme sweeteners are avoided (Col. 3). Tofu-based desserts are not recommended, except on occasion or in the case of a transition diet.

Thus the following suggestions:

Occasional Use Sweetener	Occasional Use Combinations, Thickeners or Garnishes	To Be Avoided
Sweet vegetables	Chestnuts	Sugar
Cabbage	Seeds and Nuts	All refined artificial
Carrots	Fresh/cooked/dried/fruit	sweeteners
Daikon	Azuki beans	Carob
Onions	*Kanten*/kuzu	Chocolate
Parsnips	Grated ginger	Molasses
Pumpkin	Grated peel or juices of	Honey
Squash	orange/lemon/tangerine	Tropical Spices
Amazaké	for garnish or spice*	Baking powder
Barley malt/rice syrup	Whole grain flour	Fresh yeast
Apple cider or apple juice:	(Wheat/corn)	Tofu-based desserts
cooked with kuzu or added		
as a sweetener		

* Organic particularly important here.

When making dietary adjustments in this category, we see it not only as a possible source of excess sweets, but also through pie crusts and cakes, as a possible source of excess oil or dry-baked food.

SEASONINGS

Various seasonings are used in the macrobiotic diet according to the following recommendations:

Regular Use	Occasional Use	To Be Avoided
Mineral rich sea salt	Ginger root	Fruit and wine vinegars
Tamari soy sauce	Grated raw daikon	Some spices and herbs
Miso	Brown rice vinegar	
Umeboshi plum	Sweet brown rice vinegar	
	Umeboshi vinegar	
	Mirin	
	Horseradish	

Salt

One of the most important tastes in the macrobiotic diet is salt, since the extreme yang quality of salt determines the balance or imbalance of all other dietary factors. Mineral rich sea salt is recommended since it contains substantial amounts of essential mineral elements. Mineral rich sea salt contains approximately 97.5 percent sodium chloride: commercial refined table salt however is almost pure sodium chloride—it is devoid of all trace elements and contains additives. The taste and effect of refined salt is much stronger than mineral rich sea salt and nutritionally it is very imbalanced.

Salt is necessary in cooking. However this taste should not dominate a dish but rather enhance it, by drawing out the flavor of the foods it is combined with. Thus salt or salty seasonings should be used moderately and the resulting taste should be mild.

Generally salt consumption is increased or decreased according to the following factors:

Increase	Decrease
In colder climates or seasons	In warmer climates or seasons
	For females
For males	For more mentally active people
	For elderly people
For more physically active people	For babies under 10 months (no salt)
	For ages 3–7, 1/4 to 1/3 the adult amount—
	(from 7 onward gradually increase
	to standard)

The main sources of salt in the diet include mineral rich sea salt, miso, tamari soy sauce, and umeboshi plums. Umeboshi vinegar contains sea salt and sea vegetables may also have a slight coating. Only naturally processed miso, tamari soy sauce and umeboshi are recommended. Miso and tamari soy sauce are fermented foods. The longer these foods ferment, the milder the salty taste.

Properly used, salt provides energy, improves blood quality and circulation and gives direction in life. The average salt content of the standard macrobiotic diet is four times less than the standard American diet. However since there are many ways to take salt in the diet, there is always the danger of overconsumption. We should remember the following:

- Salt is used to enhance the natural flavor of the food it is combined with.
- The use of salt should be moderate and the taste of a meal only mildly salty.
- Salt is generally cooked into the food. With the exception of adding tamari soy sauce to noodle broth at the table, neither tamari soy sauce, unrefined sea salt, nor miso should be taken from dispensers on the table. Instead, condiments are added to make subtle adjustments in the final taste of a meal.

The following is a checklist of the different ways we consume or may overconsume salt in the macrobiotic diet.

Grains: Salt is added during the cooking process, usually one pinch of salt to one cup of dried grain. Condiments should be used sparingly, on average no more than two teaspoonsful per person per day. The ratio of gomashio generally varies between 1: 8 and 1: 20—those who are taking too much salt should increase the proportion of sesame seeds. Tamari soy sauce should be simmered into a broth before serving. Prepackaged instant noodles with their sauces may be overly salty and other varieties of Japanese noodles, which usually contain salt, should be rinsed after preparation.

Soup: In miso soup, up to one flat teaspoon of miso is generally recommended per serving and this should be simmered in before serving. In other kinds of soup, a slightly higher amount of salt can be added than is used for grains for example, up to 1/4 teaspoon of salt per bowl. Prepackaged instant miso soup may be overly salty.

Vegetables: In vegetable dishes, either sea salt or miso is added during the cooking process, usually toward the end. In the case of pressed salads or quick pickles, salt should be washed off if they taste too salty.

Beans: Once more, sea salt, tamari soy sauce or miso are added during the cooking process, usually after the beans are 80 percent cooked.

Sea Vegetables: In some cases, with kombu especially, it may be necessary to brush off the salt before soaking. Once again, in the preparation of a sea vegetable dish, the salty taste, which is usually tamari soy sauce, is added toward the end of cooking.

Fish: When broiling, salt is sprinkled directly over the fish. If this method is used often it may be a source of excess salt consumption. When raw fish is consumed, the fish is usually dipped into a small side dish of tamari soy sauce mixed with wasabi. This too can be an easy way to consume excess salt. Only a small amount is necessary with each dipping.

Seeds and Nuts: These foods should be lightly salted. Store bought varieties are often heavily seasoned. They may be a source of overconsumption of salt, especially when one regularly snacks on such foods.

Snacks: Store bought crackers and chips, especially those imported from Japan, are often heavily salted.

Dressings, Sauces and Gravies, Condiments: Overconsumption of dressings, sauces and gravies, garnishes or condiments in general are a common source of excess salt.

The signs of excess salt consumption include the following conditions: excessive thirst or the taste of salt in the mouth; an excessive appetite; sleepiness; a dark color to the skin, especially around the eyes; body stiffness; loss of weight; rigid thinking.

Oil

Oil naturally complements salt. Most of the need for oil in the macrobiotic diet is satisfied within the foods themselves. Grains, beans and seeds all contain oil, as do nuts and fish. For those in good health, it is recommended that oil be used moderately in small volume. Seriously ill people may need to avoid the use of oil for a period.

Unrefined vegetable quality oil is recommended and the most frequently used type is dark sesame oil. Recommendations for the kinds of oil used are as follows:

Regular Use	Occasional Use	Avoid
Dark sesame oil	Mustard seed oil	All industrially refined oils
Light sesame oil	Sunflower oil	Cottonseed oil
Corn oil	Safflower oil	Palm oil
	Soybean oil	
	Olive oil	

Signs of excess oil consumption include an oily skin and liver and gallbladder problems.

Possible sources of excess oil include the following:

Grains: Deep-fried rice balls; pan-fried croquettes; fried rice and fried noodles; deep-fried seitan

Vegetables Dishes: Tempura style; sautéing with oil; deep-fried vegetables; kinpira style; stir-fried vegetables

Beans: Excess consumption, especially from the occasional use list; deep-fried bean products such as deep-fried tofu or tempeh.

Sea Vegetables: Excess oil used in the preparation of hijiki or arame dishes

Nuts and Seeds: Excess consumption of these foods or of nut and seed butters

Fish: Excess consumption of more fatty varieties such as eel, salmon, or mackerel. Excess use of pan-frying with oil.

Other Seasonings—*Dressings, Sauces, Garnishes, and Condiments*
This category includes important ways to balance a meal, and create the five basic tastes according to the Five Transformations.

Dressings
Dressings are most commonly used for salads, marinades, and servings of leafy green vegetables. They include:
1. *Tamari soy sauce dressings:*   These dressings combine tamari soy sauce most often with brown rice vinegar, lemon or ginger.
2. *Umeboshi dressings:*   These dressings combine the sour-salty taste of umeboshi most often with minced onions, a little sesame oil, sliced scallions or parsley.
3. *Miso dressings:*   The sweet-salty taste of miso is often combined with a dash of brown rice vinegar, grated ginger and/or sesame butter.
4. *Tofu dressings:*   Puréed tofu is often mixed with grated onions, sesame butter, umeboshi plums, sliced scallions or chives.

Dressings, if used too often, or in excessive quantities, or if too strong, can be a possible source of excess salt or oil consumption.

Sauces and Gravies
Sauces and gravies include:
1. *Dashi broth:*   A basic soup stock made with kombu and often with shiitake mushrooms as well
2. *Miso sauce:*   Made with finely sliced, sautéed vegetables and miso
3. *Kuzu sauce:*   Made with various cooked ingredients, combined with and thickened by diluted kuzu
4. *Sweet and sour sauce:*   Various finely chopped cooked vegetables cooked in a soup stock, thickened with kuzu and seasoned with sea salt or tamari soy sauce, brown rice vinegar, and either apple juice, mirin or a touch of maple syrup
5. *Bechamel sauce:*   Made from whole wheat pastry or brown rice flour, spring water, dried onion, and tamari soy sauce

Again, this category can be a possible source of excess salt consumption. Bechamel sauce used too often, can also be a source of excess flour in a form particularly difficult to digest.

Garnishes
Garnishes include:
1. Grated daikon or radish
2. Grated horseradish
3. Chopped scallions
4. Freshly grated ginger
5. Toasted nori
6. Breadcrumbs

7. Others, including wasabi, red pepper, freshly ground pepper and lemon slices

Condiments

Condiments are kept on the table, serving a similar function to salt and pepper. While the salty taste is primarily cooked into the food, minor adjustments according to each individual's personal condition and taste, can be made with condiments. The main varieties used include the following:

1. *Gomashio*—the most commonly used condiment. It is alkaline, an excellent way to absorb salt, and its amino acid content complements brown rice. Gomashio is generally prepared in the ratios of 1 part salt to between 8 and 20 parts sesame seed.

2. *Sea vegetable powders*—made from sea vegetables crushed or ground into a fine powder. Varieties used include nori, dulse, kombu, kelp, and wakame. Roasted sesame seeds can be combined as well.

3. *Tekka*—made from burdock, carrots, lotus root, Hatcho miso, and ginger— sautéed together for a long time in dark sesame oil and cooked down into a concentrated black powder. Tekka should be used sparingly since it is very yang.

4. *Umeboshi plums*—served whole, sliced, or puréed with raw scallions and onions. No more than one half to one umeboshi plum per day is recommended.

Other condiments include the following:

5. *Cooked miso*—with scallions or onions. This condiment has a sweeter, more pungent taste.

6. *Nori condiment*—prepared by cooking small squares of nori with spring water and tamari soy sauce.

7. *Shiso leaves*—green or purple colored leaves of the beefsteak plant, which are traditionally combined with ume plums in the processing of umeboshi. Shiso leaves can be chopped, roasted or combined with roasted sesame seeds.

8. *Shio kombu or "salty kombu"*—small squares of kombu soaked in tamari soy sauce for one or two days, then further covered with tamari soy sauce and cooked over a low flame for several hours. Shio kombu is very yang. No more than one or two pieces are recommended per day.

9. *Aonori (green nori)*—comes in small flakes and can be sprinkled over a meal.

10. *Brown rice vinegar and umeboshi vinegar*—can be used sparingly to add flavor to a dish. Brown rice vinegar has more downward while umeboshi vinegar more upward energy.

Condiments provide valuable sources of minerals and most are predominantly salty in taste. Some are dry, some are moist. We can consider these factors along with volume consumed, when making recommendations. Generally no more than one or two teaspoons of condiment per day is advised.

BEVERAGES

The frequency and amount of beverage intake depends upon a person's individual condition, as well as climate, seasonal and environmental factors. Macrobiotic people tend to consume less liquid than those on a standard modern diet. The general guideline is to drink only when thirsty. If one urinates more than three to four times per day it is an indication of overconsumption of liquids. If one is continually thirsty it may be a sign of overconsumption of salt or dry foods. It is wise to avoid ice cold drinks even in summer.

Beverages are recommended as follows:

Daily Use	Regular Use	Occasional Use	Avoid or Limit
Bancha tea	Grain coffee	Amazaké	Distilled water
Roasted barley tea	Dandelion tea	Nachi green tea	Coffee
Roasted brown rice tea	Kombu tea	Green magma	Cold drinks
Spring water	Umeboshi tea	Vegetable juices	Hard liquor—whiskey
Well water		Northern climate fruit juices	Highly mineralized water and bubbling water
		Beer	
		Saké	Black tea
		Mu tea	Stimulant beverages
		Soy milk	Stimulant herb teas
			Tap water
			Wine

Bancha tea is the most commonly consumed beverage. It contains little caffeine and is slightly alkaline.

Roasted barley tea has a cooling effect on the body and is commonly enjoyed served cool during the summer months.

Grain coffee should contain 100 percent cereal grains, wild grasses, beans, and other vegetable-quality ingredients. Those which contain honey, molasses, beets, figs, or other sweeteners are less desirable.

Umeboshi tea when served cool is an excellent summer beverage. Though salty, it quenches the thirst and replaces the salt lost in perspiration.

Mu tea is a more yang beverage. It provides strength and vitality and is more popular for occasional use in colder months.

Amazaké, made from fermented sweet brown rice, is quite sweet in taste and usually served hot, often with a dash of grated ginger. It may also be used as a base in desserts.

Commonly consumed vegetable juices are carrot and celery juices.

The most favored fruit juices are apple juice and apple cider. Others include grape, pear, apricot, and cranberry juice. Fruit juices should be natural products containing no additives, preservatives or additional sweeteners. Since they are concentrated foods, vegetable and fruit juices should be served only occasionally and in small amounts. The yin quality of fruit juices can be made more yang by cooking with kuzu and serving hot.

Beer and *saké* should be naturally brewed without additives, preservatives, or sugar.

Soy milk is a very yin beverage and better served only occasionally or to those on a transitional diet. Soy milk containing chocolate, carob, honey or other strong flavorings should generally be avoided.

The preceding information presents an outline of the standard macrobiotic diet. By making various adjustments we endeavor to find a diet that is suitable for each individual. Some of the broad factors that we need to consider in making adjustments include season and gender.

Seasonal Adjustments

In Chapter 2, a table of foods was presented according to the Five Transformations. These foods are listed according to the season in which they appear: the season in which they should most often be consumed. Other factors such as cooking styles, cooking time, and salt intake also need to be considered.

Spring: Energetically, spring corresponds with the tree phase—more upward energy. We thus consume more tree nature food at this time. This kind of food includes barley, wheat, wheat products, sprouts, leafy green vegetables, wild grasses, and short time pickles. Cooking styles include more light sautéing. Salt intake is reduced slightly.

Summer: Summer corresponds with the fire phase—very active energy. More fire nature food is consumed at this time. These foods include sweet corn, summer squashes, leafy greens, locally grown fruits, and tofu. More salads are also consumed, including fresh vegetable, fruit, noodle, pressed, and lightly boiled salads. Lighter cooking methods are used and salt intake is reduced.

Autumn: Autumn corresponds with the metal phase of energy, which is very yang, condensed energy. More metal nature food is consumed at this time. This kind of food includes early autumn squashes and root vegetables, hard leafy greens such as daikon greens, as well as cabbages, onions, turnips, and other round vegetables. Slightly stronger cooking methods are employed: these include nishime-style boiling, long time sautéing, and kinpira-style braising. Seasoning is stronger.

Winter: Winter corresponds with the water phase of energy transformation, characterized as floating energy. At this time we minimize cold, cool, and raw foods, and increase salt intake. There is increased consumption of winter squashes, burdock, daikon, carrots, onions, root and ground vegetables, longer aged pickles, and sweet brown rice and mochi. More oil is used, in such cooking styles as tempura, fried and deep-fried food, long time sautéing, and kinpira. As well, nishime-style boiling, baked dishes, and stews are more often prepared.

Man and Woman

Slight variations on the standard diet exist for the different sexes. Some important differences are as follows:

Males: Stronger seasoning and cooking methods; less raw food, fresh salad, fruit, sweets and desserts; greater volume and wider variety; more animal food

Females: More yin quality food and lighter cooking methods; more salads, fruits, raw food, sweets and desserts; less animal quality food; less volume of food

Four Basic Conditions

When we give shiatsu we evaluate a person's overall condition. We further evaluate the condition of each meridian and its corresponding internal organ. Both overall and meridian conditions can be classified into four basic categories. Our procedure is to follow standard dietary recommendations and make adjustments according to each individual's overall condition. We make further adjustments according to the condition of specific meridians following, or along with the general recommendations. This section concentrates on the individual's general condition. While four categories are presented they are not necessarily mutually exclusive. We may find that a person has an overall excess condition of both yin and yang factors or an overall deficiency in both yin and yang factors. Nevertheless most people tend to be a little more yin or a little more yang.

In the following guideline suggested for people in temperate regions, a checklist has been included with each condition. In these lists we see ways to make change according to each condition. It is not suggested that all changes be recommended or that all might be necessary, such decisions depend upon the extent of the condition, length of macrobiotic practice and so on. Duration of such changes are particularly difficult to suggest in such a guideline, especially since we should keep in mind that we change our diet according to climatic and weather changes anyway. As a general guide we could recommend such changes until the condition begins to noticeably change. However it is hoped through going over the suggestions one can get a "feel" on how to approach each condition to help restore a state of balance.

AN OVERLY YANG CONDITION

An overly yang condition can arise from two factors:
(1)   From excess yang. This condition is called yang jitsu;
(2)   From a deficiency of yin. This condition is called yin kyo.

1.   Yang Jitsu—Yang Is in Excess
The dietary cause of this condition may be one of two things:
1.   *The diet is too narrow.*   The individual has been eating very simply as is the case of a fasting diet of whole cereal grains, liquids, and little more. Such a person will probably have lost weight and may be low in energy.
2.   *An excess consumption of yang foods.*   This cause is the more common, consequently we will focus on it, and in addition take into consideration other factors which create yang within the standard diet.
Primary mode of change: Emphasize reducing yang.
Secondary mode of change: Increase yin.
Primary direction of change (see Fig. 18):
1.   From extreme yang, moving toward the center, reduce all forms of excess yang.
2.   From the center, moving toward yin, occasionally used foods, reduce yang factors within each food category. Increase some yin factors.
Primary dietary suggestions: Avoid commercially refined salt. Avoid or reduce all animal food, especially the more extreme varieties such as meat, eggs, dairy, and poultry. Extreme forms of yin should also be avoided or reduced. If extreme yang is reduced, there will be a slow but gradual loss of craving for extreme yin.
Other elements of change:
1.   *Salt content:*   The amount of mineral rich sea salt and salty seasonings con-

sumed should not be more, and probably less, than standard dietary recommendations.

2. *Food preparation:* Avoid roasting, grilling, baking, and other long time cooking methods. Consider reducing pressure-cooking. Employ standard or more often than standard use of steaming, boiling, and sautéing. Increase the proportion of raw food—more pressed salad, lightly salted pickles, and raw salad. You may need to suggest an overall increase in the variety of foods, cooking styles, and food combinations within standard guidelines. Those new to the macrobiotic diet may need to avoid oil, or use it sparingly, for a period. Long term macrobiotic people with this condition may need oil.

3. *Water content.* The amount of liquid used in cooking should follow standard recommendations or be slightly more.

Whole cereal grains: Avoid buckwheat until the condition noticeably changes. Cook grains with standard or less than standard salty seasonings. Consider temporarily decreasing the percentage of grains consumed. Grains may be cooked with a little more liquid and occasionally boiled. Secondary grains to be emphasized are barley and corn. Millet may be too yang to be consumed often in summer. When served, millet would best be prepared in a soft form or as a thin grain soup. More often than standard recommendations for light grains and grain products such as bulgur or long grain brown rice. One may need to increase the variety of grains consumed and their combinations with other foods. Avoid buckwheat noodles for a period. Check that a mild seasoning is used in noodle broths and that a garnish is added. One may include quick stir-fried noodles with vegetables. Avoid or restrict all baked and deep-fried flour products.

Soups: Miso: One bowl per day is sufficient or may be more than sufficient. Emphasize barley miso over soybean miso. Recommend adding standard or less than standard amounts of miso, emphasizing a very mild taste. Prepare with short time cooking. Emphasize leafy green vegetables, and avoid too many ingredients. Other: Avoid or reduce those that take a long time to cook such as grain or bean, as well as other thick soups. The cooking method of soup is to begin with boiling instead of cold water.

Vegetables and vegetable dishes: Root and round vegetables should be consumed as often as or less than standard recommendations. Leafy green vegetables should be consumed in standard or greater amounts.

Thus use standard recommendations or less often for nishime style, azuki/kombu/squash, dried daikon and kombu, root vegetables with root tops, kinpira. Follow standard recommendations or more often for boiled, pressed, and raw salad, steamed greens, quick sauté of foods (especially without oil), and seitan, tofu, or tempeh stews. Avoid or reduce miso and tamari pickles. Emphasize light, quick pickles in small amounts.

Beans and bean products: Emphasize more use of bean products. Serve beans in salads and light soups more often. Occasionally use sweetened bean dishes such as azuki beans with chestnuts, raisins, or barley malt; black soybeans with barley malt; sweet rice with azuki beans or black soybeans. Check that seasoning is mild and cooked into the beans. Avoid deep-fried bean products until the condition begins to change. Soy milk may be taken occasionally if desired.

Sea vegetables: Emphasize the use of wakame, not only in soups but also in salads. Emphasize arame over hijiki. Avoid cooking sea vegetables with oil. Avoid or reduce root vegetable-sea vegetable combinations. Avoid hijiki in summer or serve in salads. Remind to brush off the salt when using kombu.

Fish and seafood: Use only if desired and in small quantities (approximately a 4 oz serving) no more than twice per week. Recommend a white-meat fish balanced with many leafy greens.

Seeds and nuts: Emphasize that these should be lightly roasted and without salt. Limit the quantity consumed. Consume seeds and nuts more often from "less frequent use" column. Avoid or restrict nut butters and seed butters.

Fruit: Employ standard recommendations or more often. Occasionally serve fresh apple juice/cider if desired.

Snacks and desserts: Avoid or reduce dried snacks such as puffed whole cereal grains, rice cakes, crackers, and cookies.

Seasonings: Emphasize that salty seasonings should be mild and cooked into a food. Oil should be used sparingly—a dish of quick sautéed sweet vegetables and greens would be good. Pungent seasonings such as grated daikon or ginger root, and occasional lemon juice may also prove helpful.

Condiments: Minimize the use of baked and dried condiments, such as tekka and sea vegetable powder. Avoid shio kombu. Limit the amount of gomashio used to standard recommendations or less. The ratio of salt to sesame seeds in gomashio should usually be between 1:16 and 1:18. Limit the consumption of umeboshi to two or three plums per week. Recommend moist condiments such as miso with scallions or nori condiment. Employ grated daikon often.

Beverages: Avoid Mu tea. Take alcohol (beer or saké) occasionally if desired. If desired one may take vegetable juices; mild grain teas (such as mild barley tea); green magma two to three cups per week; nachi green tea two to three cups per week.

2. Yin Kyo—Yin Is Deficient

The dietary cause of this condition may be a combination of the following factors:

1. A lack of variety in the choice of foods and food preparation
2. A lack of yin styles of food preparation
3. A lack of consumption of yin foods, within standard dietary recommendations

Primary mode of change: Emphasize increasing yin.

Secondary mode of change: Decrease yang.

Primary direction of change (see Fig. 18)*:* Beginning at the center (whole cereal grains) and moving toward yin, occasional use foods, increase yin factors within each food category.

Primary dietary suggestions: Emphasize variety, freshness, and lightness, in both the choice of foods, cooking styles, and food combinations. Avoid overeating and oversnacking.

Other elements of change

1. *Salt content.* The amount of mineral rich sea salt and salty seasonings consumed should not be not more and probably less than standard dietary recommendations.
2. *Food preparation.* Emphasize the importance of consuming a wide variety of foods within standard recommendations, cooking styles, and food combinations.

Emphasize cooking fresh each day. Emphasize short-time and light cooking styles: more boiling, steaming, and sautéing. Avoid or reduce long-time cooking styles. More raw food may be necessary—more pressed salad, light pickles, and fresh salad.

3. *Water content.* The amount of liquid used in cooking should follow standard recommendations or be slightly more.

Whole cereal grains: Emphasize variety. Brown rice should be prepared on its own and together with other grains, vegetables, beans, and sea vegetables. Brown rice can be boiled occasionally. Emphasize the use of other regular use grains (especially barley and corn) as well as other occasional use grains and grain products. At times incorporate grains as salads. Use buckwheat less often. Employ standard recommendations for noodles; emphasize udon over soba and the importance of garnish with noodle dishes. Baked and deep-fried flour products not only create yang qualities of tightness and dryness but also heaviness—their consumption would be better limited. Bread should be served with liquids or steamed. One may need to suggest reducing the percentage of grains to be consumed.

Soups: Miso soup—remind of the importance of the following factors: miso should be simmered into the soup before serving; the taste should be mild; one bowl per day is adequate; it should be prepared fresh daily; it should be garnished; leafy greens should be emphasized; vary the kinds of miso soup prepared. Miso soup with sweet vegetables such as squash would be very helpful.

Other soups: Recommend tamari consommé style, emphasizing a light taste with few ingredients; split pea soup; light lentil soup; occasionally tempura in soup. One could include tofu, mochi, and ginger in soups occasionally.

Vegetables and vegetable dishes: Emphasize the primary dietary qualities recommended for this condition—variety, freshness, and lightness. Within standard guidelines, a large variety of vegetables should be consumed. They should be prepared fresh daily in a wide variety of cooking styles and food combinations. While root and round vegetables are necessary, emphasize leafy greens. Employ standard recommendations or less often for nishime style, azuki/kombu/squash, dried daikon and kombu, root vegetables with root tops, and kinpira. Employ standard recommendations or more often for boiled salad especially, as well as pressed and raw salad, steamed greens, sautéed vegetables (most often without oil), and seitan, tofu, or tempeh stews. Emphasize light, quick pickles in small amounts.

Beans and bean products: Beans need long-time cooking methods. When overconsumed, beans can make us feel slow, heavy, and dull. Since we are seeking ways to lighten this condition, it is therefore recommended to emphasize small servings, proportionately decreased consumption of beans and increased consumption of bean products. Take beans in the form of salads or soups more often. Avoid refrigerating and reheating beans: it makes them more yang. Occasionally prepare bean dishes flavored with barley malt; an azuki-chestnut-raisin dish; azuki beans with barley malt. Make more use of the "occasional use" category. Occasionally serve deep-fried bean products. Remind of the importance of presoaking beans.

Sea vegetables: Emphasize more yin forms of preparation such as arame or wakame salad, and arame with tofu. Emphasize the use of wakame. Use arame more often than hijiki. Make desserts with agar-agar.

Fish and seafood: Consume only if desired. Prepare in small quantities, no more than twice per week. Recommend either a white-meat fish balanced with a large proportion of leafy greens, or a small amount of raw fish.

Seeds and nuts: Emphasize limiting the quantity consumed. Strictly avoid nut and seed butters.

Fruit: Consume more often than standard recommendations, if desired. Emphasize fresh fruit when in season. Occasionally take apple juice/cider if desired. Occasionally use citrus fruit.

Snacks and desserts: Avoid or reduce dried snacks such as puffed whole cereal grains, rice cakes, crackers, and cookies. Avoid heavy desserts—choose desserts made of fruit over those made of grains or baked flour. Avoid pie crusts. Occasionally use amazaké. Very occasionally, use soy milk if desired.

Seasonings: Emphasize that salty seasonings should be mild and cooked into a food. Emphasize umeboshi and tofu dressings. Emphasize the importance of garnishes—vary the use of horseradish, wasabi, red pepper, lemon slices, grated daikon, and ginger juice.

Condiments: Emphasize moist condiments—miso with scallions, mildly seasoned nori condiment, or light condiments—shiso leaves. Limit umeboshi to less than two or three plums per week. Emphasize umeboshi vinegar more than brown rice vinegar. Minimize salty condiments such as tekka or shio kombu. Minimize dry condiments such as sea vegetable powders or aonori.

Beverages: Employ standard recommendations plus more consumption from occasional use categories: more green tea, vegetable juices (especially celery), northern climate fruit juices, beer and saké if desired. Avoid Mu tea.

AN OVERLY YIN CONDITION

An overly yin condition can arise from two factors:
1. From excess yin. This condition is called yin jitsu.
2. From a deficiency of yang. This condition is called yang kyo.

1. Yin Jitsu—Yin Is in Excess

Dietary causes of this condition:
1. The individual has been eating an excess of yin foods, especially extreme yin.
2. The diet is too wide. Since a yin excess condition can only arise if there is yang, it means excess yang has been consumed either recently or over long periods in the past.

Primary mode of change: Emphasize reducing yin.

Secondary mode of change: Increase yang.

Primary direction of change (see Fig. 18):
1. From extreme yin toward yin "occasional use" foods, avoid or reduce all forms of excess yin.
2. From the center—whole cereal grains, toward yin "occasional use" foods emphasize reducing yin factors in each food category. Slightly increase yang factors.
3. Recommend fish if necessary.

Primary dietary suggestions: Emphasize avoiding all forms of excess or extreme yin. Excess or extreme yang should also be avoided. Do not try to make balance by making the standard diet too yang. Yin changes to yang slowly. If the change is too quick there will be a reaction. The individual will crave excess yin once more, in order to establish a balance they will feel comfortable with. The diet therefore should not be too narrow or salty, it should contain much variety within standard guidelines. Avoid overeating.

Other elements of change:
1. *Salt content.* Consumption of mineral rich sea salt and salty seasonings should be equal to or slightly more than standard guidelines.
2. *Food preparation.* Avoid raw food. Slightly emphasize more long-time cooking methods and yang quality food choices.
3. *Water content.* Avoid cooking with or consuming excess liquid.

Whole cereal grains: Check that grains are not being cooked with too much liquid: they should not be ready for digestion until chewed fifty times or so. Use short more often than medium grain rice. The percentage of grain consumed should be the standard recommendation of at least 50 percent of the diet. Secondary grains to be emphasized are millet and buckwheat, with less consumption of whole oats. For variety, emphasize combinations of rice with kombu or azuki at times. In colder months especially, suggest baking grains more often than standard recommendations. Use "occasional use" grains and grain products less often. Check that salt content is standard or slightly increased.

Soups: Miso: Consume at least one bowl of miso soup per day but avoid large servings in order to cut down on liquids. Use leafy greens and round vegetables but emphasize root vegetables. Recommend standard seasoning or a little stronger. Cook the soup a little longer and prepare with a kombu stock occasionally. Other: Emphasize root vegetables in soups.

Vegetables and vegetable dishes: Emphasize more ground and root vegetables and long-time cooking methods. Prepare more often: nishime style, azuki/kombu/squash, dried daikon/kombu, root vegetables with root tops, kinpira, seitan/tofu/tempeh stew. Prepare standard or less often: boiled salad, pressed salad, sautéed vegetables (avoid oil), and steamed greens. Avoid fresh salad. Emphasize more salty or long term pickles such as *takuan* or miso pickles in small amounts.

Beans and bean products: Limit the consumption of tofu and only serve cooked. Beans cooked with root vegetables would be helpful. Avoid soy milk or tofu-based desserts or products. It is better to avoid occasional use beans. Emphasize cooked regular use beans over bean products. Avoid sweetened bean dishes. Salty seasoning can be slightly stronger than standard.

Sea vegetables: Slightly emphasize kombu and hijiki. Use slightly stronger salty seasoning. Combine tofu in sea vegetable dishes less often.

Fish and seafood: Employ standard recommendations if fish is desired. Sashimi (raw fish) may be consumed occasionally.

Seeds and nuts: Avoid nut and seed butters. Avoid "less frequent use" seeds and nuts. Limit the quantity consumed. Slightly stronger salty seasoning is recommended.

Fruit: It is best to avoid fruit. If craved, then fruit should be cooked with kuzu and a pinch of salt, and served in small volumes twice or less per week. As a snack one may eat dried fruit in small quantities. Avoid fruit juice—if craved mix with kuzu and serve heated. Take fresh fruit with a pinch of salt, in small quantities, if desired. Berries and melons are best.

Snacks and desserts: There may be a craving for sweets with this condition. Unless necessary, avoid being too strict. However, recommend that the sweet craving be satisfied in the following order. First, from sweet vegetables cooked to bring out the sweet taste; second, from amazaké in small quantities or cooked chestnut dishes; third, from brown rice syrup or barley malt, preferably cooked into a food; fourth, from fruit or fruit juices which have been cooked or heated.

Seasonings: Salty seasonings should follow standard guidelines or be slightly increased.

Condiments: Baked or dry condiments may be beneficial since they will help to dry out yin. However the excess use of condiments or salt will hold yin inside. The ratio of gomashio would be best between 1: 12 and 1: 14.

Beverages: Drink only when thirsty. Avoid the following drinks until the condition noticeably changes: nachi green tea; green magma; beer; saké; soy milk. Umeboshi tea and Mu tea may prove helpful if taken occasionally.

2. Yang Kyo—Yang Is Deficient

The cause of this condition may be one or a combination of the following factors:
1. A diet that lacks a center
2. The lack of yang qualities in food preparation
3. The lack of yang food consumption

Primary mode of change: Emphasize increasing yang.

Secondary mode of change: Decrease yin.

Primary direction of change (see Fig. 18)*:*
1. From the center toward yin, in each food category, increase yang factors from their present level.
2. If necessary introduce or increase the consumption of fish.

Primary dietary suggestions: Since the person needs more gathering energy emphasize more strengthening foods and food preparation.

Other elements of change:
1. *Salt content.* Consume at standard guidelines or slightly more.
2. *Food preparation.* Emphasize more yang quality food and more yang styles of cooking—longer-time cooking methods. Avoid raw food.
3. *Water content.* It may be necessary to reduce liquid consumption, including the amount of liquid used in cooking.

Whole cereal grains: Check that grains approximate 50 to 60 percent of daily food intake. If the condition is extreme, increase this percentage for short periods. Check that grains are not being cooked with too much water; they should need to be chewed at least fifty times before being swallowed. Salt content should be approximate to standard guidelines or slightly more. Emphasize short grain brown rice over medium grain. Brown rice should only be pressure-cooked or occasionally, in colder months, baked. For other grains emphasize buckwheat and millet. Whole oats and occasional use grains would be better used less often. Appropriate combinations would include the following: brown rice with azukis; baked millet and onions; grains with kombu; fried rice, occasionally in colder months; grain stews, especially in colder months. Emphasize soba over udon noodles. Occasionally use fried noodles. Consume baked and deep-fried flour at standard recommendations or less. Avoid baked flour desserts.

Soups: Take no more than two bowls per day in small quantities. Miso: Emphasize longer time cooking and the use of root vegetables. Occasionally prepare with a kombu stock. Miso content should follow standard guidelines or be slightly stronger. Use leftover rice cooked with miso soup often.

Other: Take grain soups often and azuki bean soup occasionally. Use longer-time cooking methods of soups more often. Take fish soup occasionally. Carp soup (*koikoku*) can be prepared occasionally.

Vegetables and vegetable dishes: Emphasize longer-time cooking methods, standard or slightly more than standard salty seasoning, and more root and round vegetables than leafy greens. Thus recommend standard consumption or slightly more often of nishime style, azuki/kombu/squash, dried daikon with kombu, root vegetables with root tops, kinpira, tempura and stews. Use standard or less often for boiled salad and pressed salad, sautéed vegetables, and steamed greens. Avoid fresh salad. Emphasize more salty or long time pickles such as takuan or miso pickles in small amounts.

Beans and been products: Emphasize cooked beans over bean products. Long-time cooking methods are appropriate. Use regular use beans only, especially azuki beans. Occasionally take baked bean dishes, especially in colder months, and deep-fried bean products. Limit the consumption of tofu and only serve cooked. Avoid soy milk. Avoid desserts made from tofu. Avoid sweetened bean dishes.

Sea vegetables: Slightly emphasize kombu and hijiki. Use kombu more often in grain and vegetable dishes. Follow standard salty seasoning recommendations or slightly stronger.

Fish and seafood: Employ standard guidelines, although seasoning may need to be stronger. Occasionally use stronger types of fish, such as tuna or salmon. Take fish soup more often and carp soup or salmon head soup occasionally.

Seeds and nuts: Limit the quantity consumed. Avoid nut and seed butters. Avoid less frequent use seeds and nuts, and sweetened seeds and nuts. Use slightly stronger salty seasoning.

Fruit: It is best is to avoid fruit. If craved, then fruit should be cooked with kuzu and a pinch of salt, and served in small volumes twice or less per week. As a snack, dried fruit can be taken in small quantities. Avoid fruit juice and tropical fruit.

Snacks and desserts: Limit dessert consumption to less than twice per week in small servings. The best is none, until the condition noticeably changes. Avoid tofu-based desserts and maple syrup.

Seasonings: Salty seasonings should follow standard guidelines or be slightly increased. Oil should only be used cooked into a food. Avoid pungent, spicy seasonings such as wasabi, red pepper, and lemon.

Condiments: Recommend those which tend to be drier or a little more strongly seasoned—tekka and shio kombu occasionally. Use gomashio at a ratio of approximately 1: 10 or 1: 12.

Beverages: Drink only when thirsty. Avoid the following beverages until the condition noticeably changes: nachi green tea, green magma, beer, saké, soy milk. Mu tea can be taken more often.

Chapter **4**

Meridians

The Liver and Gallbladder Meridians

Tree Nature Energy

The liver and gallbladder correspond with the tree nature phase of energy transformation. Overall, tree nature is upward energy, and like vegetation in spring or the atmosphere of morning, it represents a fast rising energy that denotes freshness and lightness. This energy is visualized in the Chinese character for East 東, of a rising sun behind a tree. Within this overall upward pattern however, tree nature also contains a downward movement characterized by its roots. Roots denote the yang aspect of this energy, while the trunk, branches, and stems, the yin.

With the physical body the liver and gallbladder are located on the right side—an indication that they are nourished more by earth's rising force, which predominates on this side. Within this overall pattern the direction of liver and gallbladder meridian flow also demonstrates an upward-downward movement. Both meridians are connected with the eyes. The liver meridian travels upward from the big toes, more on the interior side of the body, to finish at the eyes. The gallbladder meridian, which begins at the outside corners of the eyes, travels to the ears then zigzags across the sides of the head, across the outer sides of the body, and onto the fourth toes. The liver then corresponds more with the overall upward yin aspect, while the gallbladder with the more downward yang aspect of tree nature energy. Classical Chinese medicine associates the liver with the planning function and the gallbladder with decision making. Planning represents a more abstract form of vision (the ability to visualize— imagination), while decision making tends to require physical seeing and hearing, which are clearly described by the location of the gallbladder meridian. By beginning on the outside corners of the eyes one gets the biggest view—one looks to the right and left. The meridian then continues to the ears. After looking, one seeks aural information. The meridian then passes over the sides of the head—one then thinks, puts things into perspective, and makes a decision. The path of the meridian onto the feet represents the latter practical aspect.

The direction of the liver and gallbladder meridians is reflected internally by the functioning of the associated organs. The liver receives nutrients predominantly from the portal vein, which follows a path upward to the liver on the right side. The liver in turn sends blood via the inferior vena cava upward to the heart. Conversely, bile which is stored in the gallbladder, is released when needed in a downward direction into the duodenum.

---

* All macrobiotic material in this chapter (macrobiotic health evaluation, dietary recommendations, some descriptions of disorders) either comes directly from or is based on the teachings of Michio Kushi, previously published in his books, or from articles published in *East West Journal* written by his former students. References are cited in the end notes.

111

Fig. 19

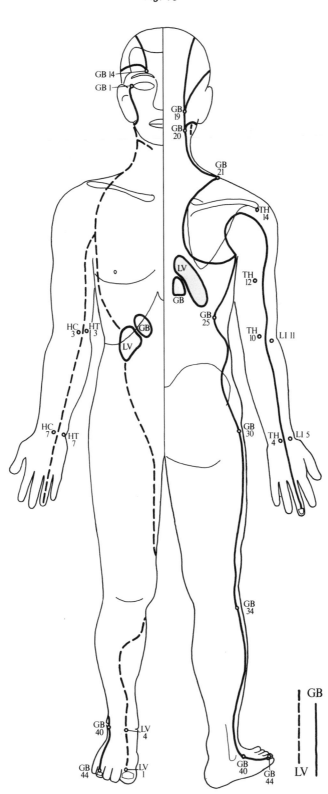

From the images we have of a tree described in Chapter 2 we can see how tree nature energy can manifest within the individual:

Roots (Yang)
Positive: Not giving up easily, unyielding, persevering, sense of endurance, persistance, resilience, sense of courage—"Holding fast to one's own roots is the foundation of courage,"[1] sexual vitality
Negative: Yang deficient—easily swayed, a "pushover," gullible, timid, indecisive, infertile, impotent, easily talked into something. Yin excess—overly impressionable, "to change like the wind," gullible, naive. Yang excess—stubborn, rigid, stagnated, rash in making decisions.

Vertical Growth Toward the Sun (Yin)
Positive: Upright, imaginative, sense of aspiration
Negative: Biased, disillusioned, sense of frustration (yang excess or yin deficient), irritability (yang excess or yin deficient)

Upward and Outward Growth of a Tree
Positive: Expressive, friendly, sociable
Negative: Inability to "branch out," unsociable, antisocial, emotionally repressed, provocative, competitive, argumentative

Spring Growth
Positive: Sense of initiative, vitality, timing
Negative: Difficulty in beginning things, sluggish and low in energy, impulsive, impetuous, rash

Overall Growth and Life of a Tree
Positive: Patient, orderly, ability to rise to the top
Negative: Impatient, "doesn't grow up," early or late maturity, immature, to stop growing mentally or spiritually

Old Age and Death of a Tree
Positive: To be firm, unyielding
Negative: Hard, dry, rigid and stubborn either physically, mentally, or in general personality

Movement of the Tree As It Responds to the Elements
Positive: Flexible, sense of rhythm, timing and coordination, responsive, resilient
Negative: Lack of flexibility and the above positive qualities

Branches of a Tree Visualized as Arms
Positive: Versatility

Branches Snap
Negative: To become angry or lose one's temper, to snap at others

To Be in the Presence of Trees
Positive: Calm, peaceful, tranquil, gentle
Negative: Loud, noticeably silent

THE LIVER MERIDIAN

According to Classical Chinese Medicine[2]
The term liver corresponds with the liver in Western medicine as well as some functions of the pancreas, and endocrine organs.[3] "The liver is the organ responsible for

spreading and regulating the ki throughout the body."[4] "Its character is flowing and free."[5] The liver is likened to the general of an army "because it maintains evenness and harmony of movement throughout the body."[6] Consequently it is the organ most sensitive to stagnation. In addition the liver is believed to store and regulate the amount of blood and it controls bile secretion. The liver is related to disorders of the eyes and vision problems, and it rules the tendons (which include ligaments and to some extent muscles). The nails, through their thickness, color, texture, and strength reflect the condition of the liver. The liver is also related to the joints, and it harmonizes the emotions. It is the most important organ with regard to women's menstrual cycle and sexuality.[7]

Problems and diseases that are commonly treated by acupuncture to points along the liver meridian include the following:

Eye diseases; insomnia; headache; dizziness; vertigo; emotional instability; sore throat; chest and rib pain; intercostal neuralgia; hepatitis; jaundice; abdominal cramps, spasms, pain and distension; hernia; impotence; nocturnal emissions; genital pain; urine retention; irregular menstruation; breast pain; abnormal uterine bleeding; prolapse of uterus; vaginal discharge; joint pain, especially of knee or ankle[8]

According to Shizuto Masunaga[9]

Masunaga defines the functions of the liver and gallbladder meridians (Fig. 19) as the "storage and distribution of vital energy." The condition of these meridians is reflected in one's eyes and nails. The liver and gallbladder meridians are also associated with the following: the iris and vision, the tendons (especially the Achilles tendon), the sexual organs and sexual response, the movement of various joints and problems in the flank region.

The primary overall function of the liver is to keep an individual full of vigor. The liver thus secures the vital supply of energy, stores nutrients, cultivates resistance against disease, and supplies, analyzes, and detoxifies the blood. The liver plans how this vital energy should be used in the body—like the command of "an army general who decides strategy."

Imbalances in the Liver Meridian are associated with the following:

Loss of vitality; sudden spurts of motivation followed by extreme fatigue; bad temper; being easily disturbed by noise; the letdown after emotional arousal; heightened emotional sensitivity; the tendency to raise one's voice; one's eyes losing their sparkle; everything taking on a yellowish tinge; dizziness upon standing; unexplainable decline in sexual performance; occasional outbreaks of fever; problems in the prostate and testicles; pain in the sacrum and coccyx; hemorrhoids; tension in the flank region; a sense of pressure in the right hypochondrium (area below rib); loss of appetite; nausea; headaches

Masunaga further identifies conditions that may arise in terms of kyo and jitsu:

- *Liver Meridian Kyo*[10]

  Cause. A loss of stamina and endurance so that even if one is motivated there is insufficient energy to persist. The reserve of nutrients in the body is diminished and the detoxification function declines.

  Mental Aspect. Lack of perseverence and a tendency to become bored; impatience and irritability; tendency for nerves to be on end; short temperedness and sudden explosive release of emotions; to be easily irritated by noise; to worry unneccesarily

Physical Aspect. Weak joints; shaky feeling in the joints when making vigorous movements; total exhaustion; tendency to have dizzy spells or to trip and fall; hardness in the Achilles tendon; things appearing yellowish; tendency toward food poisoning with nausea and vomiting; inability to gain weight; low fever lasting a long time; high fever of unknown causes; stiffness and rigidity in the muscles, which cause movements to become awkward; loss of sexual drive, and impotence

● *Liver Meridian Jitsu*[11]

Mental Aspect. Hard worker, concentrator; stubborn; tendency to never give up; to work impatiently and impulsively until exhausted; to be easily affected emotionally and to sometimes scream in a loud voice; to display emotion and then control it; to have a big appetite

Physical Aspect. Accumulated fatigue due to never-ending drive; overeating; excessive drinking; swollen chest and stomach; headaches; heaviness in the head; poor digestion; lack of exercise; dizziness due to lack of blood; high fever without cause; chills; coughing; liver organ malfunction; pulling in the anal area causing hemorrhoids; prostate problems; pain in the testicles; inflammation of the female reproductive organs; excess consumption of sugar and alcohol; forceful expression; pain in the sacrum and coccyx; total body stiffness; tightness in the hara area that feels like a rubber board; flatulence; putrefaction; to be prone to inflammations

● *Jitsu Symptoms of Other Meridians with Liver Meridian Kyo*[12]

Lung: Tendency to be constipated; stiffness in the back and shoulders; asthma

Large Intestine: Tendency to be constipated; hotness of the head; pentup energy; tired and heavy legs

Stomach: Loss of appetite stemming from liver disorders; lack of motivation to work because of lack of energy

Spleen: Dark complexion, lacking luster; heaviness in legs and general lack of energy; loss of sexual drive

Heart: A state of total exhaustion after emotional excitement

Small Intestine: Symptoms of duodenal ulcer; intermittent claudication*; facial blemishes

Bladder: Difficulty in urination; nervous strain; impotence; symptoms of poisoning; tiredness because of too much worry; hypertrophy of the prostate gland

Kidney: Excessive alcohol consumption leading to fatigue; chronic nephritis; loss of drive due to overexertion; prostatic hypertrophy

Heart Constrictor: Restlessness and inability to relax; nervousness in personal relationships; strong palpitations; hot flushes; disorders of the coronary vessels

Triple Heater: Rhinitis; stomatitis; hypersensitive peritoneum; ticklishness; tendency to get diarrhea after being chilled

---

* Intermittent claudication is a form of limping which is caused by hardening of the arteries in the legs. There is no pain or discomfort when the limbs are at rest, but after walking is begun, the pain intensifies until walking becomes impossible.

Structure and Function of the Liver[13]

The liver is the body's most important biochemical organ. It is also the largest, weighing between three and four pounds. It is located just below the diaphragm, mostly within the upper right quarter of the abdomen. The liver consists of two main lobes; a large right and a smaller left lobe. The right is further divided into three smaller lobes.

The functional unit of the liver is the lobule. There are between fifty and one hundred thousand lobules, joined together by small amounts of connective tissue. They are cylindrical structures with flattened sides. Each lobule consists of millions of liver (hepatic) cells stacked in columns which extend radially in rows from a central vein.

Blood is supplied to the liver by the hepatic artery and hepatic portal vein. The hepatic artery supplies freshly oxygenated blood, accounting for 20 percent of the liver's blood supply. The hepatic portal vein brings the remaining 80 percent from the stomach, spleen, pancreas, and intestines. At rest, about 2 1/2 pints of blood flow through the liver each minute.

Along with branches of the bile duct, branches of the hepatic artery and portal vein flow together surrounding each lobule. These branches of the hepatic artery and portal vein join together within each lobule along sinusoids (minute blood vessels) between the rows of cells. The sinusoids empty into the central vein. The central veins of the various lobules lead to a hepatic vein and the hepatic veins lead into the inferior vena cava which takes blood into the right atrium of the heart.

While the arterial blood supplies the cells with oxygen, the portal vein carries nutrients, bacteria, and old red blood cells. In turn, the liver cells secrete into the blood flowing along the sinusoids various substances required by the body. These include glucose, proteins, vitamins, fats, and most other vital substances.

Sinusoids divide the cells into rows. However, between these rows, between the columns of cells, there is an even more minute network of channels. These drain toward the periphery of the lobule, carrying bile to a local branch of the bile duct, which as stated, together with branches of the hepatic artery and portal vein, surround each lobule. There are two main bile ducts, right hepatic and left. They join into the common bile duct which connects with the duodenum at the Oddi's sphincter.

Of the more than five hundred known functions carried out by the liver, the following are among the most significant:

Carbohydrate conversion. Carbohydrates coming either directly from consumed sugar, or from digested complex forms arrive at the liver as monosaccharides (simple sugars). They are immediately converted into glucose, the body's most direct source of energy. This conversion insures that a constant supply of glucose is available for use by the brain. If the body's cells require immediate energy, the liver releases some of the glucose back into the bloodstream to meet this need. What remains of the glucose cannot be stored in its original form; it is converted into glycogen, a larger carbohydrate molecule. Glycogen can be stored, and occupies most of the liver's storage space. Glycogen is also stored in the skeletal muscle cells. When glycogen storage areas are filled up the liver transforms the remaining glucose into fat, which is stored below the skin and in other areas of the body. If it is required (when there is no sugar being ingested) glycogen and fat can be converted back into glucose. This change in state prevents the blood and general circulation from being deluged with sugar, ensuring an even sugar secretion. However there are two conditions under which sugar can get by the liver and into the bloodstream: (1) If there is simply too much sugar arriving at the liver at once, as in the case of overconsumption of simple sugars (sweets, candy); (2) If the liver has become weakened and cannot function well. In this latter way the state of the liver can contribute to low blood sugar (hypoglycemia).

Processing of protein.   Individual amino acids absorbed by the small intestine are reassembled by the liver to form various proteins. An important protein is albumin which when concentrated in the blood helps to pull fluids from the tissues by osmosis.[14] The liver also destroys worn-out red blood cells; from hemoglobin broken down in this process, the iron is stored and reutilized as are excess amino acids. Bilirubin, a golden yellow pigment is another product of this process. It is one of the components of bile which gives feces their color. If it is not excreted the skin and eyes become yellow, a condition known as jaundice. Excess amino acids are used by the liver cell for building new proteins. Or they are further broken down and converted into glucose should all other energy sources be used up. However this process produces ammonia, which is poisonous. But the liver converts ammonia into urea which is excreted by the kidneys in the urine and by the skin in perspiration. The liver also produces heparin—a chemical which prevents blood clotting inside the vessels and fibrinogen, one of the plasma proteins, which plays an essential part in the formation of blood clotting.

Fat digestion.   The liver produces bile. Bile contains bile salts produced in the liver from cholesterol (a fatlike product of the breakdown of red blood cells). Bile salts emulsify fats in the small intestine. If enough excess fat accumulates in the body it is deposited in the liver, weakening its function.

Storage.   Besides glycogen, the liver stores vitamins A, B (including B_{12}), D, E, and K. The size of certain vitamin stores of A, D and B_{12} can be so enormous that "a well nourished man can go for months without vitamin A and two to four years without vitamin B_{12} without any sign of deficiency."[15]

Destruction of poisons.   Poisons such as strychnine, nicotine, some barbiturates and alcohol are destroyed by the liver. Alcohol is neutralized by the liver at the rate of one-third ounce per hour.

Disorders Associated with the Liver[16]

An unhealthy liver can be enlarged, swollen, congested, hardened, fatty, or weakened. Specific diseases include the following:

Cirrhosis.[17]   The progressive destruction of liver tissue and the development of scarring, fibrosis, and fatty deposits. Cirrhosis is caused by the long time consumption of alcohol and according to macrobiotics of animal food, fruit juice, soft drinks, and sugar. Chronic alcohol abuse damages the liver cells making regeneration necessary, to replace them. If this repair is extensive or continues over a long period, fibrous connective tissue replaces the normal liver cells, causing scarring. Signs of cirrhosis include the following: a hard small liver, enlarged spleen, loss of appetite, fatigue, weakness, jaundice, a reddening of the palms, and development of spider naevi (networks of tiny spiderlike blood vessels under the skin). Cirrhosis may cause ascites—the buildup of fluid in the peritoneal cavity (the peritoneum is a thin layer of tissue surrounding the intestines).[18]

Jaundice.[19]   The skin, whites of the eyes, and other tissues take on a yellowish hue. Jaundice is caused by an excess of bile pigments in the body. This condition may arise as a result of hepatitis, obstruction of the bile ducts, or an excessive breakdown of red blood cells.

Hepatitis[20] (*Liver Inflammation*).   Hepatitis results in the destruction of patches of liver tissue. Hepatitis is most often caused by viruses, but alcohol, drugs, and a variety of bacterial, fungal or parasitic infections may also be the cause.

THE GALLBLADDER MERIDIAN

According to Classical Chinese Medicine
The gallbladder corresponds with the gallbladder of Western medicine.[21] "The gallbladder is a true and upright official: it controls judgments."[22] "The Gallbladder is the Fu (hollow organ) of internal purity . . . it stores pure and clean fluid . . . only the gallbladder is filled with the pure."[23] The gallbladder controls decision making. "All the other eleven Zang (solid organs) and Fu make their decisions in the gallbladder."[24]

Disorders that are commonly treated by acupuncture to points along the gallbladder meridian include the following:

Facial paralysis, brain diseases, eye diseases, night blindness, glaucoma, headache, migraine, stiff neck, deafness, ringing in the ears, toothache, dislocation of the jaw, rhinitis (inflammation of the nose), vertigo, dizziness, seizures, frozen shoulder, back pain, cystitis, diarrhea, constipation, lower abdominal pain and distension, disease of the hip joint; lower back and leg pain, sciatica, knee and ankle diseases, paralysis of the lower limb, cholecystitis (inflammation of the gallbladder)[25]

According to Shizuto Masunaga[26]
The gallbladder meridian is closely tied to the Oriental concept of gall as being the source of strength and resolve.

The gallbladder may be closely associated with the function of the endocrine system. It controls the distribution of nutrients throughout the body, and the amount and balance of digestive enzymes (including saliva, pancreatic juice, bile, and intestinal enzymes), as well as hormones from the thyroids. The gallbladder is also the organ related to decision making and it decides the course of action.

Imbalances in the gallbladder meridian are associated with the following:

Becoming overly concerned about small details; being frightened out of one's wits; losing sleep over not being able to make a decision; the eyes becoming overworked and symptoms of eyestrain; yellowing of the eyes; accumulation of mucus in the eyes; blurred vision; increased ocular pressure; not allowing enough time to eat so that the release of bile is insufficient, leading to constipation and diarrhea; the skin becomes yellowish; the joints in the legs and arms become stiff and the body as a whole becomes quite rigid; heartburn; occasional nausea in the morning; distension of the stomach; tension in the shoulders with occasional sharp pain in the side (costal neuralgia); spasms and pain in the biliary tract or stomach; hyperacidity; duodenal ulcers; coughing accompanied by phlegm.

Masunaga further identifies conditions that may arise in terms of kyo and jitsu:
• *Gallbladder Meridian Kyo*[27]
   Cause.   One is indecisive about where to focus one's energy when undertaking

something and tends to vacillate about which direction to go. One has lost vigor after great disappointment.

Mental Aspect. Fatigue after continued emotional excitement, fatigue after being pressed to make a decision; prolonged stress; fatigue from having to deal with too many details; emotional exhaustion after a big disappointment; tendency to be nervous and jittery; frayed nerves; loss of willpower; low motivation because of fatigue

Physical Aspect. Uneven distribution of nutrients in the body; symptoms of fatigue in specific areas, especially the eyes; fatigue from overuse of eyes; mucus from eyes and blurred vision; deteriorating vision; headache due to eyestrain; insufficient bile and poor digestion of fats, leading to constipation, diarrhea, or discolored stools; anemic tendency and sallow complexion; tendency to gain weight easily even when cutting down on fat; dislike of fatty foods, preference for foods with mild flavor, hyperacidity; rigidity, and pain in joints

- *Gallbladder Meridian jitsu*[28]

Mental aspect. Assumes too much responsibility; fatigued; tendency to push oneself in work; pays attention to small details; easily upset; impatient; always in a hurry for no reason; tired eyes; too much concentration.

Physical aspect. Lack of sleep, causing tired eyes; bloated stomach; loss of appetite; glassy eyes; yellowish in white part of the eye and skin; painful tearing and high pressure in the eyes; tendency to blink frequently; stiffness in extremities; stiff muscles; pain in rib cage; bitter taste in mouth; burning sensation in chest; gallstones and spasms in the gallbladder; shoulder pain; heaviness in the head; migraine headache; constipation; mucous stagnation; itching in the area of the tonsils; coughing; excessive intake of sweets; lack of sour food consumption

- *Jitsu Symptoms of Other Meridians with Gallbladder Meridian Kyo*[29]

Lung: Pulling pain in the thumbs; stiffness in pectoral muscles; phlegm

Large Intestine: Poor elimination and fecal stasis; tendency to tire easily; bloodshot eyes; vertigo

Stomach: Insufficient chewing; lack of sleep; blurred vision; car sickness

Spleen: Poor secretion of digestive enzymes; tendency to get skin rashes; stomatitis; overuse of eyes

Heart: Nervous strain; difficulty in getting to sleep; dizziness

Small Intestine: Efforts beyond one's capacity; weak intestinal function; tendency to tire easily; allergic condition; ovarian malfunction; eye fatigue

Bladder: Overwork; duodenal ulcer; spasm in bile duct; jaundice; malfunction of autonomic nervous system; deterioration of thyroid function; tiredness of eyes

Kidney: Coughing with phlegm; stiffness in back and shoulders; eyestrain; failing eyesight; mental fatigue

Heart Constrictor: Obesity; Basedow's disease; palpitations; tendency to fret and worry; fatigue from overwork

Triple Heater: Susceptibility to colds; distension of abdomen; bitter taste in mouth; restless sleep; nausea; phlegm; eyestrain

Structure and Function of the Gallbladder[30]

The gallbladder is a pear shaped pouch located on the underside of the right lobe of the liver. It is green in color and the smallest organ of the body, some 3 1/2 to 4 inches in length with a capacity of about 50 cc. Its function is to store and concentrate bile, which is produced by the liver. Bile is needed to break down fats and oils in the small intestine (fats are solid at room temperature and come mainly from animal food, oils are liquid and derived mainly from plants).

The cystic duct some 1 1/2 inches long leads from the narrow end of the gallbladder to the hepatic duct, coming from the liver. At their junction they form the common bile duct, a tube some 3 inches long which enters the duodenum at the Oddi's sphincter, some 3 inches below the pylorus of the stomach. The pancreatic duct joins the common bile duct just above the Oddi's sphincter.

Each day the liver secretes about 1,000 cc of bile, which trickles down the bile duct to the Oddi's sphincter. If this valve is closed (meaning that the small intestine is empty), bile accumulates in the duct and is forced into the gallbladder for storage. Since the gallbladder can hold only 50 cc, bile is concentrated up to twenty times. This is achieved by the structure of the inner walls of the gallbladder. They have a mucous membrane which is able to absorb water from the bile, and being folded, the walls are able to expand much like the rugae of the stomach. The wall also contains a middle muscular coat that can contract, squirting the concentrated bile toward the duodenum.

Bile is secreted when acid and fat together come into contact with the hormone secreting cells of the duodenum. The small intestine in turn secretes cholecystokinin into the blood, which causes the gallbladder to contract and the Oddi's sphincter to relax. Bile swamps the chyme with bile salts.

Bile is thick, bitter and alkaline in reaction. It consists of more than 80 percent water plus bile salts, bile acids, cholesterol, and the pigments bilirubin and biliverdin, as well as wastes and toxins filtered from the blood by the liver. Bile salts, made by the liver from cholesterol, lower the surface tension of water, enabling them to break large fat particles into tiny droplets (emulsification). In turn pancreatic secretions can more effectively act on these fats. Eighty percent of bile salts are reabsorbed at the end of the small intestine and returned to the liver to be used again. Bilirubin and biliverdin give bile its yellow-green color. They are a waste product that results from the breakdown of worn-out red blood cells by the liver. These pigments are carried in the bile to the intestines to be removed from the body. Bilirubin is responsible for the brownish color of the feces. Cholesterol, excluding water, accounts for 16 percent of the contents of bile. It is a fatlike substance present in all cells and fluids of the body and is excreted by the liver cells and cells lining the gallbladder. While it performs many necessary functions, in excess, cholesterol builds up as a plaque on the inside of the arterial walls, narrowing the space for blood to pass—atherosclerosis.

Gallstones (Cholelithiasis)[31]

Gallstones, the most common disorder associated with the gallbladder, are formed primarily from cholesterol, together with calcium and bile pigments. As a fat-like substance, cholesterol does not dissolve in water. However the alkalinity of bile and bile salts normally keep cholesterol dissolved, but if the proportion of cholesterol greatly increases or the composition of bile becomes weakened, then crystals of cholesterol are deposited in the gallbladder and stones may form. Gallstones may be as small as tiny crystals or they may be as large as one pound and they may be multiple.[32]

Gallstones can go largely unnoticed for years or they may produce bloating, gassiness, abdominal discomfort or other symptoms similar to indigestion. A gallbladder attack is often provoked by consuming fatty foods or alcohol. Pain, which can be severe, begins in the upper abdomen and can radiate through the right side up to the right shoulder blade. Such pain often occurs when a stone becomes lodged in the common bile duct and the gallbladder contracts to expel bile. This situation can lead to jaundice. In addition, fats go largely undigested and bile stagnates and concentrates in the gallbladder, irritating the walls, causing inflammation (cholecystitis). In severe cases gangrene of the organ may occur. The incidence of gallstones is four times higher in women than men—fat, fortyish, fair, and female—and its incidence increases with age. Western medicine often recommends surgical removal of the entire organ.

Macrobiotic Health Evaluation[33]

Indications of liver disorder will tend to indicate disorders in the gallbladder as well.
• *Constitutional Tendency*

Yang: If the eyes are set close together, are small in size, or tend to cross, or if the eyebrows grow close together or slant downward, there is a tendency for the liver to develop problems from becoming overly contracted.

Yin: If the eyes are set far apart, are large in size or move outward, the liver will tend to become swollen. If the eyebrows are set far apart there is a tendency for disorders to arise in the gallbladder.
• *Condition*

The condition of the liver and gallbladder can be predominantly seen in the eyes, and the area around the eyes and between the eyebrows, the nails, the skin color, and the temples.

1. *The Eyes and the Area around the Eyes*

    Yellow fatty accumulations in the whites of the eyes—similar fat accumulation in the liver

    Red or bloodshot eyes, rash or inflammation between the eyes—inflamed liver

    Red spots or styes on the eyes, eyelids and the area between the eyes—excess animal protein storage in the liver

    Watery, swollen, burning or itching sensation—overly swollen liver

    Farsightedness—contracted liver condition

    Nearsightedness—swollen liver

    Hair growing between the brows—the liver tends to be easily affected by over-consumption of animal food and oily or fatty foods, including dairy products

    Eyelids that are swollen and red or purple in color—general liver weakness due to a current excessive intake of fruits, sugar and other sweets, soda, soft drinks, tropical vegetables and alcoholic beverages

    Reddish yellow color in the pink area inside the lower eyelids—excess yang animal food consumption (poultry, eggs, dairy) along with excess yin (sugar, fruits), shows liver disorders.

1a. *The Central Region of the Lower Forehead (Between the Eyebrows)*

Vertical wrinkles—accumulation of mucus and fat in the liver; expansion or hardening of the liver. The deeper or longer the wrinkle, the worse the condition. With only one or two wrinkles, the liver is harder, with stagnation.

White or yellow patches together with vertical lines—development of a cyst or tumor formation in the liver, or stone formation in the gallbladder

Pimples, with or without wrinkles—hard fat deposits in the liver, or stone formation in the gallbladder, due to long time consumption of animal fat, including dairy products

2. *The Nails (Especially the Nails of the First and Fourth Toes)*

Ingrown—yang condition

Flared—yin

Vertical ridges—yang condition

Horizontal ridges—yin condition

White spots on the nails—indication of expanded liver condition because of excess refined sugar

Yellowing at the edges—excessive fat accumulation in the liver, possible stone formation in the gallbladder

Dry and eroding—yang condition

Brittle—yin

3. *Skin Color*

Yellowish—first appearing on the palms, but also the feet, and body overall: excessive bile secretion or other disorders of the bile functions including blockage of the bile ducts, overconsumption of saturated fatty foods (eggs, dairy food, oils and fats, together with salt as well as cold fatty foods such as ice cream)

Grayish—swollen, hard liver

Overall greenish tint—progressive development of liver cancer

Gray-blue on the cheeks—chronic liver disorder caused by excess salt, dried foods, meat, eggs, alcohol, and sugars; slow metabolism due to hardening or constriction

4. *Temples*

Green vessels—abnormal lymph circulation due to an overactive spleen or underactive gallbladder—caused by excess fluid and sugar, fats and oils, alcohol and stimulants, other yin foods and drinks

Dark color—elimination of excess sugars or from the excess consumption of salts and salt treated foods, as well as dried foods; underactive liver

Patches and pimples—elimination of excess dairy food

Red pimples/patches—excess sugar, sweets, fruits, and juices

Whitish yellow pimples—fats and oils from both animal and vegetable sources

Dark patches and pimples—excessive sweets or excessive salt and flour products

Moles and warts—excess proteins and fats together

5. *Reddish Dark Colored Lips*

Liver and gallbladder disorders due to excessive consumption of protein and saturated fats, together with excessive salts

Dietary Recommendations[34]

The liver and gallbladder are nourished predominantly by earth's rising force. This kind of energy is supplied by a diet that is light, fresh, colorful, and that contains variety, both in the selection of foods and styles of food preparation.

To restore healthy functioning certain foods should be avoided or restricted. These foods include the following:

All animal food except for occasional non fatty white-meat fish or certain shellfish such as clams or oysters. The former kind of food is high in protein, cholesterol and saturated fats. Excess consumption creates a hardened liver and a burden on the liver to process them. Oily or greasy food in general should be avoided, restricted, or used in moderation. This includes nuts and nut butters, seed butters, fried or deep-fried foods, and oily salad dressings. Vegetable oil in cooking should be used in moderation. Sugar and sugar treated foods should be avoided, since in excess they turn to fat, which places stress on the liver to process them. Refined flour and flour products are difficult for the liver to process. They also create mucus and can create a hardened, swollen liver. Vegetables, fruits and fruit juices of a tropical origin should be avoided. These include potato, sweet potato, yam, tomato, eggplant, and avocado. Spices such as mustard, pepper, and curry should be used in moderation and stimulant aromatic seasonings and drinks including coffee and black tea are best avoided. The neutralization of alcohol depends upon the liver, and it should be used in moderation. Foods containing preservatives and chemical additives should be avoided since again they create an extra burden on the liver whose job is to detoxify the blood. Chilled food, including icy beverages and ice cream, should be avoided as they tend to make fats harden thus creating the conditions for gallstones to develop.

We can then follow standard macrobiotic dietary guidelines slightly emphasizing certain foods which are especially beneficial to the functioning of the liver and gallbladder.

Grains: Barley or hato mugi, served on their own, combined with other grains or served in soups. Baked whole grain and deep-fried flour products create hardening of the liver and produce mucus if consumed in excess. *Soups:* Fermented foods are beneficial to the liver and miso soup has cleaning and detoxifying properties. Certain shellfish such as clams or oysters, known traditionally to be beneficial to the liver can be served in miso soup. *Vegetables:* Hard leafy greens such as kale, collard or mustard greens are especially recommended on a daily basis and best served steamed or boiled, retaining a fresh and crispy flavor. Broccoli and carrots are also particularly beneficial to the functioning of the liver. Ume pickles provide the sour taste. Overall, steaming and boiling are the most recommended cooking techniques and oil should be used in moderation. *Beans:* Natto and tempeh are beneficial since these foods are fermented. They can be used often. *Sea vegetables:* There could be slightly more emphasis on wakame and arame in the choice of sea vegetables. *Fish and seafood:* Mobile type shellfish such as shrimp or lobster are best used in moderation, since they are high in cholesterol. If craved, the standard recommendation of a non fatty white-meat fish is suggested. *Seeds and nuts:* Seed butters, nut and nut butters all contain a high oil content and are best consumed in moderation. *Fruits:* Standard recommendations. Citrus fruit, which belongs to the tree transformation is used occasionally as a flavoring, especially in the case of lemons, which provide the sour taste. *Sweeteners:* Barley malt may be used more often than brown rice syrup. *Seasonings:* Fermented foods such as miso and tamari soy sauce are beneficial to the functioning of the liver, as are umeboshi plums and umeboshi vinegar, used in moderation and sauerkraut. Salt and salty seasonings should be mild. *Condiments:* Shiso leaves, chives with miso, dandelion miso and scallions with miso condiments, along with wakame powder, if used in condiment size quantities, all provide nourishment for the functioning of liver and gallbladder. *Beverages:* Barley tea is appropriate, especially in the warmer months. Green magma consumed for short periods can be helpful for relaxing a tight liver, as can carrot juice, celery juice, or carrot and celery juice in small amounts.

Shiitake mushroom tea can also be beneficial in relieving liver tension. To prepare, soak one dried shiitake and cook in one to two cups of boiling water. Add one to two teaspoons of grated daikon and one teaspoon of tamari soy sauce for seasoning.

Overall one can keep the liver and gallbladder healthy by avoiding overeating, refraining from eating for at least three hours before sleep, and chewing very, very well.

Exercise Recommendations

Various exercises in Chapter 5 are especially beneficial for maintaining a healthy liver and gallbladder. These exercises include the following:

Upper hara massage—exercise 7A and B. Ideally, in a standing position we should be able to press into the liver area, up to the second phalange of our fingers, without feeling pain or hardness. By practicing abdominal massage on a daily basis you may be amazed at the effectiveness of such a simple exercise. *Self-shiatsu to the shoulders*—exercise 9. *Side stretches*—exercise 20. *Self-shiatsu exercise to the legs*—exercise 21 A(2), B(3), C(8) and D(10). *Liver meridian and gallbladder meridian side stretch*—exercise 23. *Abdominal exercise*-exercise 25(4).

The Heart and Small Intestine, Heart Constrictor and Triple Heater Meridians

Fire Nature Energy

The heart, small intestine, heart constrictor and triple heater correspond with fire nature energy. Overall, fire nature is ascending and spreading energy, as imaged by rising flames. Its energy is free and dynamic. However a more complete image needs to include the source from which fire draws its energy, from a log of wood for example. Within the yin there is yang. Within the ascending and spreading, there is a descending, clinging, and penetrating aspect, from which the ascending qualities emanate. The outward qualities of fire nature energy can be seen in an individual as brightness and cheerfulness, joy and laughter. The inward qualities correspond with the ability to concentrate and become absorbed in something, as well as emotional attachment and possessiveness. (Joy can come out of concentration—achieving a goal after years of hard work for example.)

The location and function of the heart and small intestine clearly represent these qualities. Both heart and small intestine are located according to macrobiotic theory, along the spiritual channel, the central vertical axis of the body along which the forces of heaven and earth most directly interact. While this channel is dominated by heaven's force (it is the trunk of the body's spiritual tree), both forces move along this channel. Their energies do not pass each other in the manner of cars going in opposite directions, but rather they collide, head on. The predominating energy at any

Fig. 20

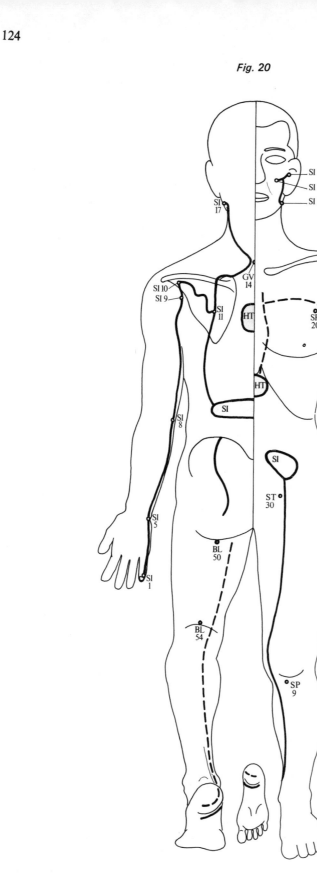

given time forces the other to recede and vice versa. Thus the motion of fire nature energy is up and down as visualized in a child jumping up and down with joy. Heaven's and earth's forces collide along this channel at seven major locations that are known as chakras.

The second or hara chakra is the midpoint or center of gravity in the body. It is the energy center of the body. Also known in Japanese as the *tanden* or Ki-Kai (ocean of ki), this point, some three finger widths below the navel, is located within the region of the small intestine where ingested food is broken down to become physical energy for the body. The physical function of this chakra reflects its more physical location in comparison with the other chakras.

The fourth or heart chakra is located in the chest region. It is the central chakra, harmonizing and balancing the functions of the other chakras, as well as each side of the body. Its function is not only physical (distributing blood) but also spiritual: Shen, the spirit or mind, is stored in the heart according to classical Chinese medicine. The heart also controls that which is fused with both physical and invisible qualities—the emotions.

Thus the heart is the center and ruler of the entire body, while the small intestine supports the function of the heart by creating physical energy. In a sense then, the image of flames mirrors the disseminating function of the heart, while the source of fuel the small intestine. This system can be seen in Zazen meditation where the breath (which ignites the flames) and mind are directed toward the tanden. Spiritual consciousness, the flames, arises from concentration on the tanden, the energy source.

The heart and small intestine also reflect the very active up/down energy of the spiritual channel in their functioning. The heart works ceaselessly throughout our entire life pumping blood. This tireless activity is stimulated by the sinoatrial node. This node, located on the heart, right in line with the spiritual channel, sends out electric impulses which keep the heart active. Moreover we see within the heart that blood first moves downward from atria to ventricle, and then upward, as the main vessels taking blood away leave from the upper part of the heart. Likewise, densely compacted and centrally located in the yang lower abdomen, the small intestine actively churns ingested food by rhythmic segmentation. This process works something like the pistons of a car. Certain sections of the intestine contract, then the sections between these contract and the former relax.

The location of the heart and small intestine meridians in the arms also reflects their internal functions. Depending upon the way one holds their arms, the heart meridian moves upward or outward, reflecting a disseminating function, while the small intestine meridian moves inward or downward corresponding with its digesting and absorbing function.

From the images of fire nature energy presented in Chapter 2 as well as the information now presented we can see how this energy manifests within the individual.

The Flames (*Yin*)

Positive: warmth; bright; cheerful; joyful; optimistic; dynamic; generous; expressive; sociable; friendly; kind; passionate; sense of compassion; sense of forgiveness

Negative: yin excess—superficial; overly excitable; haughty; pompous; overly talkative; uncontrollable; wild; reckless; scattered in one's thoughts; absent minded; overly optimistic; hysterical

Yang deficient—sad, pessimistic, gloomy, always complaining; shy and insecure in the company of others; inability to communicate or express feelings (may be yin deficient); initial enthusiasm but difficulty maintaining an interest (may also be yin deficient)

Yin deficient—feeling of entrapment

The Source of the Fuel (Yang)

Positive: insightful—getting to the heart of the matter; good ability to concentrate and become involved or absorbed in whatever one is doing; self-control

Negative: yang excess—overly possessive; emotionally attached; obsessions and compulsions; hard hearted; ill natured; resentful; sense of revenge

Yang deficient or yin excess—sensitivity to verbal communication; sensitivity to what people say about them

THE HEART MERIDIAN

According to Classical Chinese Medicine[1]

The heart corresponds with the heart of Western medicine, probably inlcuding the aorta. Some sources also include the mind.[2] The heart is the ruling organ. If the heart is strong then it can lead the movement of the other organs and coordinate the functions of the whole body. If it becomes weak and loses control, then the health of the whole body is affected. The heart stores the Shen or Spirit. "The first primitive force to generate human life is Shen and life depends on form . . . Shen is the origin of life and form is its external shell."[3] When Shen is disturbed it may manifest in excessive dreaming or insomnia, and mental problems such as hysteria or delirium. The heart rules the blood and blood vessels,[4] and controls circulation. The condition of the heart is reflected in one's complexion and tongue. Both the physical condition of the tongue and the manner of one's speech may reflect the condition of the heart.

Disorders commonly treated by acupuncture to points along the heart meridian include the following:[5]

Stiff neck; pain, paralysis or numbness of the shoulder joint, upper arm or elbow joint; heart or chest pain; angina pectoris; heart palpitations; high blood pressure; nervous anxiety; insomnia; night sweating; dream disturbed sleep; insufficient lactation; shyness; epilepsy; convulsions; anxiety; hysteria; coma

According to Shizuto Masunaga[6]

The heart and small intestine meridians (Fig. 20) occupy a central position in the body. They are associated with the functions of "conversion and integration." They regulate the function of the entire body.

The condition of these meridians is reflected in one's complexion, tongue, and the corners of the eyes.

In the Chinese classics the heart is called the "sovereign of the organs where awareness (consciousness) originates." The heart meridian works to integrate the external stimuli received by the body and to effect a response. It "converts" the input from the five senses into appropriate internal responses and thus controls the whole body as the center of ki and *ketsu* (blood and other liquid constituents of the body). It is a motivating and integrating function felt in oneself most distinctly as the beating of the heart.

Imbalances in the heart meridian are associated with the following conditions:

Nervous tension due to shock or fatigue—it produces tightness in the solar plexus area and causes one to worry excessively; obsession with the notion that one has cancer, associated with certain conditions—tightness of the tongue that causes stammering, or difficulty swallowing, and clearing the throat constantly; tendency for blood to rush to the head and for the palms to become sweaty; heart problems

Masunaga further identifies conditions that may arise in terms of kyo and jitsu:

• *Heart Meridian Kyo*[7]

Cause. One's mind is not settled and one cannot communicate with others very well.

Mental Aspect. Emotional exhaustion after some crisis, excessive stress, longstanding anxiety or nervous tension; tendency to be oversensitive and neurotic; anxiety and worrying, which affect appetite; restlessness and inability to calm down; forgetfulness, tendency to be paranoid; jittery; easily startled or very timid; tension in the tongue which causes stuttering; poor concentration, tendency toward disappointment

Physical Aspect. Feeling of tension or constriction in solar plexus; rounded back caused by weakness of muscles in abdomen; tendency toward palpitations; strong tension in the abdominal wall and a feeling of oppression in the solar plexus when pressed; nervous stomach; thick tongue coating; feeling as if something is caught in the throat; rigidity in hands; sweaty palms; tendency to tire easily; soreness and redness in corner of eyes

• *Heart Meridian Jitsu*[8]

Mental Aspect: Feeling restless and fussy; chronic tension and stiffness in the chest; trying to contain anxiety and restlessness; perpetual fatigue; tendency to stammer; stiffness in solar plexus area; thirsty; obsession with tonsillitic cancer; laughing

Physical Aspect: Pulling sensation in tongue; always clearing throat; protrusion in solar plexus and tightness in heart area; stiff body; hysteria; sweaty palms; easily perspiring; sensitive skin; shoulder pain; fever in stomach area; desire for cold drinks; cardiac nervousness; nervous stomach; heart palpitations

• *Jitsu Symptoms of Other Meridians with Heart Meridian Kyo*[9]

Lung: Feeling of blockage in solar plexus or constriction in chest; nasal congestion

Large Intestine: Low spirits; feeling of legs dragging after a big disappointment

Stomach: Feeling of heaviness in stomach causing restless sleep; loss of appetite due to shock

Spleen: Timidity and hesitancy; irregular appetite; lack of exercise

Bladder: Fatigue caused by constant tension; feeling of something caught in throat, anxiety

Kidney: Fatigue after a big disappointment; prolonged anxiety; loss of motivation, gastric ulcer

Heart Constrictor: Backache associated with excessive concern; cold sweat on the face

Triple Heater: Head feeling unclear (hazy); heaviness over the whole body

Gallbladder: Strained nerves after concentrating too hard; hotness of the head and feeling irritable, weak grip

Liver: Feeling of tension and discomfort in upper half of the body; eye irritation

Structure and Function of the Heart[10]

Not much larger than a fist and weighing about 10 ounces, the heart functions ceaselessly to pump blood throughout the body, pushing our blood through more than 1,000 complete circuits everyday of our lives. It steadily pumps about 75 gallons of blood every hour, though during strenuous activity this figure can be as high as 500 gallons.

The heart is actually two separate pumps placed side by side, united by a thick dividing wall called the septum. The walls of the heart are made of thick cardiac muscle and enclose four chambers. The two upper chambers, the atria, receive blood returning to the heart. The two lower chambers, the ventricles, send blood out into the systemic circulations. The walls of the ventricles are thicker than those of the atria. The walls of the left ventricle are the thickest because it has to pump harder than the other chambers, in order to distribute blood throughout the body.

Low in oxygen and high in carbon dioxide, dark red blood received from the body through the venae cavae enters the right atrium. The right atrium acts as a storage area for the larger and stronger ventricle below it. The right ventricle relaxes (diastolic action) causing blood from the atrium to surge into it. The atrium contracts to complete the transfer. The right ventricle contracts rapidly (systolic action), and blood is pumped upward out of the heart and into the large pulmonary artery which leads to the lungs. Within the lungs carbon dioxide is unloaded and oxygen taken up. This oxygen rich blood turns bright red. It returns to the left heart via the pulmonary vein, which enters the left atrium, by the relaxation of the left ventricle and is ready to be forced out into the aorta and around the body. Both atria and both ventricles contract simultaneously, in rapid succession, ensuring that each side of the heart expels an equal volume of blood.

The valves of the heart ensure that blood flows in one direction only. They shut automatically if blood attempts to move against the proper direction of flow. Simple rings of muscle around the inflow veins, the vena cavae and pulmonary veins, prevent backflow. The tricuspid valve is located between the right atrium and right ventricle, and the mitral valve between the left atrium and left ventricle. At the exits to the ventricles there are the aortic valve of the left heart and the pulmonary valve of the right heart. These valves ensure a one way flow of blood—from vein to atria to ventricle to artery, as the heart contracts and relaxes.

Oxygen supply to the heart is supplied by two coronary arteries, which branch from the aorta, just beyond the aortic valve. They divide and spread over the heart in a network. Three systems of coronary veins return the deoxygenated blood directly into the right ventricle. Blockage of a coronary artery results in a complete lack of blood to the area served by that artery. Heart muscle is able to survive without oxygen for up to ten minutes. Beyond that the muscles stop contracting. They die and are replaced by nonfunctional scar tissue, considerably weakening the pumping power of the heart.

The heart has its own built in mechanism which maintains the rhythmic beat independent of its nerve connections. It is known as the pace maker, a knot of tissue located on the rear wall of the right atrium. Also known as the sinoatrial node or S-A node, it is the source of bursts of electrical activity that spread through the walls of the heart like ripples across the surface of a pond. It first stimulates the atria and then the ventricles to contract.

The Circulatory System[11]

The body contains about 10 pints of blood. This blood, via the circulatory system, carries oxygen, glucose, hormones, and other essential substances to the tissues and carries away carbon dioxide and other wastes produced by metabolic processes within the cells. The heart is at the center of the circulatory system. It pumps oxygenated blood to the tissues through thick walled, muscular, and slightly elastic vessels called arteries. The largest artery is the aorta which is nearly one inch wide. It leaves the heart from the left ventricle and first travels upward. Large arteries branch from the aorta, taking blood to the neck, head, and arms. The aorta then bends and passes down in front of the spine down the middle of the body, carrying blood to the kidneys, liver, intestines, and legs. The large arteries further branch into smaller vessels called arterioles which form a network in the skin, in the muscles, and in the organs that they supply. The muscle cells in the walls of the arterioles enable them to contract, thus giving them the ability to regulate blood flow in particular regions, according to needs. Arterioles further subdivide and the blood eventually passes into minute capillaries, tubules averaging only one-twenty-fifth of an inch in length, and one-hundredth of that in diameter. The wall of the capillary is only one cell thick. The total surface area of capillary walls in the body is over 6,000 square meters. Through this immense area the exchange of nutrients and oxygen for waste products takes place between the blood and the cells of the tissues.

On the return journey of circulation capillaries join up with slightly larger vessels called venules. The venules unite to form wider and wider collecting vessels until they become the major veins that return this deoxygenated blood to the heart. The returned blood is then pumped by the heart through the pulmonary arteries to the capillaries of the lungs. Carbon dioxide is exchanged for oxygen within the lungs and the newly oxygenated blood returns to the heart via the pulmonary veins.

Veins have thinner walls than arteries and the pressure in them is lower. Veins expand and collapse to adjust to the blood volume within them. Veins contain one way cup-shaped valves which prevent the backflow of blood to the tissues. This factor along with the massaging effect of nearby muscles helps to prevent blood from collecting in the lower parts of the body.

Blood Pressure. With each contraction of the heart the pressure of the blood in the arteries reaches a peak, called the systolic pressure. It then decreases to a minimum, the diastolic pressure, before the next contraction. Blood pressure is always expressed as two figures, the first representing the systolic, the second the diastolic, in millimeters of mercury. In a healthy young adult 120/80 is average. A person is considered to have high blood pressure if the systolic pressure consistently exceeds 100+his or her age, or if the diastolic pressure is greater than 100. The lower limit for a normal adult is 80/40: below this we usually faint.

Atherosclerosis (*Hardening of the arteries*)[12]. This disease is one of the most common problems of the circulatory system in Western countries. Fat deposits accumulate within the vessel walls. Small blood cells called platelets then stick to these fat accumulations, causing scarring. From these accumulations the vessel walls become thick so that the internal diameter of the arteriole is reduced. This process often accompanies high blood pressure. It can eventually block arteries and therefore prevent sufficient blood from being pumped to various parts of the body.

Macrobiotic Health Evaluation[13]

The condition of the heart is reflected in the facial color, shape of the nose, the mouth and speech, and the hands; as well it is seen in other parts of the body such as the face as a whole, the feet, and outermost ridges of the ears.

1. *Facial Color*

   Aside from natural skin colors, various abnormal facial and skin colors reflect disorders in the condition of the heart as well as in other organs:

   Reddish color. Apart from blushing, being out in the cold or following strenuous activity, this color is caused by expanded blood capillaries beneath the surface of the skin, showing that the heart and circulatory system are overworked and expanded. Often accompanied by a puffy, swollen appearance, this color indicates that the heart muscle is expanded and loosened. The cause is excess yin: sugar, fruit, salads, spices, pastries, along with the overconsumption of fluid, including coffee and alcohol.

   Purplish. A more severe condition of the above, indicating a dangerous overexpansion of the heart muscle and of the low blood pressure that often follows. This color, especially on the tip of the nose, indicates the possibility of a sudden heart attack or stroke.

   Pale color. The heart has become very tight from overconsumption of excessive contractive foods including meat, dairy food, and salt.

2. *The Nose*

   In general, the right and left sides of the nose correspond with the same sides of the heart. The bulb of the nose reflects the heart muscle as a whole. The upper bulbous region shows the atria and the lower the ventricles. The tip generally corresponds with the coronary arteries. The nostrils show the condition of the lungs and pulmonary vessels. Pimples and patches on the nose show circulatory disorders and the location on the nose corresponds to their location in the heart. These spots show that deposits of fat and cholesterol are accumulating in and around the heart and the coronary vessels.

   Normal well-formed nose. Average length and roundness—balanced mental/physical condition including the heart and circulatory system. Normally in the Orient, tropics and among other traditional societies, the nose tends to be broader and flatter; in North America and Europe, it is narrower and raised.

   High rounded (eagle) nose—excess consumption of poultry and eggs; tendency toward aggressiveness, self-centeredness and restlessness; indication of the development of atherosclerosis and the accumulation of layers of fat around the heart muscle

   Upward tilted tip—excess animal food, especially fish and seafood, during the mother's pregnancy; tendency toward sharpness in thinking, narrowness and shortsightedness; tendency toward hardening of the arteries, especially if animal food is consumed regularly in childhood and in later life

   Pointed nose (like Pinocchio)—overconsumption of certain kinds of fruit including melons and berries; indication of weakness of the heart and an excitable nervous condition

   Drooping nose—excess consumption of fruits and salad, liquids and sweets; weakness of the heart as well as the kidney and bladder functions

Swollen nose—from a combination of the overconsumption of meat, poultry or eggs along with soft drinks, juices, sugar, some vegetables of tropical origin, coffee, and other fluids. Indicates a swollen overworked heart and circulatory system laboring to provide oxygen to the cells and tissues. Liquid is retained in the body because of excessive salt and mineral intake, primarily from animal sources. Often a sign of developing congestive heart failure.

Nose with a hardened tip—caused by the excessive intake of saturated fat and cholesterol from such sources as beef, pork, poultry, eggs, cheese, and other dairy products. Indicates hardening of the arteries and muscles and the accumulation of fat around the heart and other major compacted organs, including the liver, kidneys, spleen, prostate or ovaries. A sign that a heart attack or stroke may occur.

Cleft nose (split or indentation at the end of the nose)—caused by a nutritional imbalance, especially a shortage of minerals and complex carbohydrates during the fetal stage and childhood development. Can also be produced in childhood or later in life by an excessive intake of simple sugars (fruits, juices, sucrose, honey, and soft drinks). They deprive the body of minerals and complex sugars. Irregular heartbeat and murmur.

Crooked nose—a general imbalance in the mental and physical constitution as a result of ancestral or parental disharmony. A nose bending toward the left shows that the left side of the body, including left atrium and ventricle, the left lung and left kidney, the descending colon, and the left ovary and testicle, are stronger and more tolerant of stress and abuse than the organs on the right side. It generally shows that the father's hereditary factors or influence were stronger. Bending toward the right it shows more activity in the right chambers of the heart and other organs on the right side of the body. As well it indicates stronger hereditary factors and influence of the mother.

3. *The Mouth and Speech*

The right side of the mouth represents the right chambers of the heart, the left side, the left chambers. Swelling or looseness on one side of the mouth reflects a similar condition on the same side of the heart. A mouth that as a whole is becoming swollen or loose shows that the entire heart is becoming loose or weak. The condition of the heart rhythm and the balance between the two sides can be seen in how well the two sides of the mouth coordinate when the person is speaking and the degree of balance or imbalance of the two sides while the mouth is at rest.

Very excitable talkative person—expanded, overactive heart

Stuttering—heart murmur, hyperactive heartbeat, or other irregular rhythm

Slow stammering speech—tired, overworked heart and disturbances in the electrical impulses that activate the heartbeat

False starts and stops in speech—may show skipped or missed beats

Speaking rapidly or falling over words—hyperactive heart and a tendency to develop high blood pressure

Slow speech—more a kidney than a heart problem, signifying loose and overactive kidneys. If the voice is also watery it signifies an enlarged heart.

4. *The Hands and the Heart*

The left chambers of the heart correspond to the left hand, right chambers, right hand. Strength of the grip of each hand generally shows the strength of the chambers of each side of the heart. A weak grip indicates general weakness or deficiency in the heart muscles, while an overpowering grip indicates high blood pressure and an overactive heart. Either condition may indicate high blood pressure or atherosclerosis.

Comparing the two hands further reveals how well the chambers of each side of the heart are coordinated and the consequent efficiency of the heart's activity. If the size, shape, major lines on the palms, and other general features of the hands are very different, then the two chambers are very different. If the two hands are well coordinated, the two chambers of the heart are in general harmony: if not, some irregularity of the heartbeat may be present. There may be a tendency for the emotions and overall character to fluctuate between extremes rather than to be consistent, steady, dependable.

4a. *Complexion and Temperature of the Hands*
   Reddish pink shade or hot hands—overactive heart with a tendency toward high
      blood pressure; overconsumption of sweets, sugar, fruit, juices, spices or
      alcohol, usually in combination with animal food
   Cold, wet hands—overly expanded heart weakened by long-term consumption
      of inbalanced foods and drinks, especially icy beverages and dairy foods
   Cold, dry hands—contracted capillaries beneath the skin and in the heart as
      a result of excessive salty animal food, refined flour, and hard baked foods
5. *Other Indications*
   Excessive laughter, giggling, and humor—swollen, overactive heart from over-
      consumption of sugar, sweets, fruit, juices, salad, tropical foods, coffee, stim-
      ulants and alcohol, usually in combination with meat, poultry, dairy food,
      and eggs
   Jerky behavior—inability to sit still or find a comfortable position; frequent
      changes of residence, employment, spouse or partner; irregular heart
      rhythms and developing heart disease
   Small square toenails—developing heart troubles
   Redness on the outermost ridge of the ears—swollen and overactive heart
   Fever or excessive sweating—possible hyperactive heart
   Coldness or inability to sweat—hypoactive circulatory functions
   Cravings for burnt, bitter, dry foods, and stimulant beverages—all indicate the
      possibility of heart problems.

Dietary Recommendations[14]
To restore the heart to its healthy functioning it is recommended that certain foods be substantially reduced or avoided. These include the following: meat, poultry, eggs, milk, cheese, yogurt, and other dairy products; refined salt; sugar, honey, and other refined sweeteners; soft drinks, coffee, black tea, and other strong stimulants or aromatic beverages; refined oils of either animal or vegetable quality, mayonnaise, margarine (including soy margarine), and artificial dressings; all oily and greasy foods; spices, some herbs, and ginseng; refined flour, white rice, and other polished grains; all foods containing chemicals, additives, and preservatives; tropical foods of all kinds, including tomatoes, potatoes and eggplants (even when living in a tropical area); artificially preserved food including all canned food, frozen food, and instant food,

pesticide sprayed food, dyed food, and irradiated food. Exercise caution with vitamin and other supplements.

Further, one can follow standard macrobiotic dietary recommendations, introducing or slightly emphasizing certain foods which are beneficial for the functioning of the heart. These foods include: red millet; corn; bitter tasting vegetables such as watercress, mustard greens, dandelion greens, turnip greens, and burdock; lightly roasted sesame seeds and gomashio, which are excellent for restoring elasticity to the heart and diseased arteries; round, heart-shaped vegetables such as fall and winter squashes, radishes, onions, rutabagas, and turnips.

An imbalanced condition of the heart falls into three basic categories: an overly yang condition—overactive heart, an overly yin condition—underactive heart, and a combination of excessively yin and excessively yang conditions—irregular heart. In each of these conditions a more restricted diet is recommended until the condition noticeably changes, usually for a period of two months or more.

An overly yang condition: People with this condition have high blood pressure and usually atherosclerosis, which has resulted in fatty deposits both in the coronary arteries or other blood vessels and fatty accumulations in and around the heart muscle itself. People with this condition are susceptible to a sudden massive heart attack or stroke, which may result in immediate death.

Variations on standard dietary guidelines are as follows:

Cooking should generally be less salty and lighter. Brown rice, barley, corn and whole wheat can be consumed regularly, oats and rye occasionally. Millet, buckwheat, and bread and other baked flour products should be minimized. Soups should have a milder flavor (less miso, tamari soy sauce and salt). Leafy green vegetables should be emphasized more while root vegetables should be consumed less than average. Raw salad can be consumed occasionally and boiled or pressed salad frequently. Beans and bean products should be lightly seasoned and used more regularly. Sea vegetables should be prepared with quicker cooking styles and should have a light taste. A small volume of quick or lighter pickles can be consumed. Condiments should be lighter and used in moderation. Fish and seafood should be avoided and sesame or corn oil used only in moderation. Fruit and desserts occasionally, either dried, cooked or raw and naturally sweetened. Occasionally, lightly roasted seeds and small servings of nuts and nut butters. Shorter prepared lighter tasting bancha.

An overly yin condition: People with this condition generally have a tendency toward low blood pressure (sometimes following a period of high blood pressure) and a generally weakened congested heart. They may suffer strokes or heart attacks but are much more likely to survive them than those with an overly yang condition. Such people also tend toward lung and respiratory ailments, anemia, melancholy and depression, leukemia, and possibly lymphoma or breast cancer. They tend to be introverted by nature, appearing to others as shy, retiring, lacking in self-confidence, quiet, tired, and prone to illness.

Variations on standard dietary guidelines are as follows: cooking should generally be more salty and stronger. Brown rice, barley, corn, whole wheat berries, millet, and buckwheat can be taken regularly; oats and rye occasionally. Baked flour products, noodles, and other forms of pasta should be taken only occasionally. Soup should have a little stronger flavor (slightly more miso, tamari soy sauce or sea salt). Root vegetables should be emphasized over others, round vegetables used moderately, and leafy greens less often. Avoid raw salad but occasionally consume boiled or pressed salad. Beans and bean products should be a little more strongly seasoned and used less regularly. Sea vegetables should be cooked for a longer period and have a slightly thicker taste. A small volume of stronger pickles can be consumed. Condiments can be a little stronger in flavor. A small volume of white-meat fish or seafood can be taken occasionally. Avoid raw oil and use occasionally only dark sesame oil, in moderation. Avoid or minimize fruit. If craved, take small quantities of raisins or other dried or cooked fruit. Occasionally, lightly roasted seeds can be used. Limit the use of nuts and nut butters. Longer prepared, stronger-tasting bancha.

A combination of excessively yin and yang conditions: People in this group suffer from heart murmurs, disturbances in heart rhythms, or other abnormalities in coordination between the left and right sides of the heart. High blood pressure and atherosclerosis may also be present. They are also susceptible to oily or dry skin, alternating diarrhea and constipation, diabetes, hypoglycemia, jaundice, and lung, pancreatic, or kidney cancer.

Variations on standard dietary guidelines are as follows: the way of cooking should generally be medium, neither too long nor too short, the flame neither too high nor too low. Brown rice, barley, whole wheat berries, and corn can be used regularly; millet, buckwheat, oats, and rye occasionally; bread and baked flour products should be minimized, noodles and other pasta used only occasionally. Soup should have a moderate flavor. Choose from all temperate type vegetables but emphasize more round varieties. Minimize raw salad but boiled or pressed salad can be taken frequently. Beans and bean products should be moderately seasoned and consumed in moderate volume. Sea vegetables should be cooked to a medium degree and have a moderate taste. Condiments should be used moderately. Fish or seafood should be minimized. Occasionally use dark sesame or corn oil, only in moderation. Avoid raw oil. If fruit is craved take a small amount of dried or cooked fruit (locally grown and seasonal). Use only naturally sweetened desserts if craved. Occasional lightly roasted seeds; a few nuts and some nut butter; medium prepared, medium tasting bancha.

THE SMALL INTESTINE MERIDIAN

According to Classical Chinese Medicine[15]

Anatomically the small intestine corresponds to the small intestine of Western science but functionally it corresponds to the large intestine, since its main functions are considered to be in the absorption of water.[16] "The Small Intestine controls the Transformation of Matter and the separating of the Pure and Impure."[17]

Since we know that the coupled organ of the small intestine, the heart, is the body's emotional center, and that the small intestine meridian ends at the ear, we might consider that on a psychological level the small intestine functions to absorb what is actually said as opposed to what one wants to hear—the separation of fact from fiction.

Disorders commonly treated by acupuncture to points along the small intestine meridian include the following:

Headache; facial paralysis; toothache; eye disease; deafness; ringing in the ears; pain and stiffness in the neck; pain, numbness and aching in the shoulder joint or upper extremities; lumbar pain; epilepsy, mental disorder; malaria; vomiting; gall-stones; bronchitis; and asthma[18]

According to Shizuto Masunaga[19]

In the Chinese classics the small intestine is referred to as "the organ which receives and transforms nourishing substances." It receives food into the body and converts this into nutrients to produce blood and tissues; thus controlling the whole body by providing nutrition. The small intestine meridian aids the heart meridian by keeping ki down in the hara region to maintain calmness and composure. Strong emotions have an effect on the lower abdomen. Anger, shock, and anguish cause blood to collect in the lower abdomen and it becomes congested. This condition leads to blood stagnation which can in turn cause low back pain and chilling of the lower extremities, especially among women; thus the small intestine meridian is also related to the function of the ovaries and maintaining menstrual regularity. Two Japanese biologists, Professor Chishima and Dr. Keiichi Morishita have advanced the theory that blood is produced in the small intestine.

Imbalances in the small intestine meridian are associated with the following:

Holding things inside—not expressing anger for example; shock; stagnation of energy in the neck and shoulder area; easily becoming fatigued; often experiencing low back pain and cramps in the legs; irregular bowel movements due to problems in digestion and assimilation; imbalance in functioning of the ovaries—causing menstrual disorders, migraine headaches, and neurotic symptoms that are associated with new mothers

Masunaga further identifies conditions in terms of kyo and jitsu:

- *Small Intestine Meridian Kyo*[20]

Cause: One lacks the confidence to assert oneself and has a tendency to be shy and retiring.

Mental Aspect: Becoming too involved with details; great patience; holding in feelings; suppressing deep sorrow; wearing out one's nerves concentrating too hard; excessive anxiety and worry; a strong desire not to be outdone; tendency to be introverted; awkwardness in manner; psychological trauma

Physical Aspect: Poor intestinal function, which causes one to be thin; loose or flabby flesh; poor absorption of nutrients, causing anemia and lack of energy; constipation or diarrhea caused by poor digestion; chilling of legs and waist along with hotness of face; weakness in lower half of body, causing a feeling of heaviness from the waist down; fatigue and soreness in lower back, leading to heaviness in legs; blood stagnation; appendicitis or problems that stem from an appendix operation; susceptibility to food poisoning; stiffness and tension in back of neck; shoulder stiffness with migraine headaches; ringing in ears; loss of hearing; dysmenorrhea and gynecological problems

- *Small Intestine Meridian Jitsu*[21]

Mental Aspect: Patient; strong determination to the end; ability to hold everything in oneself; accomplishing what one sets out to do; restless; overworked; tendency not to eat slowly; restless rapid eye movement; headaches

Physical Aspect: Blood being stopped in lower abdomen because of shock; irregular circulation of blood; hip ache; stiff shoulders; giddiness; stiffness in cervical verebrae like morning stiffness; difficulty in rotation; puffiness in eyes and ears; feeling of being chilled and hot in the head; redness in cheeks; stiffness in solar plexus; stiffness and coldness in lower hara; frequent trips to toilet; poor circulation in the extremities; frostbite; poor digestion; constipation; ovary malfunctioning; poor circulation in legs due to malfunctioning of the intestinal artery near navel; lower backache due to curvature in the lumbar area; pain in the shoulders; pain in the upper teeth; lack of saliva secretion

- *Jitsu Symptoms of Other Meridians with Small Intestine Meridian Kyo*[22]
  Lung: Mental fatigue along with heaviness in the hips and legs; loss of spirit
  Large Intestine: Gynecological problems accompanied with chilling of hips and legs; congestion in lower abdomen caused by shock; dislocation of hip
  Stomach: Irregular appetite and eating too many sweets; shoulder stiffness due to dysfunction of ovaries; coldness in legs; appendicitis
  Spleen: Digestive problems caused by excessive worry; chilling of back; large amounts of gas
  Bladder: Overworking; state of shock; autotoxemia; fatigue due to overstrain of autonomic nervous system
  Kidney: Lingering fatigue after childbirth; low back pain; subject to great stress
  Heart Constrictor: General fatigue; tendency toward palpitations; stiffness in back or low back pain
  Triple Heater: Whiplash injury; lack of exercise; ringing in ears; Ménière's disease; overexertion; hardness and persistent tension in forearms; sore throat due to a cold
  Gallbladder: Lack of stamina; eyestrain; arthritis; malnutrition due to poor digestion
  Liver: Duodenal ulcer, dark spots on skin, intermittent claudication

Structure and Function of the Small Intestine[23]

The small intestine absorbs food constituents into the bloodstream. Foods are broken down into their smallest components: nutrients then cross the intestinal lining while the remains are passed on to the large intestine.

Structurally the small intestine connects the stomach with the large intestine. A tightly coiled tube more than twenty feet in length, the small intestine is located in the center of the abdomen. It is anatomically divided into three continuous sections. The 10-inch-long duodenum which connects with the pyloric sphincter, lies in the area of the solar plexus. The next section, the jejunum, is about 10 feet long. The next, the ileum some 12 feet in length, connects with the large intestine via the ileocecal valve, in the lower right quadrant of the abdomen.

The intestinal tube is less than 1 inch in diameter. Anatomists distinguish four layers in the wall of the small intestine: the mucosa (the innermost surface); the submucosa; the muscular coat; and the serosa, the outer protective layer.

The mucosa is lined with goblet cells that secrete mucus, and tiny hairlike projections called villi. The villi in turn are covered with microscopically fine microvilli which vastly increase the surface area, making "the total absorptive area of the inside wall of the small intestine of an average person about the same as a standard football field."[24]

The submucosa contains a large number of blood vessels, the muscular coat consists of two layers of muscles. The outer muscles run longitudinally and the inner in circles. Between these layers of muscles are nerves connected with the autonomic nervous system.

Food reaching the small intestine has already been acted upon by the mouth, and digestive juices (including hydrochloric acid) and enzymes of the stomach, creating an acidic fluid called chyme. Within the duodenum chyme is made alkaline. The presence of food and hydrochloric acid within the duodenum causes the intestine to produce the hormones secretin and pancreozymin, which stimulate the secretion of bicarbonate and enzymes from the pancreas. The small intestine also produces the hormone cholecystokinin which stimulates the gallbladder to contract and secrete bile. Bicarbonates are alkaline and neutralize the acid, while bile salts act like a detergent, emulsifying fatty acids into smaller particles, better enabling pancreatic secretions to work on these fats to be readily absorbed by the intestinal wall.

Chyme is thoroughly mixed with digestive juices by the activity of the muscular coat, which performs functions of rhythmic segmentation and peristalsis. In the former, the circular muscles contract and divide the tube into segments. Contraction of the muscles between these segments makes smaller segments and the first set of muscles relaxes. This churning motion takes place between twelve and sixteen times per minute and thoroughly mixes chyme with digestive enzymes, facilitating absorption by bringing the contents into contact with the villi. A wave of contraction (peristalsis) flows from the duodenum to the ileocecal valve. It arises as a result of the presence of food within the intestine.

Carbohydrates and proteins are absorbed through the intestinal walls, which are quite thin, into blood vessels that link with the hepatic portal vein. The portal vein leads to the liver where nutrients undergo further processing before being sent to other parts of the body. Carbohydrates are absorbed mainly as monosaccharides, principally glucose, and proteins are absorbed mainly as amino acids. Fats do not enter the bloodstream directly. They are largely absorbed through special ducts in the villi called lacteals, which connect with the lymph system. These eventually drain into the thoracic duct which empties into the vena cava in the upper thoracic region. Fats then travel to the liver for further breakdown or storage. Fats are principally absorbed as triglycerides.

It takes between two and four hours for chyme to travel the distance of the small intestine and it cannot enter the large intestine until its first section, the cecum, is empty.

Disorders Associated with the Small Intestine

Disorders in the small intestine cause malabsorption. Signs of malabsorption include unexplained weight loss, nutritional deficiencies, abdominal discomfort (including cramps, burning sensation, gas, and bloating), diarrhea, abnormal stools, anemia, belching, passing of rectal gas, vomiting, and nausea. In children it affects their growth.[25]

Malabsorption can arise from a number of factors:[26]

1. Ulcers, occurring especially in the duodenum. They are most likely caused by an imbalance in the production of acid versus protective mucus. Mucus production can in turn be affected by diet, stress, emotions, environment, mental outlook, and nonsteroidal anti-inflammatory drugs such as aspirin.

2. Failure in the digestive process to produce enzymes needed to break down certain foods. Lactose intolerance is an example. This is an inability to break down lactose, the sugar in milk. It is caused by the lack of lactase, an enzyme secreted in the walls of the small intestine.
3. Intestinal obstructions such as tumors, adhesions, or scarring within the small intestine, as well as strangulated hernia
4. Intestinal damage from radiation therapy, certain drugs, or injury
5. Intestinal infections. Parasites such as tapeworms, though rare, can be found in the small intestine.
6. Congenital defects
7. Intestinal paralysis. Peristaltic action ceases to function.
8. Diverticulosis; outpouchings that form in weakened segments of the intestines, especially in the duodenum and jejunum, and particularly in older people
9. Inflammatory processes
10. Bacterial overgrowth.[27] As well as within the large intestine, millions of bacteria inhabit the small intestine, usually in a state of symbiosis. They may even synthesize certain vitamins such as B_{12}. Unlike the large intestine, large numbers of bacteria within the small intestine are not found within the food contents passing through but rather live within and off the mucous coating. Overgrowth of such bacteria is prevented by peristalsis, and the presence of bile and gastric acid. If these factors are reduced, bacteria begin to multiply rapidly, reaching concentrations, at times, 100,000 times what is normal.[28] They cause gas and, because of their close contact with the inner surface of the intestinal wall, they may cause inflammation; and by their sheer number they can limit the area available for the absorption of needed nutrients.

Bile and acid secretions in adequate amounts depend upon the following:
1. Food should be adequately chewed.
2. Gastric acid must be adequate for the amount of food taken in. This will ensure that the food is digested and bacteria within the food is destroyed.
3. Sufficient time is needed between meals so that food can be thoroughly digested and levels of digestive juice restored before a new meal is introduced into the intestinal tract.

Macrobiotic Health Evaluation[29]
The constitution of the small intestine is seen in the mouth (p. 156). The condition of the small intestine is seen in the lower lip, the forehead, and the head hair.
1. *The Lower Lip*
The corners of the mouth correspond with the duodenum. The inner area of the lower lip corresponds with the small intestine.
Swollen lips or mouth drooping open—expanded intestinal condition. If also wet, diarrhea is indicated.
Swollen and dry or cracked—tendency toward constipation
Lips that are tight and contracted or a mouth held tightly pursed or the jaws clenched—a constricted intestinal condition and a tendency toward constipation
Corners of mouth dry or beginning to crack—excessive consumption of salt,

baked foods, and saturated fats, leading to a contracted and congested duodenal condition

Sores or blisters on the corners of the mouth—too much oily food, leading to an acidic or ulcerous duodenal condition.

Either expanded or contracted intestinal conditions can lead to poor absorption of nutrients, resulting in more extreme blood diseases, such as anemia or leukemia. In addition, these conditions can cause incomplete food digestion, fermentation, mucous formation, flatulence, ulcers, inflammations and eventually cancer. As well they can cause many lower body problems such as poor circulation in the legs, excess weight around the hips or varicose veins. Multiple sclerosis is another disorder that these conditions may help bring on.

2. *Lip Color*
   Clear pinkish red—healthy color
   Vivid red—expanded capillaries in the intestines with probable high blood pressure and possible intestinal inflammation or infection
   White—probable anemia and poor blood circulation
   Dark or purplish—blood stagnation
   Black spot on the lips—toxic blood stagnation; possible tumor formation
3. *Middle Area of the Forehead*
   Horizontal ridges or deep lines—swollen intestine
   Vertical lines—contracted condition
   Acne—fatty acid accumulation
   Moles—accumulation of excessive protein mucus from animal food
4. *Head Hair*
   The head hair directly corresponds with the intestinal villi.
   Oily, dry, splitting hair—similar condition of the villi
   Hair beginning to fall out—weakening of the digestive system, loss of villi, loss of absorption ability
5. *Shoulders, at the Base of the Neck*
   Hardness—intestinal blockage and stagnation

Dietary Recommendations

The standard macrobiotic diet will restore healthy functioning of the small intestine. Hard saturated fats weaken absorption ability by creating hardness within the intestine as well as putrefaction and possible bacterial overgrowth. Shellfish may create intestinal cramps. Stimulant and aromatic foods and beverages, spices and the like may create irritation and inflammation of the intestinal wall. Sugar, fruit, and fruit juices in large quantity or tropical origin, and chilled or iced beverages, can severely weaken intestinal function and once again create malabsorption.

THE HEART CONSTRICTOR MERIDIAN

According to Classical Chinese Medicine

Also called the pericardium or circulation-sex, the heart constrictor cannot be considered as an internal organ but most likely corresponds to the pericardium, coronary

Fig. 21

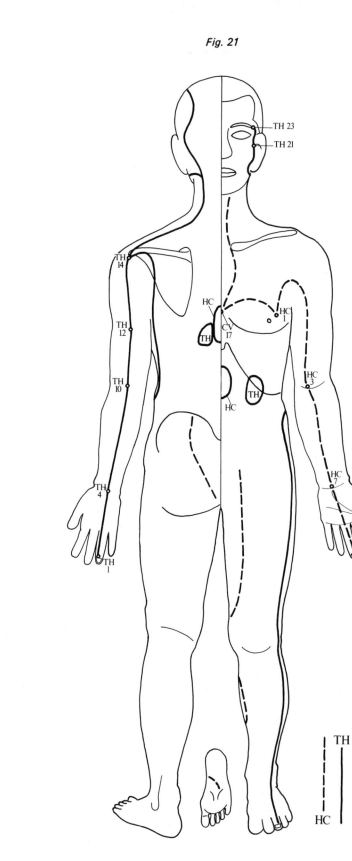

arteries, major arteries, and part of the pleural membrane.[30] The heart constrictor meridian is the external protector of the heart and has, at the same time, the function of administering the controlling action of the heart. "The pericardium is the organ from which the feeling of happiness [heart] comes."[31]

Disorders commonly treated by acupuncture to points along the heart constrictor meridian include the following:

Coughing; fullness of the chest; chest pain; palpitations; angina pectoris; epilepsy; convulsions; hallucinations; insomnia; shyness; emotional instability; schizophrenia; vomiting; nausea; hiccups; congestion of the uterus; pain of the upper arm, elbow, wrist, and fingers[32]

According to Shizuto Masunaga[33]
The heart constrictor and triple heater meridians (Fig. 21) are associated with the functions of circulation and protection. They circulate nourishing ki and protective ki to the central and peripheral areas of the body. By their process the body is integrated, filled with vitality, and able to defend itself.

Both the heart and small intestine, heart constrictor and triple heater meridians correspond with the fire phase of energy transformation. In classical Chinese medicine, the heart and small intestine are known as sovereign fire, the heart constrictor and triple heater as ministerial fire. Likened to political posts the former pair are regarded as the ruling organs, the latter as their assistants.

The heart constrictor is assigned the government post of the King's messenger. Its function is to assist the central coordinating function of the heart and to convey the will of the heart throughout the entire body. The heart constrictor is often regarded as corresponding with the pericardium, the membrane which surrounds the heart. Masunaga sees a broader view: he relates it to taking care of the actual work of the central circulatory function. This function includes the heart and pericardium, the aorta, all the major arteries and veins, the lymphatic ducts, and blood circulation which regulates the distribution of nutrients. In this way the heart constrictor is able to inhibit or stimulate the functioning of all the organs.

Just as the pericardium protects the heart, the heart constrictor meridian in like manner involves a protective function. Its role as the King's messenger involves a physical function explained above and a nonphysical function. Its nonphysical role deals with the emotions, conveying the intentions of the heart or giving expression to the emotions, since the emotions are related to the heart. "[The heart constrictor] . . . is the palace official from whom pleasure and mirth are derived."

Imbalances in the heart constrictor meridian are associated with the following:

Exhaustion from working too hard; working too long in the same position; haziness of the head; difficulty in relaxing—blood rises to the head to cause hotness of the head, while the extremities become cold; occasional discomfort in the pyloric region (area above the navel); rapid pulse; abnormal blood pressure, or pyrosis (heartburn); attacks of angina pectoris in more serious cases; insomnia; palpitations; shortness of breath; fulgurating (pricking) pain; sense of oppression in the chest

Masunaga further identifies conditions in terms of kyo and jitsu:
- *Heart Constrictor Meridian Kyo*[34]

Cause: The circulatory function declines and an excessive burden is placed on the heart because of poor posture or working in one position too long.

Mental Aspect: Great impatience without any ability to act; total exhaustion, causing one to be in a daze; restless sleep and excessive dreaming; anxiety caused by breathing difficulties; being repeatedly startled by small things; great shock which almost seems to cause a heart attack

Physical Aspect: Tendency for the throat to swell; feeling of obstruction in chest, which makes it hard to inhale; chest pains; heart problems; palpitations; shortness of breath; tendency to tire easily and inability to exercise vigorously; abnormal and fluctuating blood pressure; swelling and chilling of extremities; tendency toward gastric and duodenal ulcers; ulcers; prone to tonsillitis; heartburn; tenderness on the sternum and pectoral muscles

● *Heart Constrictor Meridian Jitsu*[35]

Mental Aspect: Restless when asleep or awake; nervous in social situations; easily excited; abnormal concentration on work; abnormal emotions; hypersensitivity

Physical Aspect: Strong palpitations and high blood pressure; palms getting hot; dizziness; easily fatigued; poor circulation; headache; stiffness in solar plexus; tightness in hara area; pain in stomach; cardiac malfunctioning; tightening in the fingers—clenched fists; colitis due to diarrhea or constipation; coated tongue

●*Jitsu Symptoms of Other Meridians with Heart Constrictor Kyo*[36]

Lung: Cardiac asthma; numbness in the toes; heaviness in the shoulders, back, and chest

Large Intestine: Hotness of head and cold legs; great tension from the neck down to the shoulders; chilling during sleep

Stomach: Poor digestion due to overwork; high blood pressure

Spleen: Exhaustion after too much mental work; gastroptosis

Heart: Fatigue coming from restlessness; ringing in the ears; hotness of head and palpitations

Small Intestine: Fatigue due to anxiety; cerebral infarction; palpitations

Bladder: High blood pressure due to stress; pyloric ulcer; labored breathing; low blood pressure or temporary high blood pressure

Kidney: Overwork and straining one's nerves; tension across the shoulders; heaviness in the chest; irritation of the windpipe leading to frequent coughing; unwilling to make an effort

Gallbladder: Basedow's disease; hardness of forearms; heartburn; pain in the back and shoulders; nervousness as a result of sudden shock

Liver: Dizziness upon standing; feeling tired all over—accumulation of mental stress and poor circulation due to impaired liver function

THE TRIPLE HEATER MERIDIAN

According to Classical Chinese Medicine
Anatomically such an internal organ does not exist. Functionally, it probably represents many endocrine functions and some of the circulatory functions, including functions of the lymphatic system.[37]

"In general terms the function of the triple heater is to circulate Qi, blood and fluid, to rot and ripen food and water, and to harmonize the digestion of solid and liquid food."[38]

The trunk of the body is divided into three parts:

The Upper Heater—above the diaphragm including the hands, head, and chest but
mainly the respiratory system

The Middle Heater—the upper half of the abdomen between the diaphragm and
navel, corresponding mainly with the digestive system, particularly the function
of the pancreas

The Lower Heater—the lower abdomen below the navel and including the lower
extremities, corresponding mainly with the genitourinary system[39]

The upper heater functions to circulate ki around the whole body and protect the
outside. The function of the middle heater is principally to take water and food and
transform it into ki, blood and fluid—into nourishment. The function of the lower
heater is in the draining and flushing of the pure and impure, and also the expulsion
of urine and feces.[40]

Disorders commonly treated by acupuncture to points along the triple heater
meridian include the following:

Headache, facial paralysis; eye diseases; stammering; toothache; sore throat;
coughing; epilepsy; fever; common cold; deafness; ringing in the ears; redness and
swelling of the ear; stiff neck; shoulder and back pain; pain or paralysis of the arms,
elbows and hands; disorder of the wrist joint and surrounding soft tissue[41]

According to Shizuto Masunaga[42]

While the heart constrictor assists the heart, the triple heater assists the heart's paired
organ, the small intestine. It is associated with the mesentery (membrane) surrounding
the small intestine and is responsible for conveying the nutrients absorbed by the small
intestine to every corner of the body.

While the heart constrictor is associated with the central circulatory function, the
triple heater controls peripheral circulation and lymphatic flow. The triple heater is
therefore associated with the skin, mucous membranes, and serous membranes which
are supplied by peripheral capillary and lymphatic networks.

In classical Chinese medicine, the triple heater is assigned the role of "the official
in charge of water works." In the body, in a corresponding manner, the triple heater
meridian regulates water metabolism.

A "heater" is an area of heat production (center of metabolic activity). The triple
heater is therefore also a traditional classification of metabolic activity in the organs
located in the top, middle, and bottom sections of the torso.

Imbalances in the triple heater meridian are associated with the following:

An inability to relate well with others and to be overly defensive and "to always
have one's guard up"—leading to overall tension and stiffness: the forearms become
tense and rigid and the fists are constantly clenched, the head often feels heavy as if it
were covered with something; oversensitive to changes in the environment—adversely
affected by sudden changes in temperature and humidity; tendency to be allergic; the
mucous lining of the nose and throat is hypersensitive and the lymph nodes swell
easily; to constantly catch colds which affects the eyes and throat; sense of oppression
in the chest, and the abdominal wall and the skin surface in general is hypersensitive,
causing ticklishness, itching and oversensitivity to pain; eczema and urticaria (nettle
rash); edema occurs readily; sometimes the arms as well as the back of the head feel
numb.

Masunaga further identifies conditions in terms of kyo and jitsu:

- *Triple Heater Meridian Kyo*[43]

   Cause: One is overprotected at home and cast out into the world unprepared. One tends to be poor at adapting oneself to one's surroundings, overly cautious, tense, and awkward, and does not have enough opportunity to get release from nervous tension. One is overprotected as a child, or neglected when love was really needed from one's parents.

   Mental Aspect: Tendency to carry a mental burden or to be overanxious; excessive worrying over trivial matters in dealing with others; tendency for thinking to be disorganized due to fatigue; a feeling of being in a daze

   Physical Aspect: Hypersensitive skin, and weakness in mucous membrane and lymphatic system; tendency toward allergic reactions in the tonsils, nose, and throat; frequent colds which take a long time to go away; headaches; ringing in the ears; dizziness, eyestrain, hotness of head, excessive discomfort with changes in temperature and humidity; feeling of constriction in chest; tension in abdominal walls; extreme ticklishness; inflammation of peritoneum, causing abdominal cramps and pain; misalignment of cervical vertebrae; and tension in the neck, numbness from the neck down to the back of the arms

- *Triple Heater Meridian Jitsu*[44]

   Mental Aspect: Extremely cautious; hypertense; tendency to clench the palms; tightness in the arms; heaviness in the head; nervous reaction to external changes in heat, cold, humidity; heaviness in chest (upper heater), stomach (middle heater), and lower hara (lower heater)

   Physical Aspect: Overcautious, sensitive, unconscious tension in the arms, stagnation in the brain, causing a heavy feeling—meninges become red; abnormal eye pressure; pain in neck, shoulder, and arms; prone to inflammations in general; lymphatic inflammations; inflammation of nasal mucosa; itchy skin; tightness in chest; poor circulation in legs; pain in rib cage; susceptibility to humidity; ticklish; inflammation in the mouth and womb; rash; peripheral circulation is not good; one's body is watery; poor gum condition causing loose teeth.

- *Jitsu Symptoms of Other Meridians with Triple Heater Meridian Kyo:*[45]

   Lung: Chest pains with a cold; pleurisy

   Large Intestine: Common cold; dizziness; fatigue in arms and lower half of body; blood stagnation in the pelvis

   Stomach: Acute gastritis; lack of exercise; feeling tired after overeating

   Spleen: Feeling ill after eating; heaviness in head from excessive anxiety

   Heart: Hotness of head and chilling of extremities: feeling of general lassitude; fatigue or strain felt in the back of the eyes; stiff shoulders

   Small Intestine: Whiplash injury; appendicitis; ringing in the ears; shoulder tension from lack of exercise; ovary malfunction

   Bladder: Allergic constitution; numbness down arms and legs; frequent urination

   Kidney: Lack of sleep or restless sleep; prone to nosebleed; blurred vision; recovery period after a cold

   Gallbladder: Tendency for protracted colds; bitter taste in mouth; nausea; eyestrain

   Liver: Hypersensitivity of peritoneum and abdominal wall, causing frequent diarrhea; tendency to be ticklish; rhinitis

Exercise Recommendations

Various exercises in Chapter 5 stimulate the fire nature energy meridians.

Hara massage: small intestine 7. (1), (2), (3); heart constrictor 7 C. Arm meridian stretches: H.C.m—10(1); T.H.m—10(3); HT.m/S.I.m 10(4). Self-shiatsu to arms: H.T.m—11(1); H.C.m 11(2); T.H.m—11(5); S.I.m—11(6). Camel Pose No. 18—HT., Side Stretches (No. 20(2))—HT. Self-shiatsu to legs: T.H.m—21 A(1). HT.m and S.I.m. Stretch—No. 22. Abdominal exercise for small intestine 25 (1), (2), (3), (5)

The Spleen and Stomach Meridians

Soil Nature Energy

In the Five phases, fire represents the zenith of energy expansion. Earth's energy then begins to wane and heaven's force becomes dominant. In the same way that ashes return to the earth, soil nature is the next phase in the Five Transformations.

Being under the influence of heaven's force, soil nature is characterized as downward energy; energy now begins to gather and materialize. However, in the evolution of the theory of the Five Transformations soil was originally associated with the center and many of the qualities associated with soil energy come from this image of center. Both center and downward are yang qualities. However, within yang there must be yin, there must be upward and peripheral qualities associated with this energy. Heaven's force moves from infinity (periphery) to a point. Soil as the center, as the most still, most directly receives the influence of heaven's force, which is associated with the mind or thought (yin) in the mind/body relationship.

More directly, soil in itself demonstrates both yin and yang qualities. Soil's yang quality is that it is solid matter. This image suggests within the individual qualities of earthiness, practicality, materialism, and sensuality. The yin quality of soil is that in itself it stores nourishment which it gives impartially to whoever needs. This is the nurturing quality of mother Earth; it is seen within the individual in like manner. These yin and yang qualities are quite interrelated. The excess of one quality may create the deficiency of the other. For example if soil becomes too yang, too tight and compacted, it will harden and be unable to nourish. Conversely, when a farmer over-works the land, soil becomes depleted or exhausted. In the same way, the individual who becomes too acquisitive and greedy loses the quality of generosity toward others, while those who are too giving often fail to take care of their own health.

The images of center and downward movement can be seen within the body on a functional level. Soil nature energy corresponds with the stomach and spleen-pancreas. These organs are located predominantly on the left side of the body, the side which is dominated more by heaven's downward force. Moreover, the process of digestion is a downward one, as food slowly progresses downward before being absorbed. Both organs perform centralized functions. The stomach chooses the food to be ingested and stores it. Thus, the other organs of the body depend upon its good judgment. The pancreas, centrally located in the solar plexus area, supplies the enzymes necessary to break this food down into nutrients that the body can use for nourishment. The stomach and spleen meridians are also centrally located. They pass along the front of the body, over the front of the torso and along the front of the legs. The stomach meridian begins just below the eye and moves downward onto the feet. This suggests a more practical function, of looking out for and acquiring food.

Fig. 22

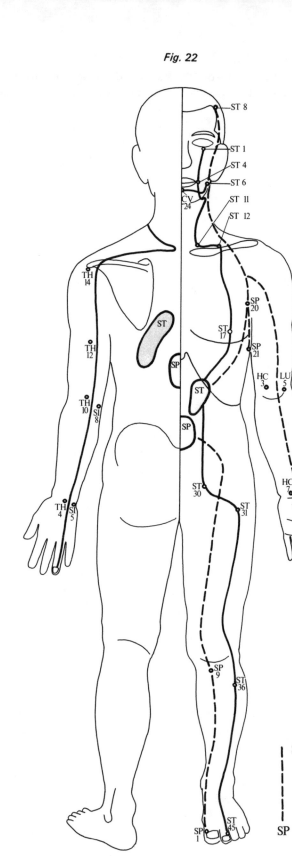

The spleen conversely, travels upward from the feet. In Masunaga's theory, the spleen meridian terminates in the head. Masunaga associated the spleen with the functioning of the cerebral cortex. The cerebral cortex is also in a way related to digestion because facts are digested by thinking.[1]

From the images of soil nature energy presented here and in Chapter 2 we can see how soil nature energy may manifest within the individual:

Soil as Center

Positive: Sense of balance, harmony, stability, clarity and direction (can see all sides); to be open, fair and frank

Negative: Unbalanced, unstable, poor sense of direction, lack of direction, aimless, confused

Soil as Solid Matter/Soil as Most Direct Receiver of Heaven's Force

Positive: Dependable, to feel solid and settled, "down to earth," earthy, grounded, practical, sense of wonder

Negative: Impractical, unsettled, "up in the clouds," silly, overly conservative, to think too much

Soil as the Storer and Provider of Nourishment

Positive: Sense of faith, confidence, security, and dependability; fertile, nourishing, nurturing, caring, unselfish, thoughtful, helpful, encouraging, self-sacrificing and persevering; accepting, impartial, modest, humble; thrifty, economical; to have a good memory; sense of taste; fertile

Negative: Inability or refusal to accept; prejudiced, suspicious, lack of trust, skeptical, cynical, apprehensive, sense of doubt, overly choosy, negatively discriminating, lack of faith—worries, insecure; thoughtless, forgetful; barren, infertile; too materialistic and acquisitive, stingy, miserly, cheap, spendthrift, poor provider; at the mercy of others.

THE SPLEEN MERIDIAN

According to Classical Chinese Medicine[2]
The spleen function most likely represents the pancreas.[3] The spleen is the principal organ of digestion.[4] It rules transformation and transportation.[5] It transforms food into nourishment (ki and blood), and is responsible for transporting this nourishment to various parts of the body. The spleen thus rules the muscles, flesh, and the four limbs; their movement (and condition) depends upon the power of the spleen.[6] The spleen governs the blood. Besides helping to create the blood, the spleen helps to keep the blood flowing along its proper paths.[7] Blood in the stool and uterine bleeding, for example, may be signs that spleen ki is weak. The condition of the spleen is reflected in the color and texture of the lips and the ability to sense different tastes. The spleen is said to be damp earth; it dislikes dampness and likes dryness.[8]

Disorders commonly treated by acupuncture to points along the spleen meridian include the following:

Abdominal distension and pain; poor digestion; insomnia and mental disorders; irregular, excessive, or absence of menstruation; dysentery, diarrhea, constipation; pain in chest, difficulty in breathing; frequency of urination and incontinence, impotence, frigidity; weakness of limbs; numbness and chilliness of leg and knee; pain and diseases of ankle joint and foot; inflammation, pain, and paralysis of big toe[9]

According to Shizuto Masunaga[10]

The spleen and stomach meridians (Fig. 22) are associated with the functions of ingestion and digestion. These functions involve the intake of food for nourishment and the process of digestion and assimilation. According to traditional Chinese medicine the spleen and stomach are together likened to the official who controls the grain storehouses.

While centered on the pancreas, the spleen meridian also includes the functions of all organs that secrete digestive enzymes (the stomach, gallbladder, small intestine, and mouth). It also relates to the reproductive glands in women (the mammaries and ovaries), and the cerebral cortex "since facts are digested by thinking." Lack of exercise and too much thinking cause a reduction in the secretion of digestive juices which in turn causes poor digestion.

Imbalances in the spleen meridian give rise to the following:

A tendency to think and worry too much as well as always feeling hungry and craving food; restlessness, associated with eating quickly and not getting enough exercise; a love for sweets and foods with a high liquid content; a constant craving for food that leads to a tendency to often eat between meals; constantly becoming drowsy and feeling like taking naps, associated with a lack of gastric juices and a mouth that is often dry and sticky; pain in the back or in the knees, which causes difficulty in sitting or standing—fluid may collect in the knee joints; distortions in the shoulder joint which often leads to "frozen shoulder"

Masunaga further identifies conditions that may arise in terms of kyo and jitsu:

- *Spleen Meridian Kyo*[11]

    Cause: One does not chew and digest things sufficiently. One lacks the perseverance to thoroughly assimilate things.

    Mental Aspect: Tendency to worry about something all by oneself; obsession with details and excessive worry; restlessness and anxiety; inclination to interfere with the work of others—cuts in on other's conversations; inability to "blow off steam" and tendency to hold things inside; overuse of the mind and underuse of the body; tendency to be forgetful; difficulty in bringing things to an end; overeating or constantly nibbling; eating too quickly and never feeling full; always sleepy

    Physical Aspect: Poor salivation and tendency for mouth to become sticky; bitter taste in the mouth; excessive thirst; preference for a lot of liquids with a meal; preference for foods with high liquid content; lack of digestive juices, causing anemia; poor discrimination of tastes; dark brown facial coloration; lack of exercise; tendency for front of legs to become cold; hard knot around navel; excessive belching and flatulence; unhealthy color in gums; tension down the whole back; plump physique with excess body fat, roughness in skin of hands and feet; cracks in the heel; knee joints are painful; nail color changes.

- *Spleen Meridian Jitsu*[12]

    Mental Aspect: Physically inactive because one spends too much time thinking; tendency not to talk to others and to remain alone; hesitant and timid; cautious and anxious; rarely exercises; mental unrest; craving for sweets; eats quickly; overeats.

    Physical Aspect: Thirsty, sticky feeling in mouth; no appetite; no appreciation for tasting foods; gastric hyperacidity; nervous stomach inflammations; overeating; obesity; heaviness in legs; no strength, stiffness in arms; tight feeling in navel area; sallow complexion; hesitancy in movement; stiff shoulders; tendency to round back; coldness in hips and back

- *Jitsu Symptoms of Other Meridians with Spleen Meridian Kyo*[13]

Lung: Poor sense of smell, with nasal congestion; effusiveness

Large Intestine: Pain in arms; constipation due to poor digestion; sensation of heaviness in legs after being chilled; thinking too much

Heart: Feeling of constraint, associated with overwork; tightness in throat; impatience; shoulder stiffness

Small Intestine: Low back pain from overstrain in childbirth; voracious appetite; pain in the heels; insufficient production of digestive juices and dryness in the mouth

Bladder: Restlessness; overeating; swelling of knees; nasal congestion; facial nerve paralysis

Kidney: Diabetes; overeating and preference for sweet foods; thinking too much

Heart Constrictor: Rounded back; great anxiety with no chance for release

Triple Heater: Lack of stomach acids, leading to anemia; sleep disturbed by obsessive thinking

Gallbladder: Difficulty in getting to sleep and restless sleep; tendency to brood over things and to overeat; indecisiveness; arthritis in knee; spasms in the bile duct

Liver: Tendency to be single-minded; excessive intake of sugar; excessive alcohol consumption; eczema

Structure and Function of the Pancreas[14]

The pancreas is a golden-yellow colored, triangle-shaped organ about 8 inches long, located near the center of the abdomen in the region called the solar plexus. Its broader end or head lies beside the duodenum and its body and tail extend to the left, up under the stomach, ending near the spleen. The pancreas is purely an organ of secretion—no food passes through it. It consists of two types of secreting tissue: an exocrine portion, which produces pancreatic juice, and an endocrine portion, which produces hormones. (Exocrine glands send their enzymes along a path to a particular location; endocrine glands release their hormones into general circulation).

Exocrine Portion. Each day the pancreas produces about 2 1/2 pints of pancreatic juice; a clear colorless liquid similar to saliva in its consistency. This juice flows along the pancreatic duct, which terminates in the common bile duct. From there it enters into the duodenum. Pancreatic juice aids in the digestion and absorption of all classes of foods in the small intestine. When chyme enters the small intestine it is acid. However the protein digesting enzymes in the small intestine work best in an alkaline condition; pancreatic juice, which is mildly alkaline, transforms the chyme to this alkaline state.

Pancreatic secretions are initiated by nervous control as soon as food enters the mouth. However, the main secretions begin when the acid chyme comes into contact with the hormone producing cells of the duodenal mucosa, which secrete the hormones secretin and pancreozymin into the blood. Secretin stimulates the pancreas to increase the rate of flow and concentration of bicarbonate (an alkalizer) in pancreatic juice. Pancreozymin increases the enzymatic content.

Pancreatic juice consists of three main enzymes, which act on all foods ingested. They are secreted in various proportions according to what type of food has been ingested. Trypsin is the main protein digesting enzyme. Amylase continues the digestion of starches begun in the mouth through the action of ptyalin. Lipase, the only fat digesting enzyme in the body, acts on the fats emulsified by the bile, breaking them down into fatty acids and glycerol, the end products of fat digestion.

Endocrine Portion. The Langerhans islets comprise the endocrine portion of the pancreas. These are tiny clusters of cells scattered throughout the organ, numbering between 200,000 and 2,000,000. They are most numerous in the tail portion. The cells secrete insulin and glucagon (anti-insulin); these hormones control the body's energy supplies by maintaining even levels of blood sugar. Insulin lowers the blood sugar level by accelerating the transport of glucose into the cells, to be burned as fuel. It also increases the rate of conversion of glucose to glycogen to be stored in the liver, or if glycogen storage spaces are filled up, as fat throughout the body. Glucagon opposes this function. It accelerates the conversion of glycogen to glucose—raising blood sugar by releasing sugar that is stored in the liver.

Disorders and Diseases Associated with the Pancreas[15]

Diabetes and Hypoglycemia. Hypoglycemia or low blood sugar is a disorder where blood sugar levels, which should remain fairly constant, drop too low. When blood sugar levels rise, the pancreas secretes insulin, which causes blood sugar to be released as energy (making us feel energetic) or converted to fat. A problem arises when insulin secretion is erratic. If secretion is slow to come then blood sugar begins to rise rapidly. When insulin finally arrives its secretion is too great and too much sugar is released into the cells. Blood sugar levels drop too low and the individual feels a loss of energy, which can lead to feelings of depression, moodiness, and negativity. However, high levels of blood sugar can be prevented earlier on. Such prevention depends on the healthy functioning of the liver, which converts glucose coming from the small intestine to glycogen to be stored and released when needed. If the liver is weak or sluggish and unable to accomplish this task then sugar can pass into the bloodstream. Another possible cause is overconsumption of simple sugars, which are rapidly absorbed into the bloodstream soon after being eaten. Complex carbohydrates by comparison are broken down slowly in the small intestine, thereby providing much less stress on the body and a slow but steady source of blood sugar. According to the macrobiotic view the overall cause of hypoglycemia is excessive yang from: the heavy accumulations of animal fat and protein, salt, and dry, baked food. Hypoglycemia leads to a constant craving of yin in the form of sweets, candies, alcohol, and stimulant beverages such as coffee.

With diabetes the pancreas has become severely weakened and is unable to secrete adequate quantities of insulin. Consequently blood sugar tends to rise to dangerously high levels, and fat and protein break down and enter into the bloodstream. This condition often leads to degeneration of tissues such as muscle, eye (in many cases leading to blindness) and nerve, or to blood-fat accumulations. This situation can lead to the potentially fatal condition called ketoacidosis or "diabetic acidosis."

According to macrobiotics, diabetes is caused by excess yin coming especially from sugar and milk products.

Pancreatitis (Inflammation of the pancreas). Pancreatitis according to the macrobiotic view, is an attempt by the body to burn away excesses in the diet that have accumulated within the pancreas, before they become more serious. Tumors, both benign and malignant, are common in the pancreas, and the chance of survival from a malignant tumor, employing modern medical approaches is grim.

Macrobiotic Health Evaluation[16]

A shorter distance between the eyes and eyebrows is yang. It indicates that the pancreas, along with other yang compact organs and glands such as the liver, kidneys, and heart tend to easily suffer disorders due to the excessive intake of yang animal food. Hair growing in this region indicates the above organs are easily affected by excess animal food along with oily or fatty foods, including dairy products.

The two major areas corresponding with the pancreas are:

1. *The Upper Bridge of the Nose*
2. *The Outside of the Temples*

    Swellings, discolorations, or other abnormal markings in these locations indicate pancreatic and sometimes also spleen disorders:

    Dark color—overburdening of the pancreas and elimination of excessive sugars including cane sugar, honey, syrups, chocolate, fruit, and milk

    Red pimples and patches—excess sugar, sweets, juice, fruits

    Whitish-yellow pimples—fats and oils from both animal and vegetable sources, including dairy foods

    Dark patches and pimples—caused by either excessive sweets or by salt and flour products

    Moles—excess animal protein and fat: indicating an overactive spleen and pancreas

    Light green color—along with whitish, reddish, or dark fatty, oily skin textures— possible pancreatic cancer

    Other areas of the body and disorders reflect problems in the pancreas:

3. *Skin*

    Excessively oily skin—overconsumption of oils and fats or disorders in fat metabolism: pancreatic disorders including diabetes

    Dry skin—an excess of fat and oil in the bloodstream: the accumulation of fat and cholesterol within the spleen and pancreas

    Yellow skin—excessive yang foods and drinks including meat, eggs, fish, seafood and salt, or from an excess of carrots, pumpkin, and squash: bile trouble and probable pancreatic malfunctioning

    Blue—excessive yang animal food and salt, along with yin—sugar and sweets, alcohol and stimulants as well as food rich in refined carbohydrates

4. *Others*

    Reddish yellow color in the pink area inside the lower eyelid—excess yang animal food including dairy, together with excess yin

    Varicose veins—excess liquid intake, including all beverages and juices as well as fruits and possibly excessive oil

Overall shiny, red, and dark nose—overactive pancreatic condition
Reddish dark colored lips—excessive consumption of protein and saturated fats, together with excessive salt
Blue-gray color in the middle regions of the white of the eye—further suggestion of pancreatic cancer

THE STOMACH MERIDIAN

According to Classical Chinese Medicine[17]

Anatomically as well as functionally the stomach corresponds with the stomach of Western medicine.[18] The stomach is called "the sea of water and nourishment and the controller of the rotting and ripening of liquid and solid food."[19] The word "sea" suggests that all the other organs of the body depend upon the functioning of the stomach for their nourishment. The stomach is considered dry earth. It dislikes dryness and prefers moisture.[20] Stomach ki moves downward while spleen ki moves upward. Thus, vomiting and belching may be signs that stomach ki is not descending, while diarrhea may indicate that the ascending function of spleen ki has been interrupted.

Problems and diseases commonly treated by acupuncture to points on the stomach meridian include the following:

Eye diseases; toothache; facial nerve paralysis; twitching of the eyelids; dribbling and salivation; asthma and bronchitis; gout; headache; morning sickness; abdominal pain and distension; stomachache; sluggish stomach; bloated abdomen; loss of or poor appetite; constipation and diarrhea; incontinence of urine; testicular inflammation; menstrual pain; prolapse of the uterus; disappearance of menstruation; disorders of the genital organs of both sexes; disorders of the knee joint including inflammation and arthritis; pain or paralysis of the lower extremities; pain or swelling of the ankle joint; high or low blood pressure[21]

According to Shizuto Masunaga[22]

The stomach meridian corresponds with the entire upper digestive tract—from the lips, through the oral cavity, esophagus, stomach, and duodenum, to the jejunum. In facilitating the functioning of these parts, the stomach meridian relates to eating, exercising, and the production of body heat. It also relates to the reproductive function in women—the development of breasts and a layer of subcutaneous fat occurring in women at puberty. The stomach meridian controls appetite, lactation, and the function of the ovaries to some extent.

The condition of the stomach meridian can be seen in the lips, the eyelids when one is drowsy, and the muscles. These muscles include the muscles of the esophagus, breasts, ovaries, fatty tissues, and muscles of the upper and lower limbs.

Imbalances in the stomach meridian appear in the following way:

Overly conscious of the stomach and appetite influenced by one's mood and the type of food; a tendency to worry over minor details and tension builds up in the neck and shoulders; the legs feeling heavy and getting cold below the knees; often yawning and tired easily; overeating associated with much belching, hyperacidity, and distension of the stomach; prone to prolonged colds with nasal congestion, rhinitis, and coughing; pit of the stomach (epigastric area) becoming hard and putting pressure on the heart, which causes pain in the cardiac region; sores appearing at the corners of the mouth and along the course of the stomach meridian, indicating inflammation of the stomach lining.

Masunaga further identifies conditions that may arise in terms of kyo and jitsu:

- *Stomach Meridian Kyo*[23]

    Cause: One is unable to accept things as they are and has difficulty in adapting to a new environment.

    Mental Aspect: Tendency to brood over things and indulge in vain regrets; appetite influenced by the type of food or one's mood; craving for cold and soft food; eating when mind is preoccupied with something else; irregular eating habits and great variation in quantity consumed; desire to lie down right after a meal; always worrying about the condition of the stomach; facial skin lacking in tone; blank facial expression

    Physical Aspect: Stomach problems or loss of appetite associated with worry; chilling of abdominal area; tightness in shoulders due to ovarian problems; tension and pain in the middle of the back; excessive yawning; tendency to have thick and heavy legs; inflexibility in muscles, wrist, and ankle joints; pain in joints; tendency toward nasal congestion and slight coughs; chilling down the front of the body and feeling cold in knees; lack of body fat; lack of stomach acids, leading to anemia; weak and sagging stomach; stomach being hard and heavy, lack of strength in abdominal muscles, causing the stomach area to appear depressed; easily fatigued

- *Stomach Meridian Jitsu*[24]

    Mental Aspect: Tendency to think too much; nervous about details; frustrated; lacking in affection; big eater; always in a hurry; overworking; neurotic

    Physical Aspect: Stomach is swollen and food is stopped in it; overeating; heaviness in stomach; vomiting; gastric hyperacidity; cold sores; poor appetite; thirsty; stiffness in shoulders; pain and stiffness in solar plexus and heart; symptoms of catching a cold/flu; poor circulation in legs; rough skin; dry complexion; belching and yawning; nasal stagnation; redness on tip of nose; tendency to become anemic; malfunctioning of female organs

- *Jitsu Symptoms of Other Meridians with Stomach Meridian Kyo*[25]

    Lung: Lack of appetite due to coughing; inability to inhale deeply

    Large Intestine: Excessive intake of cold drinks, poor appetite and complete enervation; nasal congestion

    Heart: Restlessness and tendency to eat too fast, feeling of obstruction in solar plexus

    Small Intestine: Fatigue in legs and low back; shoulder stiffness and poor appetite; stomach pain from poor digestion; pain in heels; onset of acute appendicitis; deafness

    Bladder: Gastritis or diarrhea due to nervous causes, irritability and poor disposition

    Kidney: Bitter taste and stickness in mouth, nausea after overeating; loss of appetite from overeating

    Heart Governor: Poor digestion and tendency toward palpitations, feeling of heaviness in stomach after eating

    Triple Heater: Gastritis due to overeating, stomach pains caused by chilling; overly sensitive skin as a result of exposure to the cold

Gallbladder: General feeling of fatigue and lassitude, shoulder stiffness, indigestion, and distension of stomach; low blood pressure

Liver: Excessive eating and drinking, food poisoning, gastritis as a side effect of medication; loss of appetite due to overwork

Structure and Function of the Stomach[26]

The functions of the stomach are the following:
1. To hold the large amounts of food that we eat
2. To complete the first stages of protein digestion
3. To mix all the foods with the acids it secretes
4. To pass this food on as liquid to the intestines at a proper rate[27]

The stomach is a J-shaped enlargement of the digestive canal, lying in the upper left quadrant of the abdomen, partly protected by the rib cage. The entrance to the stomach is connected with the esophagus by the cardiac sphincter. At its lower end the stomach is connected with the duodenum (the first section of the small intestine) by the pyloric sphincter. The upper, more expanded portion of the stomach, lies close to the heart, separated from it by only a thin sheet of muscle—the dome-shaped diaphragm. The lower, more contracted portion lies in the area of the solar plexus. The stomach is able to hold about 2 1/2 pints of food.

The stomach can be divided into three functional parts: the cardiac and fundic areas in the upper portion and the pyloric in the lower. The wall of the stomach consists of several layers. The innermost layer is called the mucosa. When the stomach is empty its walls tend to contract, displaying longitudinal folds known as rugae. When the stomach expands these folds disappear. The next layer, the submucosa, which surrounds the mucosa contains blood and lymph vessels and nerves. Its connective tissue binds the mucosa with the outer muscular coat, consisting of three layers of muscle: an inner crosswise layer, a central circular and an outer longitudinal layer. The combined action of these muscles enables the stomach to churn food. The outer layer, the serosa, forms a protective wall.

The process of digestion actually begins with the thought, sight, smell, and taste of food. These experiences signal the body to prepare chemically for the food to be digested. Chewing breaks food down into smaller particles, making it easier for digestive enzymes to perform their functions. In addition, saliva contains the enzyme ptyalin, which begins the first stage in the breakdown of starches. Food that is chewed well is alkaline.

Protein begins to be chemically broken in the stomach. The stomach secretes various substances for this purpose. They include the following:
1. *Hydrochloric acid.* Hydrochloric acid is produced by the parietal cells in the fundic region. It activates enzymes (biological catalysts) which are released from other cells, helps in the digestion of protein (which requires an acid environment to be broken down), sterilizes ingested food and destroys bacteria.[28]
2. *Pepsin.* Pepsin is an enzyme produced by the chief cells in the fundic region. It is responsible for the beginning of the breakdown of protein into its component amino acids (this function is completed in the small intestine).
3. *Renin and gastric lipase.* These substances perform important roles in the digestive functions of infants. Renin causes the breakup of the molecular chains of the protein casein in milk. Gastric lipase acts on finely emulsified fats such

as egg yolk, and butter and cream, splitting them into smaller particles. Both these enzymes operate best in the less acidic stomach of infants. In adults, hydrochloric acid performs the function of renin, and enzymes found in the small intestine perform the function of gastric lipase.

The stomach, which is in large part composed of protein, is prevented from digesting itself in two ways. First, pepsin is secreted in an inactive form called pepsinogen. Hydrochloric acid is necessary to convert pepsinogen into the active form called pepsin. This conversion does not occur until pepsinogen is free within the stomach. Second, the stomach cells are protected by a coating of mucous cells which form a barrier between gastric acids and pepsin, and the stomach cells.

Gastric secretion is under nervous and hormonal control and begins before food even enters the mouth. It is further stimulated by the presence of food in the stomach, initiated by the production of the hormone gastrin, which is secreted in the pyloric region when protein foods are present.

Food first enters the pyloric end and the peripheral portion of the body. As food continues to enter, it assumes a more central position and is almost completely enclosed by the food that preceded it. This manner facilitates salivary digestion. Although all food in the stomach is churned, what one eats first is largely kept separate from what is eaten later in the same meal. It remains in the layers that were formed during the meal and is not disrupted by the motion of the stomach.[29] When food is thoroughly mixed with gastric secretions and in the form of chyme, active wavelike peristaltic contractions begin around the middle of the stomach and propel the food toward the pyloric sphincter. If the duodenum is empty and the food sufficiently acid, the pyloric sphincter relaxes and a small amount of chyme is passed into the duodenum.

Emotions can substantially affect the digestive process. They can alter the muscular movements and glandular secretions. The time food remains in the stomach varies from two to six hours. It depends upon the quantity and type of food ingested and how well it has been chewed. Liquids leave the stomach within a few minutes. Fruits eaten alone leave the stomach in one or two hours. If taken along with other foods they can cause indigestion, especially if eaten before other foods, because fruits are mainly sugar and sugar stops the functioning of the stomach. Grains and vegetables stay in the stomach for much less time than either protein or fat, and fats leave the stomach more slowly than any other food. All food is finally absorbed in the small intestine. However, complex carbohydrates, principally starches (present in grains, vegetables, beans, bread, potatoes) begin to be broken down in the mouth. Protein (present in large amounts in flesh food such as fish, chicken, and meat) which takes a long time to be broken down, begins this process in the stomach. Fats (present in fatty meats, dairy foods, eggs, oils, nuts, and nut butters) are not broken down until they reach the small intestine, and it requires a long period for them to pass through. When fat or oil reaches the first part of the small intestine, the movements and secretions of the stomach are dramatically slowed and food tends to remain there. Conversely, stimulants such as coffee and spices accelerate the emptying of the stomach by stimulating gastrointestinal churning. This is why coffee is often taken after a meal. Such stimulants can also irritate the stomach walls. By stimulating acid secretion they can often cause overacidity or heartburn.[30]

For even digestion then it is advisable to eat carbohydrates first, then protein, then fat.

Disorders Associated with the Stomach

Healthy functioning of the stomach depends upon a balance between the secretions of gastric acid and mucus. Sufficient acid is necessary to digest the food but too much will corrode the walls of the stomach. If gastric secretion becomes excessive it can irritate the stomach walls and sometimes lead to ulceration. If gastric secretion is deficient there may be an increase in undesirable bacterial growth, which in turn may lead to irritation of the stomach wall. This irritation stimulates an increase in mucous production, which spreads throughout the system. This process decreases digestive power and further compromises the ability to assimilate food, which further increases the production of mucus.[31]

Another problem related to the stomach is gas in the fundic region, which is often mistaken for heart pain.

Macrobiotic Health Evaluation[32]

The mouth and lips show both the general constitution and the current condition of the individual, especially of one's digestive organs and functions. A mouth that is the same or narrower than the width of the nose indicates good constitutional physical and mental health and strength. If the width of the mouth is much wider than the nostrils, the function of the organs and glands is weak, indicating less physical and mental ability to adapt to and resist difficulties in the environment. A mouth that is horizontally wider but normal in vertical height shows the consumption during the embryonic and growing periods of both animal quality foods and refined vegetable foods (refined grains and flour products, sugar, fruits, soft drinks, and beverages). Physically this condition indicates the loss of endurance and resistance, mentally the loss of self-discipline and perseverance. A mouth larger in vertical height but not in horizontal width indicates the consumption of excessive amounts of salt along with dairy, refined grains and flours, fruits and sugar, fat and oil, soft drinks and beverages. It indicates chronic weakness of the digestive organs and functions. A mouth that is too tightly closed indicates disorders in the liver and gallbladder, or kidneys, due to excess salt, meat, poultry, and eggs. It also indicates constraints and inflexibility in material matters—stinginess, overconcern with order and cleanliness, lack of enjoyment of sensory pleasures and the inability to express emotions. A loose mouth shows disorders in the digestive, respiratory, excretory, and nervous functions due to excess consumption of raw vegetables, fruits, fruit juices, sugar and other sweeteners, drugs and medications, and the overconsumption of food and drink in general. It indicates a lack of self-control and order in matters such as appetite, finances, and physical appearance.

Overall, the constitution of the digestive system indicates more the mother's influence, her strength and condition during pregnancy.

The constitution of the stomach is indicated in the second and third toes of each foot:

Yin constitution: These two toes are longer than the large toe and may be partially or completely webbed. This yin tendency is further indicated if the mouth is considerably wider than the nostrils or if the upper lip is thick. The stomach structure tends to be more expanded. The cause is an excessive consumption of fruit, sugar, medications, and refined foods taken by the mother during pregnancy.

Yang constitution: These two toes are considerably smaller than the large toe or are curled toward the big toe, a tendency further indicated if the mouth is narrow or the upper lip nonexistent. The stomach structure tends to be tight or contracted. The cause is an excess intake of salt along with animal food during pregnancy.

The condition of the stomach can be seen in corresponding areas of the face: the upper lip and the bridge of the nose, as well as the skin as a whole and the back of the tongue.

1. *The Upper Lip*

    The left upper lip shows the upper stomach, the right, the lower stomach.

    Yin condition: The upper lip is excessively swollen or expanded. It is caused by overeating in general or overconsumption of refined grains, sugar and other sweeteners, tropical fruit and juices, and alcohol.

    Yang condition: The upper lip appears tight or contracted due to the excessive intake of meat, eggs, salt, or dry, baked goods.

    Both conditions can indicate an overacidic condition of the stomach. The tendency or presence of ulcerations may be indicated by inflammation, a blister, or discoloring on the upper lip.

2. *The Bridge of the Nose*

    Freckles or brown blotches—chronic stomach acidosis, ulcerations, hypoglycemic or diabetic tendencies, even stomach cancer; slight green shading in this area further indicates stomach cancer.

    Red color—perhaps covering the whole nose along with the upper cheeks— chronic swelling and inflammation of the stomach, spleen and lymph system, due to excessive consumption of animal protein and sugar

3. *The Skin as a Whole*

    Splotchy brown or dirty skin color—chronic acid stomach condition due to excessive fruit or sugar consumption

    Moles and warts—an acid stomach condition caused by an excessive consumption of animal protein

4. *The Near Back of the Tongue*

    Dark red color—inflammation, ulcers, potential progression toward stomach cancer

    White or yellow color or white patches—accumulations of fat or mucus in the stomach

    Blue or purple color—overconsumption of sugar, soft drinks, chemicals, alcohol, drugs, medications, and other extreme yin

    Small mushroomlike eruptions—signs of acidity, ulcerations, nausea, and regurgitation

Dietary Recommendations[33]

Soil is associated with the sweet taste and in the macrobiotic diet the principle source of this taste is whole cereal grains, usually pressure-cooked, and chewed very well. Soil being in the center of the Five Transformations implies balance. In diet, balance means avoiding extremes and using moderate cooking styles, a flame that is neither too high nor too low, cooking that is neither too long nor too short, and moderate to mild use of salt and salty products. Such suggestions are a general guideline on the standard diet to be varied according to whether the condition of either pancreas or stomach, is too tight or too weak in the case of the pancreas; too tight or too expanded in the case of the stomach.

Overly yang or contracted condition of either organ. First it is suggested to avoid extreme foods of both yin or yang categories. If the condition arises from excess yang though, then the main cause is likely to be from the overconsumption of excess animal food—beef, pork, poultry, eggs, and various types of dairy food including cheese; very salty food (refined salt irritates the stomach wall) and hard, baked flour products.

Most recommended grains are pressure-cooked medium grain brown rice and barley. All other regular use grains can also be used. However in the case of the pancreas, buckwheat and soba noodles are best avoided until the condition noticeably changes and millet may best be served in the form of a soup or in a porridge style. For both organs it is best to avoid baked flour products until the condition noticeably changes. Apart from grain soups, soups with sweet vegetables such as pumpkin or fall season squash are recommended as well as soups containing white or leafy green vegetables. Vegetable dishes should be prepared predominantly with light cooking styles such as boiling, steaming or sautéing, using a small volume of oil and the salty taste should be mild. Again emphasize white or leafy green vegetables as well as round vegetables such as pumpkin, fall season squash, and onions prepared to draw out the sweet taste. Boiled salads can be taken often. Also mildly salted pressed salads and light pickles, in small quantities as well as occasional raw salad can be served. For the pancreas, beans can be cooked with sweet vegetables and for the stomach, occasionally with a grain-based sweetener such as barley malt or rice syrup. For the pancreas the sea vegetables nori and arame are especially beneficial, while for the stomach, arame, nori, and hijiki can be used more than others. The craving for the sweet taste is best found in whole cereal grains and their products along with sweet vegetables cooked to draw out the sweet taste. Beyond this, chestnuts may be helpful as well as grain syrups such as barley malt or rice syrup. Some people with stomach or pancreatic problems may have trouble with fruit and fruit juices. However, if craved they are best served cooked or dried, or in a thin kuzu sauce.

Overly yin, expanded or weak condition. While both yin and yang forms of extreme foods may be involved, in this situation we will find that excessive yin is more the problem. Thus it is first recommended to avoid sugar and sugared food, soft drinks, spices, stimulants such as coffee or black tea, tropical fruits and fruit juices, refined flour products, alcohol, cold, icy beverages, butter, milk and cream, chemicalized food, seasonings and beverages, and oily or greasy food.

The focus of the diet should be more on the center, more on whole cereal grains and vegetables. Overall, dishes requiring longer cooking can be served more often, salty seasonings can be a little stronger and a little less liquid should be used in cooking. The main grains can be short grain brown rice, barley, and millet. Round and root vegetables can be emphasized a little more than leafy greens and longer cooking methods such as nishime and even baking from time to time can be employed. In the same way bean dishes which are baked may be appropriate if served from time to time. Bean dishes cooked with sweet vegetables can be served occasionally and it is best to serve predominantly regular use beans. Dried tofu may be more appropriate than regular tofu. Sea vegetables in the form of dried condiments such as wakame powder, or shio kombu, may be helpful and hijiki dishes emphasized over arame. For the sweet taste, sweet round vegetables are the main choice. If further sweetness is craved it is best that it be cooked into a food. Other recommendations should follow standard dietary guidelines.

Other suggestions: Chew very well, preferably until food becomes liquid in the mouth. Avoid drinking excess liquid; it dilutes acid content. Avoid eating quickly, or while concentrating on something else. Avoid oversnacking as it reduces the ability of digestive juices to build up. Eat in a calm environment. Choose cooking combinations which are simple and eat in an orderly manner—first carbohydrates, then protein, then oil.

Exercise Recommendations

Various exercises in Chapter 5 are helpful in stimulating or stretching the stomach and spleen-pancreas meridians. For the stomach these exercises include: Self-shiatsu #2 (21) and #6; hara massage #7B; and the Reclining Hero #19. For the spleen-pancreas these exercises include: Self-shiatsu #21C (6), 21D (11); hara massage #7C and the Reclining Hero #19.

The Lung and Large Intestine Meridians

Metal Nature Energy

The lungs and large intestine correspond with metal nature energy, the most yang phase within the cycle of the Five Phases of Energy Transformation. The most yang means the most gathered, the most inwardly directed, solid, condensed, and fully materialized; the most visible, clearly defined, complete, refined, and perfect.

Within the galactic cycle, this phase corresponds with the appearance of human beings, the most evolved creatures. It also corresponds with the appearance of whole cereal grains, the most modern and evolved food. In the history of civilization, this cycle corresponds with the present day, the Iron Age, a yang period of rapid change where the use of metal is prevalent and the popular music of the day is often described as hard rock or heavy metal.

Within this overall yang quality, however, there must be yin. The yin aspect of something so internalized is quite simply its surface. We should note at this stage that while the interior of a piece of metal tends to be rough, the surface can be smooth and shiny, it can reflect. However, this shiny surface usually comes about as a result of a process of refinement.

Within the physical body, both the lungs and large intestine perform yangizing functions. Air passes from the infinite expanse into the body, through smaller and smaller branches of the bronchial tree, to exchange gases with the blood, passing through the microscopically thin walls of the alveoli to do so. The large intestine absorbs liquids through its wall, to solidify waste products to be expelled from the body. Within these yangizing functions we see the yin—both of these organs are connected with the outside of the body.

This external image is further illustrated by the tenets of classical Chinese medicine which state that the lungs rule ki and that ki rules the outside of the body, and that the condition of the lungs is seen in the condition of the skin and body hair. Masunaga believes that the lung and large intestine meridians are located close to the surface of the body.

Fig. 23

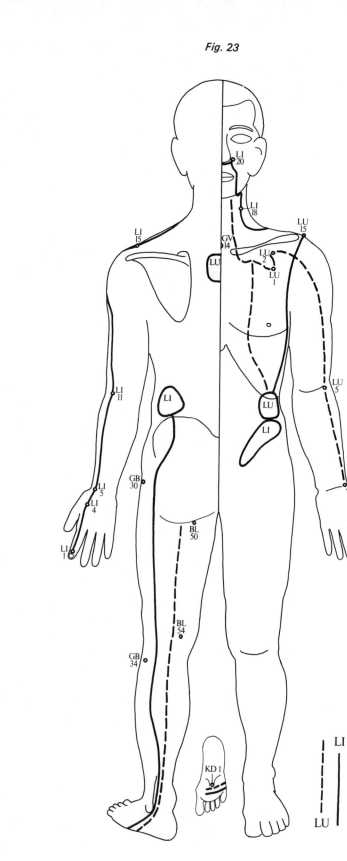

The trigrams of the *I Ching* corresponding with metal nature: Chien, The Creative and Tui, the Lake also display this yang and yin nature of metal. Containing three unbroken lines ☰, Chien represents all of the yang qualities we have mentioned. Tui however, contains a yin line on the surface ☱, symbolic of external softness and smoothness, granting the ability to shine and reflect. This trigram is also likened to a mouth, symbolizing communication and the enjoyment of food. Tui represents autumn, the time to celebrate and enjoy, following the hard work of bringing in the harvest. We could also associate it with evening meal, reflecting upon and sharing the day's experiences with our family.

Within the individual, when metal nature energy has been integrated to its fullest it would reflect in the person who is fully realized. The person stands out as a distinct individual yet simultaneously remains one with the spiritual, material, and social worlds. The individual functions in harmony with his or her total environment. Many traditional spiritual practices in the East believe that such a state depends upon the way of breathing.

Since the lungs deal with the exchange of invisible gases they manifest within the individual in a sense of oneness with the spiritual realm. By contrast, the large intestine function involves the exchange of physical substances—it manifests in the individual in his or her relationship with the material environment—mixing with and empathy for nature. Both lungs and large intestine manifest in the social realm with the individual's ability to share, mix, communicate, and exchange with others.

With the above concept along with the images of metal nature energy presented in Chapter 2, we can see how this energy might manifest within the individual.

Internalized Qualities (Yang)
Positive: sense of order, organization and self-discipline; strength of character, "solid as a rock," dependable, trustworthy, firm, responsible, reliable, realistic, independent, the ability to complete a task, the ability to self reflect

Negative: yang deficient or yin excess—disorderly, disorganized, difficulty in completing things, undisciplined; yang deficient—phlegmatic, lazy, lacking in energy, to easily tire, tendency to slump, difficulty in making or slow to make changes; yang excess—immovable, stubborn, rigid and inflexible (in body and mind), overly attached and possessive

Externalized Qualities (Yin)
Positive: the ability to share, exchange and communicate—friendly, sociable; refined, cultured, cultivated

Negative: yang excess—egocentric; yang deficient—the weight of the world on their shoulders; low self-esteem; yang excess or yin deficient—inability to get along well with others; antisocial; to build a wall around oneself.

THE LUNG MERIDIAN

According to Classical Chinese Medicine[1]
The lungs of Chinese medicine correspond with the respiratory system including the lungs, bronchioles, and trachea.[2] The lungs are said to control ki. This statement has two meanings: breath and energy. Ki is absorbed from the air through inhalation. The ki of liquid and solid food, resulting from digestion first passes to the lungs to

unite with the ki of the air to form the true ki of the human body.[3] The lungs open the nostrils, which gives the ability to distinguish odors.[4] The lungs are related to the skin, sweat glands, and body hair (regulating the secretion of sweat, the moistening of the skin and thus resistance to external causes of disease),[5] since ki controls the exterior of the body (blood controls the interior).[6] The lungs are called the delicate organ since they are the first to be attacked by disease coming from outside the body.[7]

Disorders commonly treated by acupuncture to points along the lung meridian include the following:

Coughing; difficulty in breathing; shortness of breath; bronchitis; asthma; pneumonia; common cold; whooping cough; sore throat; swollen and painful throat and neck; laryngitis; tonsillitis; chest pain; feeling of distension of the chest wall; pain in the shoulders and back; elbow swelling and pain; pain and numbness in the arm; pain and paralysis of the wrist joint; facial edema and paralysis; amnesia[8]

According to Shizuto Masunaga[9]

The lung and large intestine meridians (Fig. 23) are associated with the functions of exchange and elimination—to cope with the external environment and take in the ki of nature, as well as to eliminate those substances which have become unnecessary. The lungs take in the fine essence of air and the large intestine processes grosser materials. Both meridians lie close to the surface of the body to play the vital role of exchanging energy with the outside world.

The lungs and large intestine are associated with the following: the skin and nose (first signs of lung/large intestine meridian imbalance appear here), one's complexion, the whites of the eyes, the throat, anus, skin respiration, the pores (excretion of sweat).

Respiration is likened to the actions of a Prime Minister, who is responsible for managing external relations as well as keeping order in domestic affairs. Respiration is closely related to internal regulation while also being intimately connected with outward action. The lungs take in from the external environment the vital ki component essential for survival and refine and distribute this to activate the adaptive response of the body. Respiration is closely related with brain function and exerts a profound influence on one's state of mind.

Imbalances in the lung meridian appear in the following way:

Depression and chest congestion; a loss of vigor—one may begin to sigh; a heavy feeling in the head, and the back and shoulder area becoming stiff; becoming melancholy with a tendency to remain closed off from others; eventually, dizziness and coughing as respiratory diseases such as colds, asthma, and bronchitis set in; also gas poisoning and convulsive fits in children

Masunaga further identifies conditions that may arise in terms of kyo and jitsu:

• *Lung Meridian Kyo*[10]

Cause: One becomes isolated and closed off so that the exchange of ki with the environment is hindered.

Mental Aspect: Worry, which causes one's chest to feel blocked; an overanxious and hypersensitive emotional state; getting concerned after taking on too much work; becoming too anxious over fine details and being unable to relax and breathe deeply; a lack of spirit and motivation; exhaustion and lethargy

Physical Aspect: Hunched shoulders; shallow breathing; difficulty in breathing;

discomfort in lying on back; susceptibility to colds and coughing, especially after the upper body has been exposed to wind or cold; feverishness, with pain between the shoulder blades; tendency for the eyes to water; pale complexion; dry skin; lack of stamina; extreme fatigue; prone to overweight with elimination difficulties; inflammation in respiratory organs; lack of circulation and fatigue in thumb; physically weak

• *Lung Meridian Jitsu*[11]

Mental Aspect: Displaying resistance toward surroundings; obsessed with anxiety over small details, with inability for release; tendency to sigh and choke while breathing

Physical Aspect: Out of breath and having a cold; cough and sweat a little; prone to nasal congestion; constipation; coughing pain in chest; shoulder pain; bronchitis; asthma; mucus; thumb sensing a pulling pain; chest muscles tight

• *Jitsu Symptoms of Other Meridians with Lung Meridian Kyo*[12]

Stomach: Tendency toward prolonged colds; coughing, and fatigue or heavy feeling in legs; lack of energy and constriction in chest

Spleen: Worrying, causing heaviness in chest; shallow breathing, and food stagnation in upper digestive tract after eating

Heart: Emotional collapse; to feel thoroughly absent-minded; continuous tension leading to a feeling of growing oppression in chest

Small Intestine: Fatigue of hands and arms leading to shoulder stiffness; diarrhea as a result of a cold; respiratory disease; poor digestion and absorption of nutrients

Bladder: Loss of sleep due to coughing, chilling of upper body, fatigue due to hypertension, mental and physical overwork; fits of asthma

Kidney: Difficulty in breathing; coughing and phlegm causing tightness in chest; prolonged exposure to wind; listlessness because of worry

Heart Constrictor: Dizziness due to hypertension; mental and physical overwork

Triple Heater: Feeling of heaviness in the head with congestion of blood; tendency to catch colds; bronchitis

Gallbladder: Lack of vigor due to shoulder stiffness and fatigue; timidity and constricted breathing; general fatigue and dejection

Liver: Loss of stamina due to overwork, thick phlegm; strain in back and shoulders with fever; lack of energy as a result of shock

Structure and Function of the Lungs[13]

The lung meridian corresponds with the respiratory system, the lungs and the air passages leading into them. The purpose of respiration is the release of energy in the body. Oxygen from the atmosphere is needed by the cells of all tissues to liberate energy from the nutrients absorbed. In turn, the cells release carbon dioxide, a gaseous waste product of metabolism that needs to be expelled. Both of these functions take place within the lungs in partnership with the heart and circulatory system, where gases are exchanged between the circulating blood and the air inhaled.

The lungs are paired spongelike structures, each approximately the size of an open hand. They lie on each side of the chest, enclosed and protected by the rib cage and separated by the heart, blood vessels, and esophagus. The left lung is slightly smaller and narrower than the right and is comprised of two lobes, while the right has three.

The area bounded by the rib cage is called the thoracic cavity. The diaphragm, a thin but tough sheet of muscle, forms the base of this cavity. Each lung is enclosed in a double layer of fine membrane called the pleura. The outer pleura is closely attached to the walls of the thoracic cavity and the upper surface of the diaphragm. The inner pleura is attached to the lungs. The area between inner and outer pleura, the pleural cavity, contains a small amount of fluid preventing the lung and chest wall surfaces, which are in almost direct contact, from adhering during breathing. The ribs, parallel with each other in the shape of bucket handles, are connected with the spine and sternum (breastbone) in a hingelike manner and can move slightly up and down. The intercostal muscles lie between the ribs. Together with the movements of the diaphragm, they play a major role in the breathing mechanism.

Air enters into the nose and mouth, passes through the pharynx (throat), then into a short passageway called the larynx (voice box) and then into the trachea (windpipe). Located within the cheeks and forehead, the sinuses give resonance to the voice and empty mucus into the nose. Just beyond the junction of the oral and nasal passages, the air passage bends forward slightly as it enters the larynx. The esophagus, the tube through which food passes, continues downward behind the larynx. When food is being consumed, the top of the larynx is closed off by a cartilage plate called the epiglottis. Extending beyond the larynx is the trachea. At the level of the sternum, the trachea divides into left and right main bronchi, which accompanied by the left and right pulmonary arteries, enter each lung. Each bronchi branches and further branches, into twenty divisions. As the airways become smaller, they become bronchioles, then terminal bronchioles, dividing the air into about 30,000 separate jets within the gas exchange zone. In the walls of the bronchioles small air sacs called alveoli appear. The alveoli form clusters and at maturity a pair of lungs contains about 300 million alveoli.

Alveoli are the leaves of this bronchial tree. They appear bubblelike, and have extremely thin walls, which expand and contract with inhalation and exhalation. They present a total area fifty times that of the body surface. This surface area ensures that blood and air come into contact, that balance is maintained between the rate and depth of breathing and the flow of blood through the lungs. It is through the microscopically thin lining of the alveoli and the walls of the tiny blood vessels surrounding each alveoli that blood and oxygen come into contact, that the exchange of gases takes place. The blood capillaries are so fine that only one red corpuscle at a time can pass through the capillary vessel and pick up oxygen and dump carbon dioxide, taking less than a second to do so. Oxygen is taken up by the pigment called hemoglobin in each corpuscle and delivered to the left side of the heart by the pulmonary veins, from where it is distributed throughout the body. Conversely, the pulmonary arterioles deliver oxygen depleted or veinous blood to the alveoli to be replenished.

The entire respiratory tract is lined with a mucous membrane and ciliated cells. The mucous membrane acts to moisten the air and adjust it to the body's temperature. In addition it traps impurities such as dust particles, bacteria, and viruses, that are enveloped and destroyed by the white blood corpuscles of the body's lymph glands, the tonsils and adenoids, which are located within the pharynx. Millions of microscopic hairlike structures called cilia project from the ciliated cells within the mucous membrane. In constant movement, they act together to propel the film of mucus that is being continuously produced, from the bottom of the lungs toward the throat.

Impurities are moved up and out of the lungs, either into the nasal passage, where they can be sneezed, or to the throat where they can be swallowed or coughed out.

The quality of mucus, a natural secretion of the mucous membranes lining each lung, is of prime importance in their functioning. According to the macrobiotic view and certain other approaches to natural healing this quality is affected when certain undesirable foods are consumed and need to be excreted. If the normal routes of excretion (lungs, skin, bowels, kidneys, and menses) are unable to function properly, the waste products are converted into mucus, to be eliminated in that form. In other words, mucus now becomes a form of excretion, and in this state can have a profound effect upon the health of the lungs. Within the nasal passages for example, if the quality of mucus becomes too thick or viscous and dries out, it might adhere to the cilia and mucous membrane. Crusts build up and microbes begin to invade, often leading to a cold. On the other hand, when the quality of the mucus becomes too liquid, it drips down around the cilia, which are unable to move this thin mucus. This condition leads to a watery nasal drip and possibly, inflammation.[14]

Thus, in summary, we need to consider the following factors when evaluating the condition of the lungs: the lungs should be elastic; air passages should be clear, allowing easy access of oxygen to the alveoli; the quality of the mucous lining is extremely important to the proper functioning of the lungs. The lungs as an entity expand or contract; the muscles surrounding the bronchi expand or contract; the tube wall itself can dilate or contract—when the tube wall swells, the air passageways become narrower.

Breathing.[15]   For air to flow into the lungs, the pressure inside must be less than atmospheric pressure. This state is achieved by increasing the volume of the lungs. Inhalation occurs when the structures surrounding the lungs expand and pull the lungs along with them. The resulting suction draws air into the lungs from the upper airways. Exhalation is caused by simply relaxing. The elasticity of pulmonary tissue allows the alveoli to close so that in normal breathing the air flows out passively.

There are two basic types of breathing: chest breathing and diaphragmatic breathing. In the West, chest breathing is the more common. In this type, the chest wall expands, which causes the lungs to expand. The upper and middle portions become filled with air but the lower portion is somewhat neglected. However in an upright position most of the blood is in the lower, gravity dependent areas. Thus air is not mixed thoroughly with the blood.

In diaphragmatic breathing, during inhalation the chest walls remain relatively motionless but the diaphragm moves downward. In a relaxed state, the elasticity of the alveoli causes the lungs to contract to their normal size. This in turn causes the diaphragm to bulge upward into a dome shape, since the diaphragm is connected to the lungs through the pleural layers. Upon inhalation, however, the diaphragm flattens out, increasing the volume of the chest cavity vertically as opposed to horizontally in the case of chest breathing. This movement causes pressure on the abdominal organs, so the abdominal wall needs to expand to reestablish the volume for the organs. For complete exhalation beyond the position at which the diaphragm is at rest, the abdominal muscles contract, pressing the abdominal organs upward against a relaxed diaphragm. This causes it to rise upward beyond its resting position, compressing and emptying the lung more completely than could the natural movement of the diaphragm alone.[16] Since the air is mixed more thoroughly with blood, diaphragmatic breathing is more efficient than chest breathing.

Some Disorders of the Respiratory System

Shortness of breath (dyspnea) and emphysema.[17]   The 300 million alveoli create a tremendous surface area for blood and oxygen to come into contact. Shortness of breath arises when this area is reduced; the individual compensates by breathing more rapidly. Reduction arises from the breakdown of the lining of the delicate walls of the alveoli. An area that once consisted of multiple small chambers appears as a visible hole in the lung tissue. There are two basic causes: (1) smoking, which is a yang cause and (2) artificially chemicalized food, such as ice cream, soft drinks, and frozen fruit juice. In this latter yin cause, the alveoli dilate and fuse, and the lung tissue as a whole becomes loose. (Another cause is anemia, in which the blood lacks sufficient hemoglobin to transport oxygen.) Emphysema is a more serious condition that gradually develops over a number of years. The elasticity of the lungs, which helps hold the airways open, is reduced; the smaller airways collapse on expiration, making it impossible to fully exhale stale air. The most affected group of sufferers are men between the ages of fifty and seventy who have been heavy smokers. According to macrobiotics, the consumption of extreme foods and drink is an important influence as well. Air pollution is also a contributing factor in many cases. Since the heart has to work harder, emphysema can lead to heart problems; the heart may enlarge which eventually leads to heart failure.

Bronchitis (Inflammation of the airways).[18]   Bronchitis is a disease of the trachea and bronchi, the yin section of the lungs. This condition is accompanied by fever, coughing, and chest pain. It may be acute as when it arises with colds, or chronic, when it continues for months, and returns each year, lasting longer each time. In chronic bronchitis, the airways become narrowed and partly clogged with mucus that is not moved along as it normally is by the cilia. Air has trouble entering and leaving the lungs. According to macrobiotics this condition is caused by the overconsumption of such foods as cold drinks, fruit, ice cream, and sugar. Since tobacco smoke has a tendency to destroy the cilia, it too can be a contributing factor.

Asthma.[19]   With asthma there is a hyperactive response of the breathing tubes. The bronchial tubes narrow both through spasms of the bronchial tubes and swelling of the bronchial tissues. Mucus clogs the smaller tubes and stale air is trapped. According to macrobiotics asthma is often associated with many years of overworking the kidneys, resulting from the repeated overconsumption of fluid. Asthmatics can become sensitive to many things: air pollution, paint and paint thinners, hair sprays, perfume, cleaning fluids, dust, room deoderizers, changes in the weather, pollens and grasses, animals such as dogs and cats, feather products, and food allergies—to milk, nuts and nut butters, chocolate, eggs, and fruit juice for example. The macrobiotic approach sees asthma as caused by a combination of excess yin and excess yang. It considers that healing requires a contraction of the bronchial tubes through limitation of the intake of liquid, fruits and fruit juices, as well as excess salt, dry baked products, and other tightening foods.

Macrobiotic Health Evaluation[20]
The constitution of the lungs is indicated by the nostrils. Well-developed nostrils

indicate strong lungs; small nostrils, weak lungs.

The condition of the lungs can be seen in the cheeks and the whites of the eyes.

1. *The Cheeks*

Cheeks with well-developed firm flesh devoid of wrinkles or pimples indicate sound respiratory and digestive functions. Drawn, overly tight flesh sometimes with vertical lines indicates restriction of the chest muscles, blood flow, and alveoli function. This yang condition is most often caused by excess salt, chicken and/or fish consumption, as well as dry or baked foods, or smoking. Flesh which is loose or puffy or flabby indicates a yin condition of fat and mucous accumulation caused by an excess of sugar, fruit and fruit juices and refined flour products. Swollen cheeks indicate the accumulation of liquid within the lungs.

The color of the cheeks and various markings further indicate the condition of the lungs:

Red or pink cheeks. Except during vigorous exercise or when out in the cold, this color indicates abnormal expansion of blood capillaries and a hyperactive condition of the lungs, caused by the overconsumption of yin foods and drinks including fruits, juices, alcohol and excess liquid in general, and also sugars, drugs, spices, and stimulants.

Milky white cheeks. The accumulation of fat and mucus, caused by the following: overconsumption of dairy products (cheese, milk, cream, yogurt), or tofu and other soybean products; excessive intake of flour products and fruits or ice cream produces a similar color with a pinkish shade; the overconsumption of salts may also cause a whitish or grayish color.

Pale color. A generally anemic condition due to imbalanced nourishment that often indicates tuberculosis.

Purple color. If appearing in a large area like a shadow, it indicates serious weakening of the respiratory organs due to overconsumption of sugar, chemicals, drugs, and medicines. In small areas it indicates blood stagnation or internal hemorrhage in the lungs.

Green shade. Progression of cancer

Pimples. The elimination of excessive fat and mucus caused by the intake of animal food, dairy, oils, fats, and sugar; indicating a heavy accumulation of mucus and fat in the lungs; whitish pimples—milk and sugar, yellowish—cheese, poultry, eggs

Oily skin. Caused by excess oil or fat consumption, disorders in fat metabolism and overeating in general, which lead to fat and mucous accumulation in the lungs

Dark spots. Indicating fat and mucous accumulation in the lungs and often the beginning of a cyst or tumor

Freckles. Elimination of simple sugars—honey, refined white, fruit, and milk sugars; causing harm to the respiratory organs

Hairs. Fine small silver hairs indicating overconsumption of dairy products and a lowered capacity of the lungs

Beauty marks. Indicating a past fever that led to diseases such as pneumonia and bronchitis

Moles. Indicating the elimination of excessive protein, either from concentrated sources or from overeating in general, especially of carbohydrates and fats

2. *The Whites of the Eyes* (*Sclera*)

The outside upper quadrant of each eye shows the condition of the lungs: right eye, right lung; left eye, left lung.

Bloodshot eyes. Caused by expanded blood capillaries from excess yin foods and drinks

Red spots. Blood clots or circulatory stagnation in the lungs

Dietary Recommendations[21]

Avoid extreme yang foods such as meat, poultry, eggs, dairy products, and even seafood if the condition is serious. Animal foods contain hardened fats which create a buildup of fat and mucus in the lungs. Avoid baked and refined flour products since these along with dairy foods are mucous forming. Avoid food and beverages from the yin category, including sugar and all other sweets, fruits and fruit juices, spices and stimulants, alcohol and drugs, as well as artificial, chemicalized, and refined food. Of these foods, those that contain sugar will turn into fat. Fruits and fruit juices, coffee and alcohol, expand the lungs, creating more rapid and superficial breathing patterns and consequently an unpeaceful state of mind.

To alleviate lung problems it is recommended to follow standard dietary guidelines with the following emphasis:

Emphasize brown rice over other grains. Restrict the consumption of baked flour products since they can be mucous forming. Follow standard vegetable recommendations, emphasizing greens such as broccoli, kale, mustard greens, and the leafy green tops of carrots, turnips and daikon, as well as watercress. Lotus root is beneficial for all kinds of lung disorders and helps to ease breathing. Lotus root can be boiled, prepared in a nishime style or cooked with sea vegetables, especially hijiki. It can also be prepared as a pickle or grated fresh. In this latter way it can be helpful for coughing. Lotus seeds which can be cooked with grains or sea vegetables are also helpful for the lungs. Pickles that have been aged a long time are preferred. If the lungs are weak, condiment size qualities of pungent foods could be used to tonify the lungs. These include ginger, radish, daikon, and scallions. For an overactive condition emphasize lightly cooked white vegetables such as turnips, cabbage, cauliflower, cucumber, and celery. Hijiki, arame, and kombu are preferred sea vegetables. Fruit intake is best limited and best served dried or cooked, in small volume. Nuts and nut butters should also be limited.

Other suggestions. Avoid excessive smoking and polluted air. For lung disorders, scrub the whole body daily, with a towel dipped in hot ginger water and squeezed tightly, including the chest and abdominal area, until the skin becomes pinkish in color. It helps improve circulation, energy, and breathing. Since smooth functioning of the lungs is aided by the smooth functioning of the large intestine, it is wise to pay attention to the health of this organ.

Certain exercises in Chapter 5 are beneficial for the lungs. These include deep breathing #8, meridian stretching #10 (5); Self-shiatsu #11 (3), hara massage #7A (1)(3), the Bow Pose #16, the Camel Pose #18 and abdominal exercise #25.

Abdominal Breathing[22]

Choose a quiet location. Wear loose comfortable clothing and remove any jewelry.

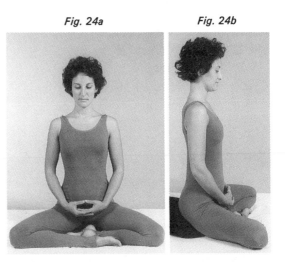

Fig. 24a   *Fig. 24b*

Sit on the edge of a cushion in lotus or half-lotus position, or cross-legged. The cushion will elevate your buttocks making it easier to keep an upright spine.

Straighten your spine. Extend your neck so that your nose and tanden are on one vertical line. Fold your hands, with the left on right, resting in your lap. The eyes can remain half-closed with vision focused on the tip of the nose (Figs. 24a, b). Closing the eyes may be helpful for the beginner.

Exhale with the mouth wide open. Keeping the thoracic cage as still as possible throughout the entire breathing process, inhale slowly through the nose. (The tip of the tongue is touching the roof of the mouth and the mouth is closed.) With your mind's eye follow the breath downward, all the way to the tanden. The abdominal muscles are relaxed during this process. Hold the breath for fifteen to twenty seconds by slightly tensing the abdominal muscles and pressing the diaphram downward.

To exhale, first contract the anus and lower abdomen, then the upper abdomen. With the diaphragm pressing downward this motion will exert pressure on the diaphragm which will in turn ensure the maximum amount of air expired. Throughout the exhalation count in your mind the number one, lasting as long as the exhalation (Uuwaaannn . . .).

At the end of the exhalation stop breathing entirely, momentarily. Then begin the process again. Repeat, counting up to the number twenty-five. Relax. Perform some abdominal massage to help loosen any tension you might feel in that area. Some leg stretches may be necessary. Then try again for another twenty-five breaths.

Inevitably thoughts will arise. To stop a train of thought, simply draw your attention back to the breath. Follow the breath with your mind's eye throughout the entire breathing process as much as possible.

The Large Intestine Meridian

According to Classical Chinese Medicine[23]

The Large Intestine of Chinese theory corresponds anatomically with the large intestine. In its function it corresponds partly to the small intestine, partly to the large intestine and rectum.[24] "The Large Intestine controls the Transmitting and Drainage of the Dregs."[25] (It absorbs liquid from the chyme passed on by the small intestine, and solidifies the stools which it excretes.)

Problems and diseases commonly treated by acupuncture to points along the large intestine meridian include:

Toothache; sore throat; pain and swelling of the throat and pharynx; tonsillitis; laryngitis; fever; diarrhea; constipation; stomach rumblings; abdominal pain; hemorrhoids; difficulty in breathing; swelling of the chest; pain, tightness and stiffness of the shoulder, back, and arm; tennis elbow; wrist pain; nosebleed; nasal sinusitis; ringing in the ears; headache; facial paralysis; hypertension; convulsions in children[26]

According to Shizuto Masunaga[27]

In classical Chinese medicine the large intestine is called "the official of transmission"—its role is to transmit the will of the Prime Minister in practical action. Thus the large intestine aids the lungs. Its function is to process and eliminate waste from food substances taken into the body. This action serves to clear obstructions of ki flow.

The large intestine is affected by withholding emotions or keeping one's feelings to oneself. When the large intestine meridian function is impaired there is difficulty in finding psychological release. Since this tendency is often accompanied by shallow breathing, lack of exercise aggravates the problem. This condition leads to physical symptoms of constipation, chilling of the extremities (poor circulation), and too much blood going to the head causing hotness of the head and dizziness.

Imbalances in the large intestine meridian are associated with the following symptoms:

Loss of motivation and an insufficient intake and elimination of ki due to lack of exercise—eventually leading to diseases of the respiratory tract (including nose, throat, tonsils, windpipe), chills and rigors, chilling of the lower abdomen and diarrhea; pale complexion, pale and sensitive skin susceptible to infection; hemorrhoids; bloodshot eyes; pain and difficulty in moving the thumb; feeling of weakness or pain in one's back

Masunaga further identifies conditions that may arise in terms of kyo and jitsu:

• *Large Intestine Meridian Kyo*[28]

Cause: Lacking of initiative and openness

Mental Aspect: Problems with personal relationships and lack of friends that can be trusted; inability to adequately express oneself to others; loss of motivation after a disappointment; depending on others instead of taking initiative

Physical Aspect: Prone to nasal congestion and dry coughs; hypersensitivity in upper respiratory tract, which causes coughing; tendency to exercise very little; not breathing deeply; tendency toward diarrhea, especially when eating hard to digest food; chilling of lower abdomen and extremities; lack of strength, pain in arms and hand (especially in line with the thumb); lack of vitality in face—pale complexion and skin aging quickly; thigh joint not normal

• *Large Intestine Meridian Jitsu*[29]

Mental Aspect: Always dissatisfied, no friend to confide in

Physical Aspect: Does not excrete properly—constipation but occasional diarrhea; lower abdomen swollen; hemorrhoids; headaches causing flushed complexion—rushing blood to one's head; running nose; nasal congestion; nosebleeding; prone to tonsillitis; coughing; swollen throat; tendency to overeat; lack of exercise; itchy skin; epilepsy; tendency to catch cold; whitish eyes; shoulder pain; stiffness in chest and arm muscles (along the large intestine meridian).

• *Jitsu Symptoms of Other Meridians with Large Intestine Meridian Kyo*[30]

Stomach: Chilling during sleep; heaviness in stomach from chilling; too little exercise for the amount of food consumed; diarrhea; empyema

Spleen: Dryness and stickiness in mouth; frozen shoulders; shallow sleep; poor digestion and diarrhea; eating too fast; preoccupation with lack of exercise; restlessness and discomfort in hips

Heart: Impatient yet unable to act; low back pain; mental fatigue; sudden shock making one unable to stand

Small Intestine: Hardening of the arteries causing the legs to be anemic; hypersensitive skin; poor intestinal absorption; elbow pain; lack of exercise causing poor digestion

Bladder: Listlessness from continuous tension; nervous diarrhea; chilling of legs

Kidney: Constipation due to lack of exercise; fatigue of kidneys due to poor excretion; diarrhea due to nervous causes

Heart Constrictor: Chilling of extremities with hotness of the head; tendency to have palpitations

Triple Heater: Prolonged colds, swelling of gums; inability to open mouth widely; toothache

Gallbladder: Eyestrain from overuse of hands; low back pain resulting from chilling; overeating and indigestion; poor digestion due to working too hard

Liver: Tendency to be constipated; jerky finger movements; eczema; hemorrhoids; allergic rhinitis; sneezing

Structure and Function of the Large Intestine[31]
The functions of the large intestine are:
1. To absorb water and nutrients through the intestinal wall
2. To solidify waste products to be expelled from the body as feces
3. To synthesize important vitamins

The large intestine is a hollow tube some 5 feet in length and 2 1/2 inches in diameter, three times the width of the small intestine. It consists of seven continuous sections: cecum, ascending colon, transverse colon, descending colon, sigmoid colon, rectum, and anal canal. Just beyond the connection with the small intestine at the ileocecal valve, the cecum begins. It is a blind pouch from which, at its lower end, the appendix extends. The open end of the cecum joins the colon, a long tube which forms the greater part of the large intestine. The first part, rising toward the liver is called the ascending colon. The colon then turns left at the hepatic flexure and this section, the transverse colon, extends horizontally across the abdomen. It rises slightly on the left side near the spleen, where it turns downward at the splenic flexure to become the descending colon. At the level of the left hip the colon turns inward toward the center, the sigmoid colon, where it joins with the rectum, a passage some 5 inches long. The last 1 to 2 inches of the rectum is known as the anal canal. The exterior opening, the anus, is held closed most of the time by the anal sphincter muscle.

A mucous membrane lines the inner wall of the colon, which is smooth and devoid of villi. A muscular coat, consisting of circular internal and longitudinal external muscles, surrounds the mucous layer. The muscular walls contract in sections, thus creating a large number of bulbous pouches called haustra. These give the intestine a puckered appearance and create an enormous capacity for expansion.

The fluid passing into the large intestine is called chyme: it consists of water, undigested food particles, and secretions from the small intestine. A maximum of 2 cc is passed into the large intestine at a time. Most water is extracted in the cecum and first part of the ascending colon. (Consequently the driest part of the stool is usually in the sigmoid colon.) Chyme fills the haustra while they are relaxed and stretched. The wall then contracts and the contents move into the next haustra. The large intestine lacks the kind of wavelike peristaltic action of the small intestine. Its main form of action consists of a strong movement known as "mass peristalsis," which pushes the contents toward the rectum. This movement usually arises after a meal when there is the pressure of food within the stomach. Mass peristalsis causes the cecum to empty in readiness for newly digested food. The nerve supply to the large intestine is sparse. Consequently an individual may not become aware of a serious problem until the condition is quite severe.

There are three main aspects to consider in the functioning of the large intestine: bacteria, mucus, and dietary fiber.

The upper digestive tract is relatively free of bacteria, which are either destroyed or paralyzed by acid secretions from the stomach. However, they are needed for proper functioning of the large intestine and they grow there profusely. Over 400 different varieties of bacteria have been identified in the intestines and the number growing there actually outnumbers the cells of the body.[32] They weigh over 3 pounds and constitute as much as 30 to 50 percent of the dry weight of the feces.[33]

The relationship between the bacteria and the individual, when proper, is one of symbiosis. The bacteria are provided with a home and nourishment, and in return they help to break down the food. There are two predominant strains of bacteria found in the colon: lactobaccillus and coliform bacteria (E. Coli). The colon needs an acid environment to function properly. Lactobaccilli produce lactic acid, a natural antiseptic which maintains this acid environment. Lactobaccilli feed off carbohydrates. Conversely, coliform bacteria feed more off protein. The protein produces ammonia, which neutralizes acidity, thus creating a more alkaline environment. This environment kills lactobacteria and creates a breeding ground in which parasites and harmful bacteria can proliferate, producing putrefaction and gas, causing infections, and excreting substances which are irritating and toxic. Such a situation can cause inflammation and chronic diarrhea. Inflammations in turn can cause spasms, cramps, and pain.

In contrast, lactobacilli perform a number of useful functions:

1. They aid in breaking down fiber and so create a proper texture for the stool.
2. They synthesize certain vitamins: vitamin K, which is necessary to help the liver manufacture substances used in the blood clotting process and some B vitamins including vitamin B_{12}.[34]
3. They maintain suitable conditions for the intestinal wall.
4. They minimize putrefaction.
5. They control the content of mucus in the stools.

The microbe culture growing in the colon is unique to each individual. Even two people eating the same diet can develop a different intestinal flora. And within the colon different bacteria inhabit different areas. The kind of flora which grows depends not only upon the kind of food digested, but also upon our overall health and emotional state. The flora is affected by the microbial population of our external environment as well.[35]

In the standard macrobiotic diet there are a number of fermented foods consumed which contain lactobacilli. These include miso, tamari soy sauce, natto, and pickles. In Japan these foods were traditionally produced at home. In such a situation, the bacteria that created fermentation in these products were the bacteria living in that local environment. Some of these same bacteria came to grow within the intestine, thus creating an harmonious exchange between the internal and external environments.[36]

Ideally the colon should contain 85 percent lactobacteria and 15 percent coliform bacteria. However in our modern society these figures are often reversed.

Mucus is a secretion of the mucous membrane lining the upper digestive tract. It keeps the surfaces of the intestinal wall moist and lubricated and aids in the smooth flow of waste products through the bowel. It also helps to protect the intestinal lining and prevents potentially harmful substances from penetrating deeper into the body.

According to macrobiotics and certain other approaches to natural healing, residue from foods that cannot be properly absorbed or assimilated by the body's cells is eliminated as waste via the mucus as well as through other forms of excretion (breath, kidneys, perspiration). These foods include all kinds of dairy, baked and fried flour products, flesh foods, highly refined foods, and synthetic chemicals; general excess and imbalance in the diet is another source. This type of mucus differs from the normal secretion of the body in a healthy non-toxic state. It has a tendency to dehydrate and due to its increased viscosity often accumulates on the intestinal wall.

Dietary fiber is that part of the food which is not digestible. It holds moisture, providing a bulky mass which increases the ability of the intestines to move its inner contents along. It also aids in supporting a plentiful population of lactobacteria in the intestinal tract. Animal food such as meat, eggs, dairy, fish, as well as refined flour, sugar, and other processed foods, lack fiber and can also be mucous forming. When food containing little fiber is consumed, the residue that reaches the colon is not easily moved along. The longer the material remains in the colon, the more moisture is absorbed from it. It becomes dryer and more compressed, creating greater difficulty for elimination. As moisture is absorbed, the mass of residue becomes more sticky and together with discharged mucus tends to adhere to the colon wall.

These feces build up in pockets or can coat the entire wall of the intestine, creating toxic accumulations which lead to poor circulation and fatigue. The absorption of vital nutrients slows down in proportion to the amount of incrustation and this accumulation becomes a breeding ground for unhealthy bacterial life forms. It leads to autointoxication as the blood capillaries pick up toxins seeping through the bowel wall and spread them to all parts of the body. The longer food remains in the colon the greater the chance of putrefaction and since the temperature within the colon is around 98.6°F, putrefaction within takes place more rapidly than externally.[37]

The time that food takes to travel through the digestive tract can vary greatly. Seventy-two hours or less is more normal and less stressful to the gastrointestinal tract. In countries where people eat only unrefined foods—food with plentiful dietary fiber, the time can be as short as four to six hours. The average Englishman takes seventy-seven hours to pass his food, while the English vegetarian forty-nine hours, and a rural African eating mainly corn and beans thirty-five hours.[38]

A toxic condition within the colon can cause a number of profound distortions in its shape:[39]

Ballooning. Feces back up and accumulate, stretching the colon to enormous proportions, often three to four times the proper cross sectional diameter. Only a small channel remains open through which waste matter can pass. This condition, which often occurs in the sigmoid colon, creates pressure on the intestinal wall and may lead to a hernia.

Diverticular Disease. Diverticula are small pouches or saclike protuberances from the intestinal wall. When the diet lacks fiber or bulk, the colonic muscles must work extremely hard to force the feces through the organ. Where there is weakness in the muscle fibers a hernia occurs. Feces accumulate within these pouches and bacteria begin to breed. They become a source of inflammation and overall, a degenerative condition develops.

Collapsed Colon. Due to a lack of muscle tone in the colon wall sacculations close in upon themselves. In a spastic colon one or more sacculations remains in a constant state of contraction. In either case the colon may have one-third or less the proper cross sectional diameter.

Prolapsed Colon. The transverse colon sags or droops and can exert pressure on the bladder, uterus, or prostate.

Redundant Colon The colon becomes so elongated that it folds back on itself, thus restricting the passage of feces.

Macrobiotic Health Evaluation[40]
The constitution of the large intestine can be determined from an overall view of the lips (see p. 154).

The condition of the large intestine is revealed in the lower lip, especially the peripheral areas, as well as on the forehead.

1. *The Lower Lip*
A swollen lower lip signifies a swollen yin condition of the large intestine. It indicates irregular bowel movements, usually constipation from a combination of excessive yin and yang foods. However if the lip is wet it indicates diarrhea. This condition also shows enteritis or inflammation of the intestinal tract. An extremely contracted yang lower lip shows overconsumption of meat, dairy foods and eggs, and blockages or fecal buildup along the insides of the intestinal wall.

Discolorations on the lower lip indicate specific disorders. A white or pale color indicates either that the blood capillaries may be abnormally constricted, or a deficiency in hemoglobin, or stagnation and slowness of blood circulation—it shows weak metabolism of nutrients and anemia. Whitish patches indicate fatty mucous deposits in the colon. Vivid red indicates that the blood capillaries and tissue are abnormally expanded and that blood circulation is faster, signs of infections or inflammation. A yellowish shade around the edges of the lips shows hardening of fatty deposits in the large intestine and blockages in the liver and gallbladder. Blue or purple shades show the stagnation of feces and blood in the colon. Dark reddish spots show stagnation of blood. A green shade around the mouth probably indicates colon cancer.

2. *The Forehead*
The right part of the forehead shows the ascending colon, the upper forehead the transverse colon, and the left part the descending colon. Swellings, discoloration, patches, pimples, or spots indicate where fat deposits, ulcers, or cancerous growths are developing in the colon.

Other Considerations

General skin color. The following are all early warning signs of overactive intestines and general digestive troubles: a purplish shading from the overconsumption of extremely yin foods and beverages; a brown shade from excessive yang animal food and yin tropical vegetables and fruits; yellow, white, hard fatty skin from the excessive consumption of eggs, poultry, cheese, and other dairy foods.

Large intestine meridian. Large Intestine 4, the pressure point in the fleshy part between the thumb and index finger, can, with pressure indicate the condition of the large intestine; right hand, ascending colon; left hand descending colon. A green or bluish hue may indicate colon cancer.

Dietary Recommendations[41]

Avoid or reduce all mucous forming foods, especially refined flour and all forms of dairy food as well as all kinds of animal food, and even fish and seafood if the condition is serious. Avoid or reduce extreme forms of yin food such as greasy, oily or fatty foods, sugar, sugar-treated foods and beverages, soft drinks, tropical fruits and vegetables, various nuts and nut butters, spices, stimulants, and aromatic foods and drinks.

Introduce fiber in the form of whole cereal grains, vegetables (especially roots and leafy greens), beans and sea vegetables: also include fermented foods such as miso, tamari soy sauce, pickles and natto, which promote the growth of good quality intestinal flora.

More specifically, follow standard dietary guidelines, slightly emphasizing the following if there are problems in the large intestine:

Consume a variety of grains but emphasize brown rice. For an overly contracted condition avoid buckwheat until the condition noticeably changes. Minimize baked and deep-fried flour consumption, even oatmeal, since these foods are mucous forming. As a good quality fermented food miso soup is recommended daily together with hard leafy greens as the main vegetable ingredient. For troubles with the ascending colon slightly emphasize leafy vegetables over root vegetables, as well as lighter, quicker cooking methods which emphasize freshness and crispness. For the transverse colon leafy and round vegetables such as cabbages, onions, pumpkins, and squashes may be used almost equally, employing medium-style cooking techniques, neither too short nor too long. For problems in the descending colon and rectum, round and root vegetables should be emphasized. Vegetable dishes which are beneficial for the large intestine include kinpira, and dried daikon and kombu. Beans and bean products should not be consumed in large volume. If there are problems with gas, check the way that beans are being prepared. Sea vegetables are beneficial to intestinal functioning. The kinds used should be alternated, emphasizing hijiki and arame. Miso scallion condiment and sautéed whole dandelions served in condiment size amounts are beneficial. Pickles in small amounts are helpful for aiding digestion. Fruit and fruit juices, served raw, easily create a cold condition in the intestines and can severely weaken its function. Fruit consumption should be minimized. When served, cooked temperate climate fruit in small volume is recommended, especially if prepared with kuzu. Avoid cold beverages as they have a paralyzing effect on the intestines.

For the purposes of cleansing, strengthening, and revitalizing the intestinal tract a much simpler diet emphasizing brown rice may prove helpful. This diet consists of pressure-cooked brown rice served with either umeboshi plum or gomashio (1: 12 or 1: 14), and with toasted nori. Along with brown rice one or two cups of miso soup and one or two dishes of cooked vegetables may be consumed everyday. This diet should not be continued longer than two weeks without proper supervision of a macrobiotic counselor and/or medical professional.

Other Recommendations. Avoid eating to capacity, chew very well, and refrain from eating for two to three hours before bedtime. Keep the abdominal region warm. Scrub the whole body daily with a hot towel; doing this will activate the circulation of the blood and general energy, promoting better digestion. Moderate daily exercise improves appetite and digestion. Certain exercises in Chapter 5 are especially beneficial for the large intestine. These include: hara massage #7 (1)–(3); meridian stretching #10 (2); and Self-shiatsu #11 (4) and #21B (4). Abdominal exercise #25 is most beneficial.

The Kidney and Bladder Meridians

Water Nature Energy

The kidneys and bladder correspond with water nature in the Five Phases. Michio Kushi describes water nature as floating energy. It is that transitional or dissolving phase between energy descending and energy rising. Since water seeks the lowest level this energy is expressed horizontally. This horizontal quality is further indicated by the position we take at night (a water correspondence) where in sleep we return to the floating world of dreams. Overall, images of water are of softness and weakness—yin. However, water can be hard and it can also be powerful—yang. In the same way, we can think of water in terms of stillness (yin) and movement (yang). Thus water nature has both yin and yang qualities and paradoxically the yang quality of power can be within the yin quality of softness or weakness.

Within the human body, the kidneys and bladder occupy yang locations—the kidneys toward the back of the abdomen in the lower thoracic and upper lumbar region, and the bladder directly behind the pubic bone. In like manner, the kidney and bladder meridians are in yang locations. Both traverse the legs—the kidney meridian moving up the yang interior of the legs and onto the (yang) center of the chest, terminating just below the collar bone. The bladder meridian begins on the inside corners of the eyes, travels over the head, down each side of the spine and onto the legs, ending on the little toes. Moreover, the kidney meridian begins on the sole of the foot at a point called Yū-Sen (bubbling spring), the most direct contact of all meridians with the earth, suggesting the drawing in of earth's force, which we can relate with movement and the horizontal expression of energy—will and drive. Conversely, the bladder is the last organ to receive the remains of metabolism, granting it the ability to monitor the functioning of the various systems of the body, a quality control or supervisory function. This characterization is further indicated by the beginning location of the bladder meridian beside the eyes, its length (the longest of all meridians) and the wide path that it takes. While the kidney meridian provides the get-up-and-go, the bladder meridian functions to see that all is in order.

From the above as well as the images of water nature energy presented in Chapter 2 we can see how this energy may manifest within the individual.

Fig. 25

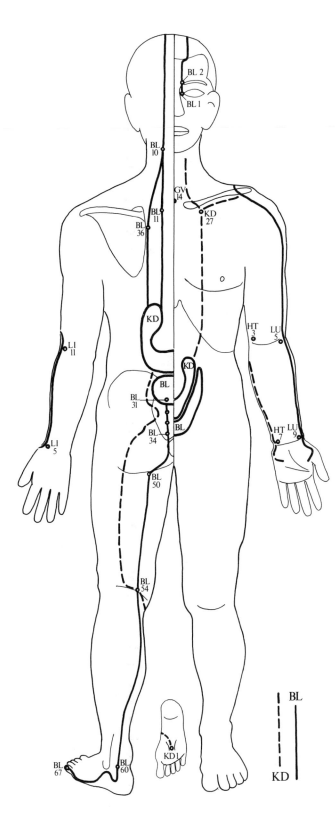

The Power of Water

Positive: The river at its mouth (yang; yang excess)—reserves; stamina; drive; motivation; "get-up-and-go"; endurance; will; aggression; resourcefulness; sense of power—uncontrollable; sense of continuity

Negative: The river as it begins (yin; yang deficient)—superficial, "doesn't know what one wants"; not staying on one path for any length of time; aimless; lack of assertion; hesitant; timid; overly cautious; uncertain; fearful; not moving around enough—tendency to stagnate

Water Seeks the Lowest Level (*either yin or yang*)

Positive: humility; "ability to get to the bottom of things"; to know deep down inside what one wants—one's true vocation; sense of mystery; feelings; emotional depths

Negative: subservient, to allow oneself to be pushed around

Water as a Medium (*either yin or yang*)

Positive: resourcefulness, adaptability—"to go with the flow"; easy to get along with; to be a good mixer, communicator, go-between; symbolic of travel

Negative: overly agreeable—says what you want to hear; imitative

THE KIDNEY MERIDIAN

According to Classical Chinese Medicine[1]

The kidneys correspond anatomically with the kidneys of Western science, but in function correspond with the adrenal glands and the endocrine glands, including the pancreas.[2] The kidneys are considered "the root of life" because the kidneys store Jing. Jing is the source of life and individual development.[3] It consists of two parts: (1) The Jing of reproduction—the basic substance possessed by male and female, that enables the human species to reproduce; (2) The Jing arising from ingested food and water—a basic nourishing substance that maintains the life and movement of the body.[4] Thus the kidneys store the potential for life and therefore rule birth, growth, and maturation. (Jing decreases in both vitality and quantity with age.)[5] In turn the other organs of the body depend upon the kidneys for their existence. The kidneys comprise two aspects, the Fire of the Gate of Life and Kidney Water. The kidneys control water in the body in all its various forms and kidney fire is responsible for initiating the movement of this water and its transformation into different states. By ruling birth, growth, and maturity, the kidneys control the bones and marrow. The bones include the teeth. The marrow includes the brain. The kidneys grant the ability to hear and they correspond with the hair on the head. The kidneys are also the "root of ki"; they enable the air taken in by the lungs (the lungs are "the foundation of ki") to actually penetrate deeply—completion of the inhalation process.[6]

Disorders treated by acupuncture to points along the kidney meridian include the following:

Mental disorders; coma; hysteria; shock; vomiting; nausea; diarrhea and constipation; sore throat; asthma; tonsillitis; toothache; coughing and chest pain; sterility in women; abnormal menstruation; prolapse of uterus; uterine bleeding; cystitis; impotence; nocturnal emission; frequent urination; incontinence of urine; disorders of the genital system; spermatorrhea; palpitations; high blood pressure; difficulty in breathing; lumbar pain; paralysis of the lower extremities; pain in the ankle and at the bottom of the foot[7]

According to Shizuto Masunaga[8]

The Chinese classics refer to the kidneys as "strong and capable ministers from whom technical ability and expertise are derived." The bladder is likened to "a governor of a state capital from which the water flows." Thus the kidneys were understood as the organ which facilitates the work of the other organs and enables them to perform their various functions. The bladder was like a local governor, who works to adjust the supply and demand in outlying areas. Therefore the kidney and bladder meridians (Fig. 25) act like supervisors over the functions of the other organs.

The kidneys and bladder include the functions of the adrenals and autonomic nervous system, as well as that of the reproductive organs. Together, these organs perform the functions of supplying vital energy and purifying body liquids.

The kidneys work to regulate the constituents of the body fluids and supply essential components to all parts of the body, and control the whole body through hormonal regulation. These functions also relate to sex hormones and one's response to stress (the adrenals). The kidneys purify the blood by isolating and eliminating those substances poisonous to the body. The right kidney, "the fire of life gate" reflects the condition of the adrenals and the endocrine system. Dysfunctions are associated with fatigue and also with hotness of the head. The left kidney the "water kidney" reflects the condition of water metabolism and regulates urine formation. Dysfunctions are associated with edema and chilling of the extremities.

Imbalances in the kidney meridian are associated with the following:

Psychological states of phobia or excessive fear, and easily startled; a tendency to be anxious and work compulsively, but with a lack of perseverance to finish what is started; a tendency to overdo things and to overreact to everything; tendency of the skin to be dark, lacking in tone and prone to swelling; the lower abdomen and back often feel cold and cramps in the leg are also common; the head may feel heavy with lack of sleep, but still there is an inability to sleep soundly; the abdomen hard and the arms and legs may feel hot; greatly reduced ability to grasp firmly in the morning; a bitter taste in the mouth or a strong odor in the mouth, and the skin susceptible to infection and eczema; frequent nosebleeds.

Masunaga further identifies conditions in terms of kyo and jitsu:

- *Kidney Meridian Kyo[9]*

Cause: A tendency to overdo things and to reach a state of total exhaustion by working too hard

Mental Aspect: Unabating anxiety or sense of emptiness; lack of perseverance and motivation, easily startled and fearful of the slightest thing; lack of composure; restlessness; continual stress at home or work from which there is no escape; loss of determination and drive

Physical Aspect: Dark complexion lacking luster; puffy skin lacking in resiliency; chilling sensation extending from the lower abdomen and hips down the legs; frequent urination or sparse urination; overwork and loss of sleep for extended period; body heavy with fatigue as if weighted down; bad breath; hormonal deficiency; excessive sexual activity; loss of sexual drive and impotence; weak and brittle bones; tendency to trip and fall; tension and hardness in waist area; tightness in rectus abdominis muscle

- *Kidney Meridian Jitsu[10]*

Psychological: Too eager for success; in a hurry; workaholic; restless; constant complaining; too much attention to detail

Physical: Blackish color in face; vomiting; blood in the saliva; prone to nose-bleeding and fainting; heaviness in the head; inflamed throat; thirsty; poor hearing when drugs are taken; ringing in ears; stiffness in back; tightness in torso muscles; abnormal hormone secretion; densely colored urine; bitterness in mouth; bad breath; prone to inflammation; fatigue from overwork; swollen hands and legs; bleeding nose

- *Jitsu Symptoms of Other Meridians with Kidney Meridian Kyo[11]*

Lung: Pulmonary emphysema; copious phlegm; chilling of upper half of body

Large Intestine: Stiffness and tension in the legs from chilling; leg cramps as a result of back strain

Stomach: Hotness of head; oversensitivity to cold; hyperacidity; gastritis due to overwork; overeating

Spleen: Dry mouth from poor salivation; low back pain; cracks in the heels

Heart: Insomnia despite physical fatigue; headaches; stiffness in neck and shoulders; bleary eyes

Small Intestine: Fatigue after childbirth or stagnation of blood in lower abdomen; tiredness due to stress; abnormalities in hormone secretion

Heart Constrictor: High or low blood pressure; angina pectoris; swelling of arms and legs; overwork and failure to rest

Triple Heater: Tonsillitis; hotness of head; hypersensitive skin; oversensitivity to cold; allergic constitution; susceptibility to infections; poor peripheral circulation and excretion of liquid

Gallbladder: Difficulty in getting to sleep; restless sleep; swelling of face and extremities, especially in the morning; nausea

Liver: Drug abuse; insect bites; liver disorders; infectious hepatitis

Structure and Function of the Kidneys[12]

The kidneys are paired bean-shaped organs, each about 4 inches high, 2 inches wide, and 1 inch thick. Joined with surrounding structures by a layer of fibrous connective tissue, they are located toward the back of the abdomen on each side of the spine, half above and half below the lower ribs.

The primary function of the kidneys is to purify the blood and discharge toxic waste in the form of urine.

Each kidney consists of an outer pale layer called the cortex, and a darker colored core, the medulla. Located in the center of each kidney is the renal pelvis. The renal pelvis connects with a thin walled tube, the ureter, which leads into the bladder.

The chemical filtration unit of the organ is the nephron, of which there are over one million, densely packed into each kidney. Each nephron is about 1 1/4 inches long and less than 1 mm in diameter. The nephron consists of a cup-shaped structure called the Bowman's capsule and a tubule. The tubule is a long coiled hollow tube that weaves from the cortex into the medulla and back again, finally linking with a urine collecting duct which leads into the renal pelvis.

The kidneys receive about 25 percent of the blood pumped out by the heart with each beat via the renal arteries. Each day approximately 2,100 quarts of blood pass through the kidneys (over 2 pints every minute) and over 180 liters of fluid are filtered.

Within the kidneys the renal arteries divide up repeatedly, eventually forming arterioles each of which lead to a Bowman's capsule. Within the Bowman's capsule the arteriole splits up into tiny walled capillaries which form a ball called the glomerulus. The capillaries reunite to form the arteriole which leaves the capsule. This arteriole forms branches and, along with a network of other blood vessels, surrounds the tubule.

Blood is forced into the Bowman's capsule under pressure. Through the extremely fine mesengial membrane of the capillary walls, water, glucose, salts, amino acids, vitamins, and urea, pass into the tubule, while protein molecules and blood cells are retained. Within the tubule numerous adjustments to the composition of the blood are made, valuable nutrients are returned to the bloodstream, and waste products concentrated to the maximum. Ninety-nine percent of the fluid is reabsorbed back into the bloodstream by the network of blood capillaries surrounding each nephron. Excess water and waste products remain in the tubule to be discharged as urine.

Functions carried out within the tubule include the following:

1. *Water balance and water and salt conservation.* Nearly all water and most salt is reabsorbed. Over 60 percent of the body's weight is water. Sixty percent of this water is intracellular, while the rest, mixed with salts, is present in a bathing solution between the cells or in other body fluids. Since it is essential that cell volume remain fairly constant and that bathing solutions be maintained at exactly the correct concentrations, the kidneys function to (1) conserve water and salt and (2) ensure a steady water balance—that the amount of water leaving the body is the same as that which entered. Salt content is maintained within 2 percent of a norm. When body fluids have decreased by 1 percent of body weight, the sensation of thirst arises, which induces us to drink. When water loss reaches 10 percent of body weight the cells can no longer function and death is imminent.

2. *The kidneys regulate the acidity of the blood.* The pH is maintained at a constant level.

3. *The kidneys produce urine.* Urine is a water solution of urea, salts, and other soluble wastes. Over 95 percent of urine is water. Of the remaining, 60 to 90 percent is urea, a toxic substance resulting from the breakdown of protein. Salt content usually results from excess in the diet. The average amount of urine passed each day is 1,500 cc.

The Adrenal Glands. The kidneys are assisted in their functioning by the adrenal glands, which lie in contact above each kidney. The adrenals consist of an outer portion, the cortex, and an inner, the medulla. The cortex secretes hormones which help regulate the following functions: water and salt metabolism; carbohydrate, protein and fat metabolism, electrolyte balance and distribution of water in the tissues; muscular and reproductive activity; resistance to stress. The medulla secretes hormones which are involved with other functions: basal and also carbohydrate metabolism; stimulation of the body into activity (through the hormones adrenalin and noradrenaline). The cortex controls more the functioning of the parasympathetic nervous system while functions of the medulla tend to stimulate the sympathetic nervous system—including the fight or flight reflex.

Disorders Associated with the Kidneys

Kidney problems involve principally two processes: (1) The passing of fluids through the capillary wall; (2) Accumulation of waste products within the kidneys.

Nephritis (Inflammation of the nephrons).[13] Nephritis can be acute or chronic. The tubules can become swollen, congested or inflamed. Since the process of urine formation involves the concentration of waste, these substances tend to be found in higher concentrations in the kidney tissues than elsewhere. They potentially can provide a constant source of irritation to the delicate kidney structures. These products include urea and other wastes of metabolism, drugs, and stimulant beverages such as tea or coffee, which act as diuretics. Diuretics increase kidney activity to rid them of the effects of these stimulants. While according to macrobiotics diuretics and drugs are yin, urea is usually the end product of protein metabolism. Urea may be yang in the case of an animal food based diet, or yin in the case of vegetable food.

Edema. When an excess of solid wastes cannot pass through the minute holes within the capillary walls, water retention and chronic swelling develop. Most often the excess fluid builds up in the legs, producing periodic swelling and weakness.

Hypertension (High blood pressure). The condition of the kidneys may be the source of hypertension. The blood pressure needs to be high enough to allow the kidneys to work. Any cause of diminished blood flow through the kidneys will cause the kidneys to release a hormone, angiotensin, which enters the general bloodstream and heightens general blood pressure. Causes of diminished blood flow through the kidneys are as follows:

Kidney constriction (yang): from excess salt and/or animal food especially cheese; kidney swelling (yin); caused by excess liquid; kidney stagnation: caused by the build-up of waste products; atherosclerosis of the kidney arteries.

Kidney Stones.[14] Kidney stones are formations of urea, calcium and phosphates. They can bring on extreme pain by a blockage of the normal flow of urine that causes stretching of the ureters and renal pelvis. The ureter wall is irritated to a degree that it goes into a spasm; this spasm is experienced as pain. Next, urine builds up in the pelvis, and as the pressure increases, the spasm usually also increases. According to macrobiotics, kidney stones are formed primarily from the long term consumption of foods high in fat, particularly when chilled or frozen, for example ice cream and yogurt, as well as beverages that create coldness within the body such as orange juice, soft drinks, and iced water.

Overall, kidney disease primarily affects people in mid to late life. We normally have large reserves of kidney function, to the extent that most people with problems do not experience actual physical symptoms until more than 90 percent of kidney function has been lost.[15]

THE BLADDER MERIDIAN

According to Classical Chinese Medicine

The bladder of Chinese medicine anatomically corresponds more with the urinary bladder, but functionally corresponds with the entire genitourinary system, including the urinary bladder, urethra, ureter, and kidney.[16]

Disorders commonly treated by acupuncture to points along the bladder meridian include the following:

Eye diseases; facial paralysis; headache; dizziness; sinusitis and rhinitis; epilepsy; tonsillitis; insomnia; aching of the shoulder joint; pain on the top of the head; abdominal pain; gastric pain or ulcer; gastrointestinal disorders; lack of appetite; nausea; vomiting; chronic diarrhea; high blood pressure; stroke; angina pectoris; palpitations; chest pain; respiratory diseases; diseases of the liver and gallbladder; genitourinary diseases; nocturnal emission; impotence; spermatorrhea; irregular menstruation; cystitis; lumbar pain; pain of the back and lower extremities; paralysis of the lower extremities; sciatic neuralgia; diseases of the knee joint; malposition of the fetus[17]

According to Shizuto Masunaga[18]

The bladder meridian is associated with the autonomic nervous system through the pituitary gland, which functions in conjunction with the entire endocrine system. Therefore the bladder meridian controls the reproductive function and the uterus, as well as the organs of elimination; these collect and excrete liquid waste products after the filtration (purification) of body fluids.

Imbalances in the bladder meridian are associated with the following conditions:

A large amount of nervous tension and overreaction; the muscles down the back often rigid while the lower back area feels weak; painful sensations in the inside corners of the eyes (next to the nose), headaches, or a throbbing sensation in the back of the head; varied symptoms caused by dysfunctions in the autonomic nervous system; a creeping sensation up and down the back, or excruciating pain in the lower back; oppressive headaches from the back of the head to the arch of the nose; at times, the back twisted by pain and contraction in the muscles; occasional chilling sensation extending from the lower abdomen down to the legs, and either increase or decrease of the frequency of urination—sometimes leading to cystitis, in which the lower abdomen feels distended and painful with a full bladder, and a feeling of urine retention persists after urination

Masunaga further identifies conditions in terms of kyo and jitsu:

• *Bladder Meridian Kyo*[19]

Cause: The whole body is out of balance, and although one feels the need to do something, one has no stamina to act.

Mental Aspect: Fatigue after extended period of stress; fretting over little things; easily startled; tendency to overreact; anxiety and fear which causes one to break out in a cold sweat; anxiety and restlessness; mental instability; neurotic tendency; complaints of general malaise

Physical Aspect: Nasal congestion; discomfort in the base of nose; heaviness in the head; pain down the back; palpitations; profuse sweating; dizziness; distension of stomach; sciatica or low back pain; hypersensitivity to cold; chilling in the lower abdomen and the legs; pain and heaviness in hips and legs; difficulty in bending backward; ticklishness; dysfunctions in the uterus or bladder; frequent urination or sparse urination; dribbling urination; poor urinary excretion causing body to swell slightly; malfunctioning in the womb; flabby skin

• *Bladder Meridian Jitsu*[20]

Psychological: Constant continuous tension—nervous stress, due to worrying over trivial details, restlessness, oversensitive

Physical: Strained back; stiff neck pain in lower cervical and thoracic vertebra;

heaviness in the back of the head and over the eyes; tightness in the back of the leg; nasal congestion; frequent urination; inflammation or pain in bladder or prostate area; strained autonomic nervous system; rushing blood to one's head

- *Jitsu symptoms of Other Meridians with Bladder Meridian Kyo*[21]

    Lung: Inability to express one's thoughts; sighing; tension in the thumbs; bronchitis

    Large Intestine: Feeling of distension in lower abdomen associated with nervous tension; sciatica

    Stomach: Weak stomach due to nervousness, chilling of extremities, heaviness in stomach resulting from worry

    Spleen: Poor appetite from thinking too much; poor digestion due to chilling; neurosis

    Heart: Insomnia from shock or excessive stress; nervousness and irritability, leading to poor absorption of nutrients

    Small Intestine: Impatience; being overworked; fatigue after shock; weak function of intestines; autointoxication

    Heart Constrictor: Hotness in hands and soles due to circulatory imbalance; pain down the back and hips; eyestrain; tendency for eyes to water; back stiffness

    Triple Heater: Chilling caused by distension of the lower abdomen; general swelling; uterine discharge; dysfunction of autonomic nervous system

    Gallbladder: Costal neuralgia; mental fatigue; constant worrying and over-sensitivity; eyestrain; bedwetting

    Liver: Extreme fatigue; fever; hemorrhoids; cramps in the Achilles tendon; restlessness and periodic irritability; impatience

Structure and Function of the Bladder[22]

The bladder is an egg-shaped muscular sac, lying toward the front of the pelvic cavity, directly behind the pubic bone. Its function is to store urine coming from the kidneys via the ureters, two tubes each averaging 10 1/2 inches in length and 4 to 5 mm in diameter. Urine is passed from the bladder to the outside of the body via the urethra. The urethra is a duct measuring about 1 1/2 inches in length in females, and 8 to 10 inches in males. Urine is prevented from leaving the bladder by internal and external sphincter muscles.

The bladder is folded into rugae like the stomach, allowing it to stretch to an average maximum capacity of 700 to 800 cc of urine. However when the contents reach about 400 cc the sensation of bladder fullness arises, the desire to urinate is stimulated, and the internal sphincter muscle relaxes. If the external sphincter muscle is relaxed urine can be expelled. However this action is under conscious control and urination can be prevented until the bladder becomes fuller.

Some of the main problems associated with the bladder are the following:

Incontinence (Inability to retain urine).[23] This condition is due to weak or poorly developed sphincter muscles. According to macrobiotics it is likely to be caused by an excess of yin foods. Other causes may be psychological, or neurological abnormalities such as M.S., spinal cord trauma, or birth defects.

Retention (Inability to expel urine).[24] This condition may be due to the loss of muscle tone in the bladder, anemia (according to macrobiotics either from a yin or yang cause), or obstruction in the urethra, such as that caused by pregnancy in women or an enlarged prostate in men (yang cause). In more chronic cases the cause may be bladder stones (again either yin or yang cause). Retention more commonly affects males and can cause extreme pain.

Cystitis (Inflammation of the bladder).[25]   Cystitis is also known as urinary tract infection (U.T.I.). U.T.I.'s are the second leading cause of visits to the physician in the United States affecting women far more frequently than men. The reason is that the urethral opening in women lies in close proximity to anal and vaginal sources of infectious agents, making the migratory journey of these microbes to the bladder much shorter and easier than in a male. The infection is usually caused by a bacteria, most often E. coliform, which is present in the intestines.

In males, cystitis usually occurs secondary to some other abnormality such as prostate enlargement or stones. Urine is usually sterile and the bladder lining resistant to the development of infections. However, if the bladder does not completely empty, the contents can provide an excellent breeding ground for bacteria to grow.

Cystitis may be chronic or acute and is characterized by a painful and frequent desire to urinate. The urine may be bloody, foul smelling and/or cloudy.

From the macrobiotic view the cause of cystitis is the condition of the body that allows these bacteria to breed, generally coming from excess yin such as coffee, tea, fruit juices, alcohol, chocolate, and spices.

Macrobiotic Health Evaluation[26]

Constitution: The constitution, or innate strength of the kidneys, is seen in the ears. The larger, the thicker, the lower set on the head, the larger the lobes, and the flatter against the head, the stronger the kidneys and the overall constitution of the person.

Condition: Overall, the condition of the kidneys will reflect the condition of the bladder. Problems of the kidneys can basically be divided into two categories: (1) Too yang—too contracted or tight, causing restriction in blood flow and the discharge of waste; (2) Too yin—too swollen or loose. The kidneys have become weakened and sluggish.

The condition of the kidneys can be seen in the area underneath the lower eyelid, the skin, the ears, the hair, and other sites as well. Areas coresponding to the kidney appearing on the right side of the face show the condition of the right kidney, on the left side the left kidney.

1. *The Area Underneath the Lower Eyelid*

    Eyebags often appear in this area. There are two main causes:

    A pooling of liquid—the eyebag appears watery and swollen. The kidney tissues are swollen and there is frequent urination due to the excessive intake of any kind of liquid.

    Pooled mucus—the eyebag appears fatty and swollen. There is fat and mucous accumulation in the kidney tissues. Chronic eyebags indicate that mucous accumulation is developing in the ureters, the wall of the bladder, the ovaries, Fallopian tubes and uterus, and in and around the prostate gland, creating bacterial activity, inflammation, itching, vaginal discharge, ovarian cysts, and eventually the growth of tumors and cancer in these areas. Small pimples or dark spots show that accumulated mucus and fat in the kidney tissues is forming into kidney stones.

Both kinds of eyebags indicate the decline of physical and mental vitality.

In addition, various colorings around the eyes indicate different conditions.

Dark color—excess yang condition, contraction of the kidneys and exhaustion of the adrenal and gonad hormones; caused by excess salt, roasted, baked, or dried foods or the result of excessive sexual intercourse; stagnated metabolism in the kidneys and excretory system, the ovaries, testicles, and reproductive functions, and a high level of toxicity in the blood due to inadequate detoxification of the kidneys

Yellowish—excess cheese or dairy food consumption or excess consumption of root and round vegetables (carrots, pumpkins, squash); temporary disorder of kidney and excretory functions

Grayish—malfunction of the kidneys due to metabolic stagnation caused by the excessive intake of heavy, fatty animal food, and the overconsumption of salt and other yang foods

Other indications include:

Tight and drawn in this area—overcontracted kidneys

Swollen and puffy—expanded condition

2. *The Skin*

Wet skin—overconsumption of liquid; overworked kidney condition

Oily skin—overconsumption of oils and fats or disorders in fat metabolism; stones forming in the kidneys

Rough skin due to overconsumption of protein and heavy fats—fat and mucous accumulation in the kidneys

Doughy skin—fat and mucous accumulation in the kidneys due mainly to the overconsumption of sugar, dairy, and refined flour products

Brown skin—kidneys and excretory disorders from excess yang animal food and salt along with yin sugar and sweets, alcohol and stimulants as well as foods rich in carbohydrates

Dark skin—kidney, excretory, sexual and hormonal disorders due to excess yin, including sugar and sweets, fruits and juices, drugs and chemicals

Eczema—massive elimination of excessive fats caused mainly by the intake of animal food, especially cheese and other dairy, or eggs cooked with butter; accumulation of fat and cholesterol in the kidneys

3. *The Ears*

Red—excessive contraction of the kidneys; excess salt or animal foods

Oily—overworked kidneys due to excessive fat or oil intake

Moles or warts on the ears—animal protein; mucous deposits in the kidneys

Pimples or lumps—accumulations of fat and perhaps stones in the kidneys

Deafness—associated with fatty congestion in the kidneys

Excessive Discharges of wax—possible fatty accumulations in the ureters

Ringing in the ears—discharge through the kidneys of some extreme form of yin

4. *The Hair*

Hair loss shows a weakening of the kidneys.

5. *The Sole of the Foot*

Pain or hardness when pressing KD.1 (Yū-Sen) indicates kidney disorders.

Calluses in the region of KD.1 represent an effort on the part of the kidneys to discharge excess mucus, protein, and fat through the kidney meridian in the foot. This condition is caused especially by flour products, fats and oils, and sugar and sweets.

6. *Urine*

   Healthy urine is light gold or yellow in color. Darker urine indicates excess salt consumption. Urine that is lighter in color is caused by too little salt or a diet that is too yin. Normally we should urinate three to four times per day.

7. *Upper Part of the Forehead*

   This area corresponds with the bladder. Lines or ridges here indicate troubles with the organ.

Dietary Recommendations[27]

Both kidney and bladder disorders can be either overly contracted (yang) or overly expanded (yin) and the cause of both organ's conditions is similar. Excessive salt consumption is the prime cause of an overly contracted condition; but excess fat, mucus, and the waste from protein and fat metabolism, especially the hard saturated fat of animal food, can also be influential factors. An overly expanded or weak condition can arise from the buildup of toxic waste, again from protein and fat mucous accumulation, from the residue of medicinal drugs, or from the consumption of excess fluids including water, fruit juices, and alcohol. Coffee can severely weaken the kidneys and iced beverages can contribute to the formation of stones. All of these kinds of foods are best avoided.

Foods that are beneficial to kidney and bladder function, of either yin or yang condition, include buckwheat, beans as a general food category, particularly azukis, and sea vegetables. These foods can be prepared in more yin or more yang ways according to the condition to be treated. For example, buckwheat, which is quite yang, might best be served in combination with another grain, or as a soup or a salad for the person whose kidney/bladder condition is too yang. For the same condition, azuki beans could also be mixed with grains or prepared as a soup. Bean products instead of long-time cooked beans may be a better choice. Arame and hijiki are more appropriate sea vegetables for the kidneys and nori for the bladder. For example, for the bladder nori could be best served as a condiment, which is somewhat moist. Overall, for a yang condition cooking methods should be lighter and shorter time with a moderate to very mild use of salt and a little more liquid.

For an overly yin condition longer-time cooking methods should be employed with a little less liquid and a moderate salty taste. Buckwheat could be served more often as a main dish. Vegetable dishes such as nishime would be more appropriate as well as more emphasis on root vegetables. Regular-use beans and the regular method of cooking may be emphasized over bean products. Kombu in the form of a condiment, shio kombu, could be helpful. Beverages and liquids should be reduced—drink when thirsty.

Beyond these suggestions it is advised to follow standard macrobiotic recommendations.

Exercise Recommendations

Certain exercises in Chapter 5 are beneficial for balancing the energy flow along the kidney and bladder meridians. These include the following: Self-shiatsu #4, #21B (5),

#21D (9), #21D (14), the Plough Pose #1 (5), the Cobra Pose #17, and the Forward Bend #24. In addition, the kidneys should be kept warm. A cotton band called a *haramaki* is commonly worn in the Far East for this purpose. Finally, from the location of the beginning of the kidney meridian on the sole of the foot we can see the importance of movement. Moderate physical activity should be incorporated into one's daily life.

Chapter 5

Self-shiatsu Exercise Program[1]

These exercises have been drawn from various sources including Dō-In, self-shiatsu, hatha yoga, Oki yoga, and the martial arts, as well as my own personal experience. Through morning week-day classes over the past four years I have endeavored to develop a program that is comprehensive and easy to begin and practice for most people. The goal was to create a sequence so that one exercise would naturally lead into the next. For the practitioner this program complements the exercise gained through giving shiatsu. Moreover self-shiatsu is a good way to discover the location of the meridians as well as directly experiencing the effects of one's own massage. For the receiver these exercises will intensify and reinforce the benefits gained from shiatsu. Self-shiatsu can also be performed with yoga poses. After doing an *asana*, perform self-shiatsu along the meridians being stimulated by the pose, and then repeat the *asana*. It is surprising how helpful it can be to gain greater flexibility.

Since most exercises are quite simple in structure, their effectiveness depends upon regularity and intensity of practice. The best results come from a daily routine, preferably in the early morning. While it is beneficial to test oneself, it is advisable not to overexert. Begin with the exercises and repetitions you can do comfortably and gradually build up over time.

If you are out of condition, certain exercises, particularly the yoga poses, may cause undue discomfort the following day. They may even be dangerous for some people. These exercises include: Shoulder Stand 1(4), Plough 1(5), Shoulder and Neck Stretch 12, Bow 16, Cobra 17, Camel 18, Reclining Hero 19, and Forward Bend 24. If you have doubts about performing any of these consult a qualified yoga instructor for assistance.

To perform all exercises takes about ninety minutes. If you have only ten or fifteen minutes, do numbers 1 through 10 plus some abdominal exercise. With exercises that require movement to either side, begin by moving to the easier side first. However, repeat more times on the difficult side. In exercises that require forward spinal movement, always move from the hips not the shoulders. Simultaneous movements are shown with both hands on the body. Alternate movements are shown with one hand raised to the maximum and the other on the body. Use the following technique for breathing: as you prepare for the pose allow the abdominal muscles to relax and inhale deeply as though the breath were sinking into the tanden. Hold the breath momentarily and breathe out slowly as you perform the pose.

1. Rolling Exercise

1) Sit comfortably with legs crossed, one leg extended slightly forward (Fig. 26). Focus on some object ten feet or more in front of you.
2) Roll back onto the shoulder, on the side of the closer leg (Fig. 27).

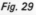
Fig. 26   Fig. 27   Fig. 28

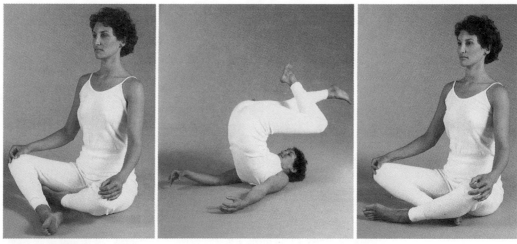

Fig. 29   Fig. 30

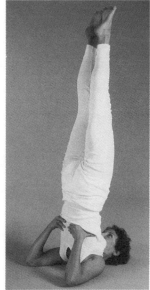

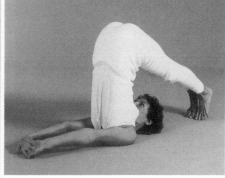

3) Without the head touching the floor, shift your weight to the other shoulder and roll forward on that side. Return to the sitting position with the other leg extended forward, once again focusing on the object in front of you (Fig. 28). Repeat 20 to 30 times. This exercise, a popular warm-up for Aikido training, is an easy way to get your energy moving. It will limber up the spine, create a positive attitude and with regular practice, aid in strengthening the *hara*.

4) Shoulder Stand

Following the last roll back, bring your body into a shoulder stand, legs straight, with Achilles tendons alternatively stretched or relaxed (Fig. 29). Hold the pose momentarily. By pressing your palms into the lower back area, extend your body vertically, moving from one shoulder to the other, until all body weight is focused on your shoulders.

5) The Plough

Bring the legs over your head so that the toes touch the floor with the arms extended and fingers interlaced, facing away from the back (Fig. 30). Focus on keeping the legs straight and stretch the sacroiliac joints and coccyx up toward the ceiling. Hold through any discomfort by rocking from one shoulder to the other.

Center the focus on the spine and gradually extend it from neck to sacrum. Hold momentarily then sit seiza.

Seiza is the traditional Japanese way of sitting. In seiza one feels stable, centered and relaxed. Initial discomfort will gradually disappear with practice of this exercise program. In the beginning, such discomfort can be relieved by placing a thin cushion behind the knees.

2. Dō-In

In this section we apply simple tapping motions by raising loosely clenched fists 8 to 10 inches from the body. Dō-In causes energy to be drawn to the surface. It warms us up. Sitting comfortably in seiza, make loosely clenched fists.

Head

Fig. 31

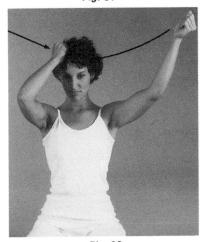
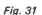

1) On each side of a center line from hairline to base of skull, apply gentle alternate tapping motions in 9 to 10 places on each side (Fig. 31).
2) Repeat in like manner over the temples and around the ears, in 7 to 8 places on each side.
3) Tilt the head forward and slightly to the side. Apply tapping motions to the base of the skull in upward motions 10 times or so (Fig. 32). Repeat on the other side with the other hand.
4) Over the forehead, from a center line toward the temples, apply Dō-In simultaneously 10 times or so (Fig. 33).
5) With open palms, gently slap the face 10 to 15 times simultaneously on both sides (Fig. 34).

Fig. 32   Fig. 33   Fig. 34

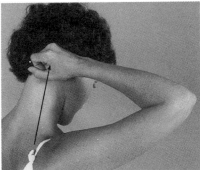

Fig. 35

Then gently brush across closed eyes 3 times (Fig. 35).

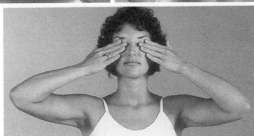

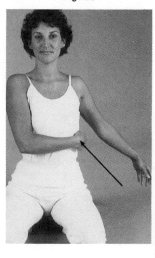

Fig. 36

Chest

7) From lower to upper, side to center of chest make 5 or 6 horizontal lines and give Dō-In to 5 places on each line (Fig. 36). All the while open the chest and keep the spine naturally straight.

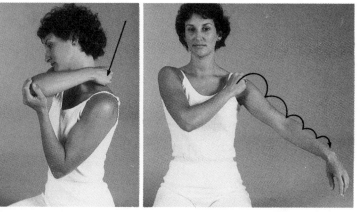

Fig. 37   *Fig. 38*

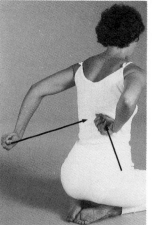

Fig. 39

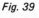

Shoulders

8) Continue across the left shoulder 15 to 20 times (Fig. 37).

Arms

9) Continue down the outside of the left arm, toward the wrist in 5 places (Fig. 38). Repeat twice.

10) Turn the arm over and do likewise. Repeat steps 7 through *10* in mirror image on the right side.

11) Clap hands 10 times or more.

Back

12) Lean forward slightly from the hips, keeping your chest open. With the back of loosely clenched fists make alternate tapping motions down each side of the spine from the base of the shoulder blades, in 5 to 6 places each side (Fig. 39).

13) Continue onto the hips, alternately tapping 7 to 10 times each side (Fig. 40).

Legs

Divide the upper legs into 3 sections: outside, outside of center, inside.

14) With loosely clenched fists, begin on the outside line (gallbladder meridian—GB. m) (Fig. 41). Apply simultaneous tapping motions in 5 places toward the knee. Repeat twice.

15) Continue on the outside of center line (stomach meridian and tripler heater meridian—ST. m and T.H.m) in like manner.

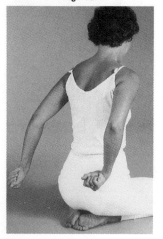

Fig. 40

16) Continue on an inside line (spleen meridian—SP.m) in like manner (Fig. 42). Change position. Open your legs at the knees with feet nearly touching.
17) Apply tapping motions on a deeper inside line (liver meridian—LV.m) toward the knee in 5 places (Fig. 43). Repeat twice.

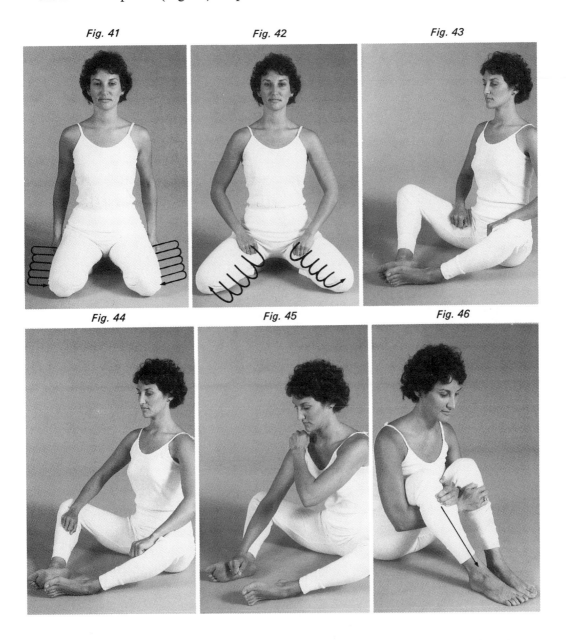

Fig. 41   Fig. 42   Fig. 43

Fig. 44   Fig. 45   Fig. 46

18) Continue on the inside lower leg from knee to ankles in 5 places (Fig. 44). Repeat twice.
19) Continue onto the feet, alternate tapping 10 times or so to each foot (Fig. 45).
20) Draw the knees together and apply simultaneous tapping motions down the sides of the lower legs (GB.m).
21) Open your knees and feet a few inches. From behind your lower legs, weave

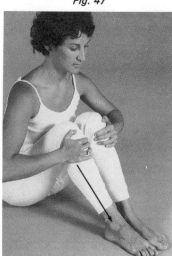

Fig. 47

both hands so that the fingers of each hand are resting on the outside front of the opposite leg, just below the knees. Lightly stretch the knees apart and exhale as you apply simultaneous pressure to the ST.m, from knees to ankles, in 6 to 7 places (Fig. 46). Repeat. Finish by applying pressure with your middle fingers to ST. 36, where you began. The T.H.m runs parallel with the ST.m, approximately 1 inch further to the outside. Shiatsu can be applied here in like manner.

22) Lean forward. Give heel of palm pressure from the bony extensions just below the knees down the sides of the legs (GB.m) to the ankles, in 7 to 8 places (Fig. 47). Repeat. Return to seiza.

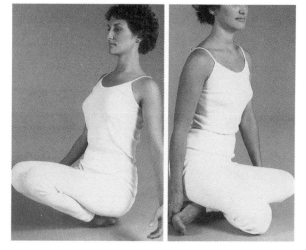

Fig. 48   Fig. 49

3. Exercising the Ankles and Knees

Sit comfortably, knees together, with arms by your sides and back naturally straight. Raise your knees 10 to 12 inches from the floor (Fig. 48). Hold momentarily and return to seiza. Repeat 5 times. The last time hold for a half a minute or more, extending as your body wants to extend. Come into a kneeling position and place the lower left leg behind your right knee. Inhale. While exhaling, sit down and hold the position momentarily (Fig. 49). Come up and inhale. Tucking the leg close behind the knee, once more sit down while exhaling. Repeat. Then repeat twice on the opposite side.

Regular practice of these exercises will aid sitting in seiza, by keeping the ankles and knees flexible.

4. Shiatsu to Lower Legs

Assume a semi-kneeling position. With arms free of tension, place the heels of your palms in the center behind your knees, fingers facing each other

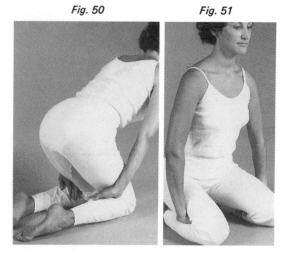

Fig. 50   Fig. 51

(Fig. 50). Apply fairly strong pressure simply by sitting down (Fig. 51). Release by raising your body, then slide your hands to the next point. Continue from knees to Achilles tendons, in 5 to 6 places.

5. Toes

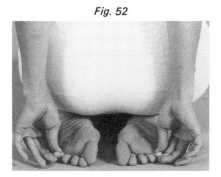

Fig. 52

Ki energy easily stagnates in the fingers and toes since these are turning points for direction of ki flow along the meridians. Massage to points in these areas greatly helps to alleviate pain and stiffness in the limbs.

Firmly pinch the top and bottom of each toe with the index fingers and thumbs, beginning with the little toes (Fig. 52). Stretch each toe away from the foot by leaning your upper body slightly forward.

6. Upper Leg-ST.m

The ST.m follows a line slightly to the outside of center. With broad angle elbow pressure at a diagonal to the upper leg, give shiatsu from hip to knee (Fig. 53), in 3 to 4 places. Repeat. Left leg, left elbow; right leg, right elbow.

Fig. 53

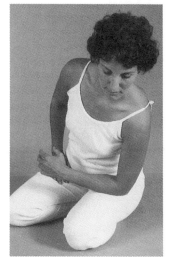

7. Hara Massage

Hara massage takes only 3 or 4 minutes, yet if practiced regularly it has extremely beneficial effects. By reducing stiffness and deeply accumulated hardness, our energy center (which is what the hara is) becomes more supple and ki flow more balanced and harmonious.

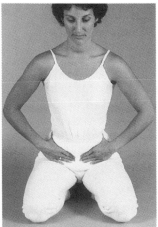

Fig. 54

Lower Hara

1) Sit comfortably in seiza with index fingers and thumbs on your waist.

2) Breathing normally, apply pressure with your fingertips to the lower abdomen, inward and downward in outward moving spirals (Fig. 54).

3) To relieve deep stiffness, inhale. Focus your mind on the area of stiffness. Upon exhalation apply deep pressure with your fingertips and hold. Once more inhale and upon exhalation apply deeper pressure and hold. Once more, repeat.

Upper Hara

Divide the rib cage into three areas: A. lower; B. middle; and C. center.

Fig. 55

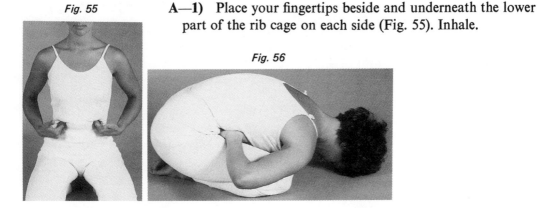

A—1) Place your fingertips beside and underneath the lower part of the rib cage on each side (Fig. 55). Inhale.

Fig. 56

2) Upon exhalation, keeping the chest open and moving from your lower back, bring the shoulders to your knees (Fig. 56). You will find in this position that the abdominal muscles are more relaxed. On both sides, simultaneously apply deep pressure underneath the lower section of the rib cage, in forward, backward, sideways, and circular motions.
3) Once more inhale. Upon exhalation apply deeper pressure and hold. Repeat, applying even deeper pressure. Overall, the lower area relates to the lungs, however deep discomfort on the right side may relate to the gallbladder.
4) Maintaining the same position, point your fingers toward the waistline. Inhale. Upon exhalation apply kneading pressure downward toward the waistline and then upward, then again, deeper. Return to seiza.
B—Place your fingertips beside and underneath the middle section (Fig. 57). Inhale. Upon exhalation repeat steps *2* through *4* as above. These areas relate to the liver on the right side, and stomach and spleen on the left.

Fig. 57   *Fig. 58*

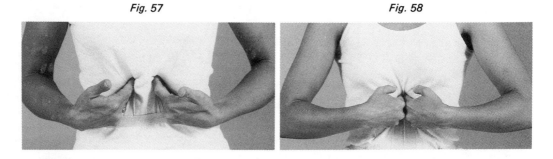

C—Place your hands, back to back, in the central area between the sternum and navel (Fig. 58). Inhale. Repeat steps *2* through *4* as above. The pancreas is located in this area.

8. Deep Breathing

Sit in seiza. Interlace your fingers with palms facing the floor (Fig. 59).
1) Inhale as you make an arc, raising your hands above your head, palms facing the ceiling. Throw strength into your hara and focus your vision on the hands as you gain maximum vertical stretch (Fig. 60).

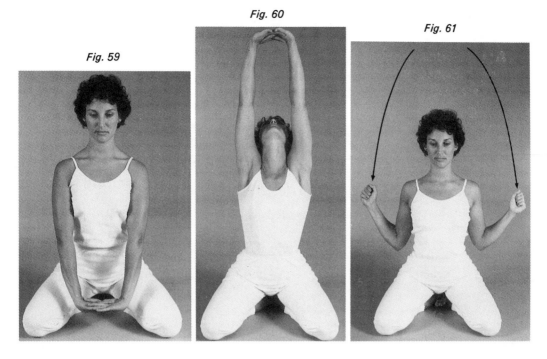

Fig. 59

Fig. 60

Fig. 61

2) Look to the front and hold the stretch for 10 seconds or so as you relax into it.

3) Slowly exhale as you keep the chest open, and move your arms downward on the same plane as your back (Fig. 61).

4) Continue until your elbows touch your sides. Then bring your hands to your sides also. Relax. Repeat at least twice more. Harmonize exhalation and downward movement so that both finish together.

9. *Rotating the Neck, and Self-Shiatsu to the Shoulders*

Sitting in seiza with arms by your side, slowly rotate your head 5 times counterclockwise, 5 times clockwise. Only neck and head should be moving, while your body remains fairly stationary.

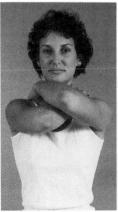

Fig. 62

Cross your bent arms, with elbows outstretched, directly in front of you, one above the other (Fig. 62). Your fingertips are resting on the shoulders on each side of the neck (Fig. 63).

(i) Inhale and raise the arms slightly. (ii) While exhaling, focus your attention on the shoulders, lower the elbows and apply

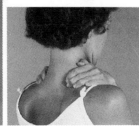

Fig. 63

pressure across the shoulders, from neck to arms in 4 to 5 places, 3 times. If you feel stiffness in any particular area, inhale. While exhaling, apply deep but brisk and repetitive pressure. If you feel weakness, hold on that point throughout the exhalation, and repeat.

10. Arm Meridian Stretches and Wrist Stretches

In seiza, spread the knees a little more than hip width apart. Assume a kneeling position and place the palms on the floor with the fingers facing you (Fig. 64). Inhale.

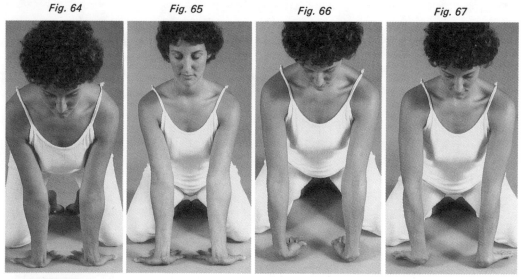

Fig. 64   Fig. 65   Fig. 66   Fig. 67

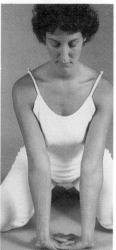

Fig. 68

1) **H.C.m (Heart constrictor meridian) stretch.** While slowly exhaling, return to seiza, maintaining palm contact with the floor as much as possible (Fig. 65). Hold for a few moments. Then, while inhaling, return to the kneeling position, and repeat. If you are supple in this position extend your hands further forward.

2) **L.I.m (Large intestine meridian) stretch.** Turn the palms over so that the back of the hands are on the floor (Fig. 66). It is important not to bend the arms, even if it means not sitting down. Repeat twice as above.

3) **T.H.m (Triple heater meridian) stretch.** With the wrists together as above, turn the fingers away from each other at a 45 degrees angle (Fig. 67). Repeat twice as in step 2.

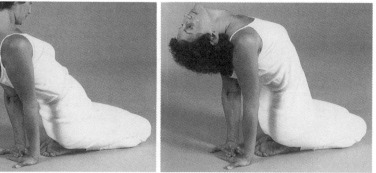

Fig. 69   Fig. 70

4) HT.m (Heart meridian) and S.I.m (Small intestine meridian) stretch. Interlace the fingers and invert the hands so that the palms are on the floor, the palms facing you and little finger side of the palms facing away (Fig. 68). Repeat twice as in steps *2* and *3*. To intensify, stretch each palm to the floor alternately and/or extend the arms further forward.

5) LU. m (Lung meridian) stretch. In seiza with knees together, place the hands behind your back with fingers interlaced as above (Fig. 69). Place the heels of the palms by your feet. Inhale and allow your abdominal muscles to relax. Upon exhalation, roll your head backward and extend the chest forward and upward, while pressing the palms against the floor (Fig. 70). Hold momentarily and repeat.

11. Shiatsu to Arms, Hands, and Fingers

Using the left knee for support, rest your left forearm in front of you, with the right palm over your left. Imagine 3 lines: inside, which is closest; center; and outside.

1) HT.m. With your right knee, beginning just below the elbow, apply shiatsu along an inside line in 3 to 4 places toward and onto the wrist (Fig. 71). Repeat.

2) H.C.m. Raise your body slightly; move forward a little and give knee shiatsu down the center of the arm, as above.

3) LU.m. Raise the thumb side of your left hand and repeat as above, along an outside line, twice (Fig. 72).

4) L.I.m. Turn the palm over and repeat twice as above, along an inside line from the elbow (Fig. 73).

Fig. 71

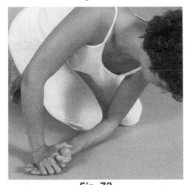

5) T.H.m. Extend your arm forward slightly. This time apply elbow shiatsu down the center of the arm (Fig. 74). Draw your elbow toward you slightly as you proceed.

6) S.I.m. Return to seiza with the lower left arm across your chest. Give thumb shiatsu along an outside line in 6 to 7 places, from elbow toward and onto the wrist (Fig. 75).

7) On the back of the hand imagine 3 lines between the knuckles. Continue with thumb pressure from

| Fig. 72 | Fig. 73 | Fig. 74 |

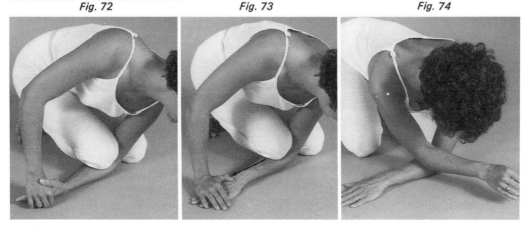

wrist to finger along each |line, in 3 places. Then give thumb shiatsu to L.I.4 between the index finger and thumb.

8) Take the little finger between your index finger and thumb. Apply strong squeezing pressure to the sides of each phalange, stretching the finger from the hand as you proceed. On the points beside the nail apply pressure 3 times (Fig. 76). Then repeat to the top and bottom of each phalange in the same way.

9) Repeat the above steps on the other fingers and thumb.

10) Turn the palm over. Along 3 lines: inside, center, and outside, give thumb pressure from fingers to wrist in 3 places, twice to each line.

11) Repeat mirror image, steps *1* through *10* on the right arm.

12) Finish by interlacing the fingers and stretching away from you and then toward you (Figs. 77 and 78).

13) Repeat the arm meridian stretches of section 10, steps *1* through *5* once more to see the increase in flexibility.

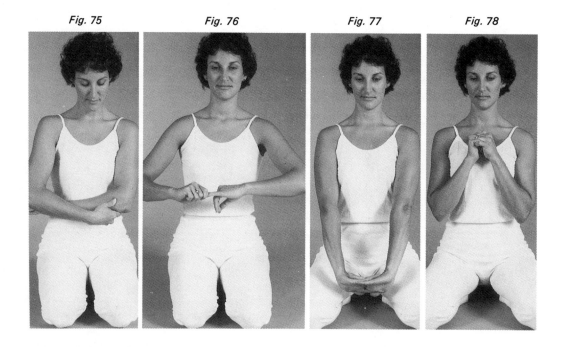

| *Fig. 75* | *Fig. 76* | *Fig. 77* | *Fig. 78* |

12. Stretching the Shoulders

Begin in seiza with your hands behind your back, fingers interlaced. Assume a kneeling position and then place the top of your head on the floor (Fig. 79). Your back should be naturally straight: arms and palms face the ceiling. Inhale.

1) While exhaling, extend the arms over your head as far as is comfortably possible. Hold momentarily and inhale. Upon exhalation, try to extend a little further forward. Repeat at least once more and hold.

2) Keeping the rest of the body fairly stationary, move your arms to the right side. Repeat as above twice. Each time you extend, look for the direction of maximum stretch. Return to the center position and repeat on the left side.

3) Upon returning to the middle position, roll further forward, stretching your

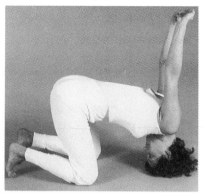

Fig. 79

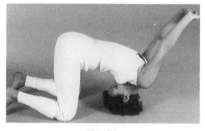

Fig. 80

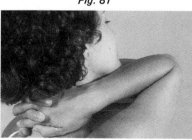

Fig. 81

neck. Inhale. Upon exhalation further extend the hands over your head (Fig. 80). Hold. Repeat twice more. Those with stiff necks should perform this last exercise with hands by the sides of their head.

4) Return to seiza. Interlace your fingers and place them at the base of the skull. Draw your head onto your hands and rotate in semi-circles across the arc created by your interlaced fingers (Fig. 81).

5) In seiza, place the fingertips on your shoulders (Fig. 81). Briskly extend your arms with a flicking motion spiraling outward, 10 times (Fig. 83).

6) With your arms by your sides, finish by shaking hands vigorously for 30 seconds or more so that your whole body moves.

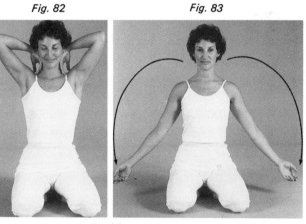

Fig. 82   Fig. 83

13. Rotation

Sitting in seiza and maintaining an upright posture, simply rotate the arms to your sides 10 times in each direction (Fig. 84).

14. Knees and Hips

The purpose of this exercise is to gain flexibility in the knees and ease of movement from the hips while practicing shiatsu.

Sit in seiza with arms extended horizontally in front, one hand on the other (Fig. 85). Inhale. While exhaling, lower your hips

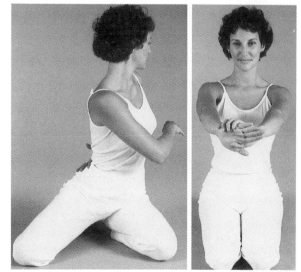

Fig. 84   Fig. 85

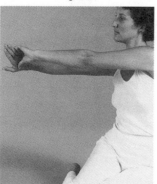

Fig. 86

to one side with arms facing in the other direction (Fig. 68). Then move to the other side. Throughout, your knees should remain together and on the floor. Repeat briskly 5 to 10 times on each side.

15. Spinal Twists

1) Sit in seiza with knees together and inhale. Lean back, placing your left hand on the floor. Keep the chest open and feel a stretch from the knees to your left shoulder (Fig. 87).

Fig. 87

2) Upon exhalation, bring the right arm across your body so that both hands are resting flat on the floor. Hold momentarily, then inhale. Upon exhalation, extend. Hold. Repeat at

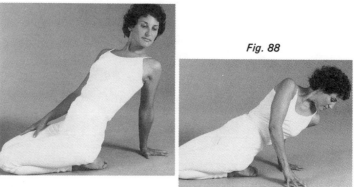

Fig. 88

least once more. This time, with normal breathing hold for 30 to 60 seconds, extending as your body wants to extend. Your head should be facing the floor on a line passing between the knees, which are still together (Fig. 88). Repeat on the right side.

Fig. 89

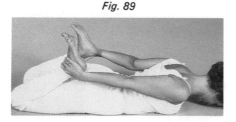

3) To intensify the stretch, come up on your toes and perform the exercise as above.

16. Bow Pose

This exercise opens the chest while stretching the lung meridians in the arms.
1) Lie on the stomach, legs no more than hip width apart, palms by your sides.
2) Bring the feet to the buttocks and grasp your ankles (Fig. 89). Inhale.
3) While exhaling, pull the legs back so that the chest rises and opens (Fig. 90). Look straight ahead and keep the knees fairly close together. Hold for 30 seconds or so. Breathing normally, extend as your body wants to. Relax. Repeat at least once more, holding even longer.

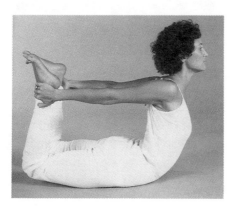

17. *Cobra Pose*

This exercise will bring energy to the kidneys and reproductive organs.

1) Lie on your stomach, legs together, forehead to the floor and palms by the shoulders (Fig. 91). Inhale.

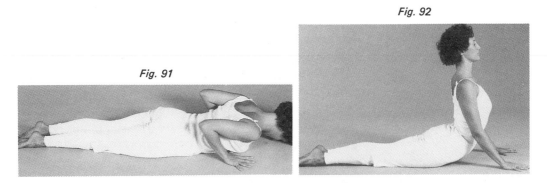

Fig. 92

Fig. 91

2) While exhaling raise your upper torso, keeping the hips on the floor as much as possible (Fig. 92). Contract the buttock muscles to protect the lumbar vertebrae from being pressed together, and extend the torso vertically. You should feel the focus of the extension in the lower dorsal spine, above the lumbar region. Look directly ahead and keep the chest open, shoulders relaxed. Hold for 30 seconds, then relax. Repeat at least once more, holding even longer.

18. *Camel Pose*

This exercise opens the chest and is therefore beneficial to the lungs. It also stimulates the ST.m in the upper legs. If you overexert in this exercise you may have pain in the lower back region on the following day.

1) Get comfortable in a kneeling position with knees hip width apart. Drop your torso backward. Place the left hand on the sole of your left foot: right hand, right foot (Fig. 93). Let your head drop back in a relaxed manner. Inhale.

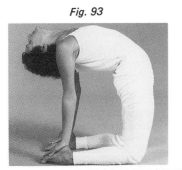

Fig. 93

2) Upon exhalation, extend the hips forward and sternum vertically. Then hold. Once again inhale and while exhaling, extend. Hold. Repeat. This time hold the posture for 30 to 60 seconds. Breathe normally and extend as your body naturally wants to. Relax in a posture similar to Figure 56 only with the arms by the sides. Repeat steps *1* and *2*.

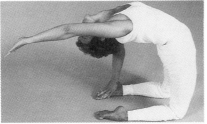

Fig. 94

3) To increase the stretch—while exhaling, raise one arm above the head and hold; then repeat with your other arm (Fig. 94). This pose will stimulate the HT.m in the arms and draw energy to the heart region. If the heart is weak it may also strain it, so perform with caution.

Fig. 95

19. Reclining Hero Pose

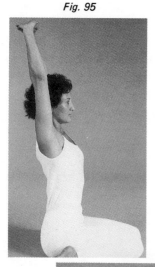

1)   Sit with buttocks between your legs, knees together. Interlace the fingers and while inhaling raise the arms above your head and extend vertically (Fig. 95). Relax into the stretch, then while exhaling bring the arms to your sides.
2)   From the above position lie down with arms extended above your head. Relax in this position for up to 1 minute, keeping the knees together and on the floor (Fig. 96). This exercise stimulates the ST.m in the upper legs. To get up from this pose, make a fist and place below the lumbar vertebrae; use it to propel the body upward.
3)   If you feel pain in this posture perform the following upon returning to seiza. Place the palms on the floor and

Fig. 97

Fig. 96

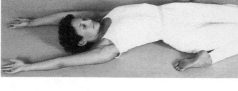

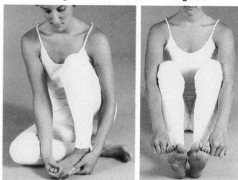

extend your legs back, stretching one leg at a time (Fig. 97).
4)   Return to seiza and give shiatsu to the backs of the lower legs and toes (Exercises 4 and 5).
5)   Sit with your feet in front, heels on the floor.
6)   Give thumb shiatsu to each foot on 6 lines from toes to ankle. Begin with the left foot, giving support with your right hand. The first 4 lines are above the 4 smaller toes, slightly to the little toe side above each one. Beginning above the little toe, give shiatsu in 4 to 5 places,

Fig. 98   Fig. 99

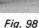

toward the ankle (Fig. 98). Repeat in like manner above the next 3 toes. Repeat on a line between the second and big toe, and then on a line along the inside of the big toe.
7)   Repeat in mirror image on the right foot.
8)   Bring the feet together. Grasp the little toes between your index fingers and thumbs. With firm, squeezing pressure to the sides of the toes, rotate and stretch the toes away from the feet (Fig. 99). Repeat simultaneously on each other pair of toes.
9)   Return to seiza and give elbow shiatsu along the upper leg, holding wherever you still feel pain (Exercise 6).
10)   Repeat the exercise again and hold for longer. You should feel some of the stiffness and tension to have subsided.

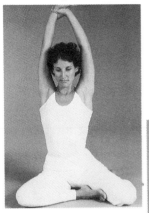

Fig. 100

20. Side Stretches

1) Sit in a half-seiza posture with your left leg extended backward. Take the right hand in your left; while inhaling, raise both arms above your head, extending vertically as much as possible (Fig. 100).

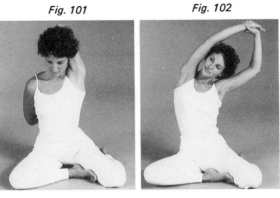

Fig. 101   Fig. 102

2) While holding your breath, let the abdominal muscles relax so that the breath appears to sink into the lower abdomen. Drop the left arm over your shoulder and grasp the left hand with your right from behind (Fig. 101). Upon exhalation lean forward from the lower back, stretching your left arm vertically as much as it is comfortably possible. Keep the chest open and do not look down too far. Hold for a few moments, inhale, and upon exhalation extend further forward, hold, then extend. Then hold for 30 seconds or so and then repeat. This exercise stimulates the HT.m.

3) Once more inhaling, raise the arms above your head. Upon exhalation, keeping your torso nearly vertical to the floor, stretch the arms to your left side and hold momentarily (Fig. 102). Release. Raise the arms above your head once again, extend vertically and inhale. After relaxing momentarily, repeat again twice. Repeat mirror image on the right side. This exercise stimulates the GB.m and TH.m in the torso.

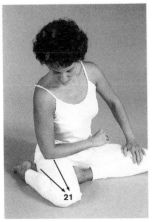

Fig. 103

21. Shiatsu to the Legs

Sit in the same half-seiza posture with your right leg extended backward.

To simplify meridian location, compass directions will be used: N (north); N.E. (northeast); N.N.E. (north of northeast), etc. North is front, east is right side.

A. Right upper leg

1) *T.H.m:* Over the N.E. section of the leg, by simply leaning your body forward, apply broad flat elbow pressure from hip to knee in 3 to 4 places (Fig. 103-1). Repeat.

2) *GB.m:* On the most easterly line, apply pressure as above (Fig. 103-2).

B. Right lower leg

3) *GB.m:* Place the left hand on your right knee. Fro[m] the bony extension below the outside of the knee (the head of the fibula), apply thumb pressure along a most easterly line to the ankle in 7 to 8 places (Fig. 104). Repeat.

4) *L.I.m:* On a line parallel with the GB.m but beside the fibula, two thumb widths closer to you, apply thumb shiatsu as above.

5) *BL.m* (Bladder meridian): In like manner, apply thumb pressure down the center of the calf muscle to the Achilles' tendon in 3 to 4 places.

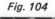

Fig. 104

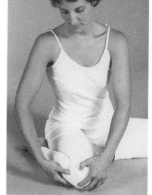

Fig. 105

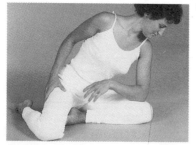

C. Left upper leg

6) *SP. m* (Spleen meridian): Along a line approximately 1 1/2 inches from the lateral side of the leg, give elbow shiatsu toward and onto the knee in 3 to 4 places (Fig. 105).

7) *S.I.m:* Down the center of the upper leg, apply shiatsu as above.

8) *LV.m* (Liver meridian): Below the gracilis tendon in the upper leg, apply shiatsu as above. To facilitate shiatsu here, position your elbow on the upper point before leaning your body considerably forward to apply pressure (Fig. 106).

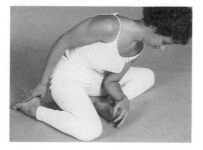

Fig. 107

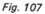

D. Left lower leg

Place your right hand over the bottom part of the lower leg.

9) *KD.m* (Kidney meridian): From behind the knee (KD. 10) apply shiatsu with your left elbow just over the calf muscle in 3 places. Repeat.

10) *LV.m.* Repeat as above, deeply, on a line immediately anterior to the calf muscle (Fig. 107).

11) *SP.m.* From the knee, repeat as above, immediately in front of the LV.m, beside the tibia. Change your support: the left elbow now rests above your left knee (over SP. 10). With your right elbow continue down the SP.m to the ankle in 3 to 4 places (Fig. 108). Repeat. Continue onto the arch of the foot in 2 to 3 places. Repeat.

Fig. 108

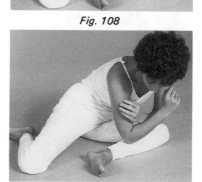

12) Support the left foot with the left hand. With your right thumb and index finger pinch and stretch each toe away from the foot, beginning with the little toe (Fig. 109).

13) Come into a kneeling position. Imagine 3 lines: inside, center, and outside. Beginning on the outside line from toes to heel, give thumb shiatsu in 4 to 5 places on each line.

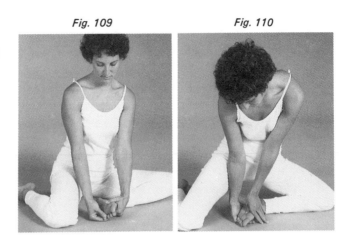

Fig. 109   Fig. 110

14) Place your thumb over "Yū-sen" (KD. 1). Inhale. Upon exhalation apply pressure and hold (Fig. 110). Inhale again. Once more apply pressure and hold. Repeat. Repeat steps *1* through *14* in mirror image on the other side.

22. *Heart Meridian and Small Intestine Meridian Stretch*

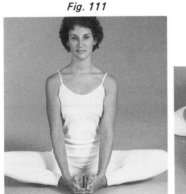

Fig. 111

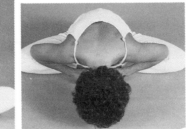

Fig. 112

1) Sit with your knees apart, feet together, spine naturally straight. Interlace your fingers and place the hands around the toes and feet (Fig. 111). Gently rock from side to side to get comfortable in the position. Inhale.

2) Upon exhalation, extend your body forward from the lower back and bring your knees to the floor (Fig. 112). Hold momentarily, then inhale. Repeat this process at least 4 more times. Following the last exhalation, hold for up to 1 minute, breathing normally. Allow your body to extend as it wants to. Attempt to place your knees and chest on the floor.

23. *Liver Meridian and Ballbladder Meridian Stretch*

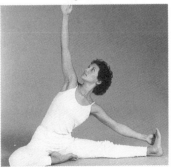

Fig. 113

1) Sit with the left leg extended to the side, Achilles tendon stretched. Place the sole of the right foot against the inside thigh of the left leg. With your back on a plane perpendicular to the floor, grasp the left foot with your left hand.

2) As you inhale, raise and extend your right arm vertically above your head (Fig. 113).

3) As you exhale, lower the right hand to your left

foot and hold (Fig. 114). Inhale. Upon exhalation, extend a little more. Hold momentarily, inhale and repeat, then again hold, inhale, and extend. Upon the last repetition hold for 30 to 60 seconds or more. With normal breathing, extend as your body naturally wants to extend. Repeat in mirror image on the right side.

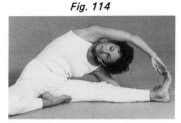

Fig. 114

Fig. 115

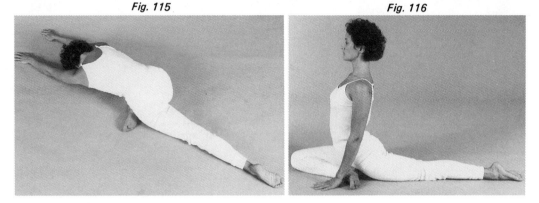

Fig. 116

4) Repeat again on the left side. This time hold for up to 2 minutes. Close your eyes and focus on the areas of tension. Breathing normally, extend as your body wants to.

5) Return to the original position. Extend the bent leg another 12 inches or so forward. Roll your body over the bent leg and extend the arms above your head, chest on the floor (Fig. 115). Gently rock from side to side, stretching the muscles through the buttocks area and the inside leg. Continue for 30 seconds or more.

6) Then place the hands by your sides, a little more than hip width apart. Raise your upper body in a similar way to the Cobra position (Fig. 116). Hold for 30 seconds or more.

7) Repeat steps *4* through *6* on the right side.

24. *Forward Bend Kidney Meridian and Bladder Meridian Stretch*

Fig. 117

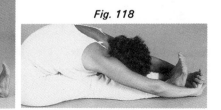

1) Sit with spine erect, legs extended, Achilles tendons stretched. Interlace your fingers.

2) As you inhale, raise the hands above your head. Hold while relaxing into the stretch (Fig. 117).

3) As you exhale, lower the arms to your feet (Fig. 118). The movement should be from the pelvis and hips, not shoulders. While holding, once more inhale. As you exhale, extend. Hold, then repeat once more, this time holding for 30 seconds or so.

Fig. 118

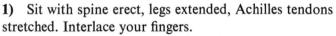

4) Repeat the exercise again, this time holding for up to 2 minutes.

25. Abdominal Exercise

Fig. 119

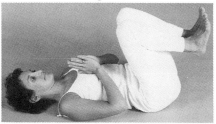

Fig 120

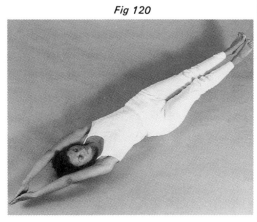

It is best to do one or more abdominal exercises each day, alternating from day to day.

1) Lie on your back. Bring your knees to your chest

Fig. 121

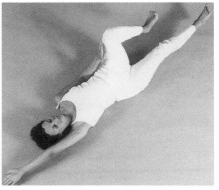

about hip width apart and your hands over your chest as if in prayer (Fig. 119). Inhale. As you exhale, extend your legs and arms away from each other horizontally. Finish the extension with both hands and knees a few inches from the floor, arms and legs straight, Achilles tendons stretched (Fig. 120). As you inhale, return to the beginning position. Repeat 20 to 50 times. Try to harmonize one cycle of exhalation with one complete extension. The slower the exercise is performed the stronger the effect. This exercise will benefit more the large intestine.

Fig. 122

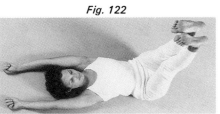

Fig. 123

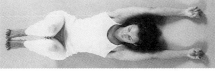

Fig. 124

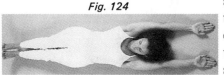

A variation on the above exercise: Bring the arm and leg together on one side, the arm and leg on the other side extended (Fig. 121). Inhale. Extend the contracted side without touching the floor and contract the extended side. Repeat 15 times each side.

2) Lie on your back, Achilles tendons stretched. Extend the arms above your head, shoulder width apart, and make loosely clenched fists. Slowly inhale as you raise the legs to a 90 degree angle (Fig. 122). Remember to keep the legs straight, Achilles tendons stretched. Hold momentarily. Bring the knees together to your chest (Fig. 123). As you exhale extend the legs horizontally a few inches from the floor (Fig. 124). Exhalation and full extension should finish together. Without the feet touching the floor, repeat the exercise 10 to 30 times. Upon the last extension, hold your feet a few inches from the floor to the count of 10 or 15 before relaxing.

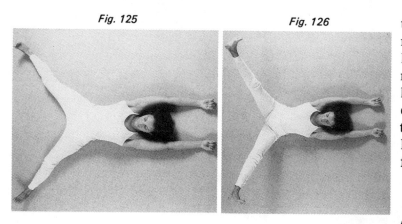

Fig. 125

Fig. 126

This exercise tends to strengthen more the lower hara. To strengthen more the upper hara repeat this exercise in reverse: that is bring your legs to the chest first, then vertically,

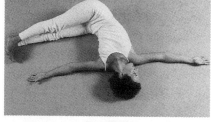

Fig. 127

then in an arc to within a few inches of the floor.

3) To further strengthen the lower part of the lower hara, including reproductive organs, begin Exercise (2) with your legs apart, Achilles tendons stretched (Fig. 125). Slowly inhale as you raise the legs to a 90 degree angle (Fig. 126). Hold momentarily and then do either of the following procedures:

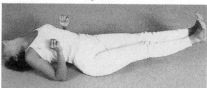

Fig. 128

(i) Lower your legs to the starting position just above the floor as you exhale. Repeat up to 20 times.
(ii) Bring the knees together to your chest (see Fig. 123).

As you exhale, extend your legs horizontally as in Exercise (2). Upon full extension once again begin the exercise with legs apart. Repeat 10 to 30 times.

4) To stimulate the liver-gallbladder and stomach-spleen-pancreas, employ the following technique:

Lie on your back with arms extended to the sides, legs together extended, Achilles tendon stretched. As you inhale, raise your legs to a 90 degree angle. Upon exhalation, lower your legs at right angles to the torso, to the left side (Fig. 127). Hold momentarily a few inches from the floor. You should now be looking toward the right side. While inhaling raise your legs to a vertical position and while exhaling extend to the right side, your head facing to the left side. Repeat on each side 5 to 10 times.

5) A more vigorous exercise that stimulates heart-small intestine and lungs-large intestine is the following:

Lie on your back with legs extended, Achilles tendons stretched. Arch the back so that the top of your head is on the floor. With the elbows by your sides, make loosely clenched fists with the lower arms pointing toward the ceiling. Inhaling, raise your legs about 10 inches from the floor (Fig. 128). Upon exhalation, briskly lower your legs 6 inches. With a short inhalation, raise the legs and with short exhalation lower them. Repeat the exercise, pumping briskly 30 times.

A variation on this exercise is the legs apart as in Exercise (3), for similar effect to Exercise (3).

Finish by lying on your back, arms by your sides palms up, and eyes closed. Relax completely for 1 or 2 minutes.

Chapter 6

How to Apply Zen Shiatsu Pressure

The goal of shiatsu is to strengthen the receiver's innate healing power. We can achieve this by balancing the flow of ki energy along the meridians. The function of the Zen Shiatsu practitioner is to initiate the movement and redirection of ki. Shiatsu is stationary pressure to a point—the pressure of heaven's force. There is a distinct method in applying shiatsu pressure: how to press is equally if not more important than knowing where to press. The purpose of this chapter is to review these most important principles regarding the application of pressure.

1. Relaxation

Heaven's force is more predominant at night or when we are still. At these times we tend to draw in more of heaven's force, while in the daytime or when moving, we draw more on earth's force.

Heaven's force promotes relaxation. In such a state we restore our energies: we revitalize. Since it is predominantly the pressure of heaven's force, shiatsu promotes relaxation. Shiatsu is even more effective when we establish a relaxed environment before beginning. Conversely, tension acts as a barrier. The body closes up to either giving or receiving. Shiatsu is in the main a one-way transfer of ki from giver to receiver. As the giver extends ki, that which is given is replenished by universal ki. Since shiatsu induces relaxation the giver is able to connect with the receiver's ki, from which the physical body arises.

Let us look at the principle of relaxation for the giver and receiver.
• *The Receiver*
Shiatsu should be practiced in a warm, quiet, pleasant environment. Since shiatsu is best practiced on the floor, one will need a *futon* and a small firm pillow. A thin cushion for the giver to kneel on may also be helpful. For receivers with a stiff neck it may be helpful in the supine position to place a thin cushion under their chest; cotton sheets and a cotton thermal blanket to cover the receiver may also be useful. It is advisable for the receiver to wear loose, comfortable natural fiber clothing, preferably with long sleeves. Clothing is worn to reduce the friction which occurs with direct skin contact, especially in the warmer months, when the body perspires. Moisture would cause uneven pressure, since the giver's hand would not be able to slide smoothly from one point to the next. The receiver should refrain from eating at least three hours before shiatsu and from drinking stimulant beverages on the same day.

It is important that the receiver be kept warm. In shiatsu, energy moves to the center, often leaving the extremities cold. If the body is cold it is likely to become tense, preventing the exchange of ki. Since a room is coldest at floor level, we should pay special attention to heating.

For those who are talkative, allow them to speak for a while but discourage conversation once shiatsu is well in progress. It is ideal if the receiver closes his or her eyes, remains silent and simply focuses on the giver's touch.

To test if the receiver is relaxed, lift a limb and then let it gently drop. If it remains in the air, explain to the receiver the importance of letting go—to lay back, close their eyes, do nothing, and hopefully enjoy.

• *The Giver*

In posture, there are two important indications that the giver is relaxed. First, the body's weight is on the underside, which means that posture follows heaven's force, the force of gravity. The shoulders are relaxed, the arms fall naturally to the sides: the posture is stable and more than likely both knees are on the floor. The back is naturally straight. Second, energy is focused in our hara, more specifically at the tanden. There is a tendency for Western people to center in their chest but with practice one can learn to center in the hara.

In giving shiatsu the first consideration is to make the massage as enjoyable as possible. If not, the receiver will be unable to open up to our shiatsu. This is not to say that there will be no pain. However, there is good pain and there is bad pain and there are ways of minimizing even good pain. Bad pain arises from faulty technique, such as slipping off a muscle or applying excessively strong pressure. Good pain lasts momentarily, remaining well within the threshold of endurance.

Some people will find their first shiatsu massage to be a little uncomfortable. Probably it is simply because they are not familiar with the quality of shiatsu pressure. One can assume a better response with subsequent treatments. However it may take three or four sessions until a receiver fully opens up to the benefits of shiatsu.

When we give shiatsu there are three things to consider: our posture; our supporting hand; and our moving hand. To explain in detail we need to introduce the next principle.

2. Principle of Support

Masunaga interpreted the Chinese character for person 人 as two people supporting each other. He would also often talk of "skin-ship" in an age of crowded solitude. In-shiatsu, he pointed out, the receiver depends upon our support, while we in turn, literally depend upon them for supporting our own body weight.

When we pray we unite our hands to establish a feeling of oneness within ourselves. When we give shiatsu, in like manner we *always* apply both hands, to establish a sense of oneness between giver and receiver. It is a sense of oneness we take for granted until it is not there, in much the same way that we may not realize the oneness of a healthy mind and body until illness arises.

Though we apply both hands to the body each performs a different function. Our left hand is dominated by heaven's force: a force moving to a point. In other words, this force promotes stability. In shiatsu the left hand is usually stationary, supporting the right. Since the right hand is dominated by earth's force, it is the moving hand. However since heaven's force is far greater than earth's force, we can see that the supporting hand is actually of more importance than the moving one. An important rule to remember is that we always apply the supporting hand before the moving one. In the movements of our two hands once more we can see the two axes, vertical and horizontal. In actual practice it is not always possible for the left hand to support;

however we adhere to this principle as much as possible and nearly always one hand will support while the other moves.

Let us now look at the first two principles from a practical point of view.

• *Posture*

The giver first needs to establish a posture which is comfortable to work in. Seiza (Fig. 148) can be considered the standard posture. It is the most stable and centered. In this posture we move from our lower back, not from our shoulders. The back is naturally straight and there is no tension in our limbs. Like the test for the receiver, if someone were to lift and then drop an arm, it would naturally fall to our side, following the line of heaven's force.

There are numerous variations on seiza which we can apply. The following are some of the most common:

(i)   Seiza on toes (see Fig. 166). The purpose of this posture is to gain extra height and leverage.

(ii) Seiza with knees at various distances apart, on toes or not (see Fig. 149)—to vary our height.

(iii) Seiza with one knee pointing forward, the other at an angle of 45 degrees or more (see Fig. 155)—to gain even greater leverage than when we are just on our toes. The further away the outside leg, the greater the leverage.

(iv) Seiza with one knee on the floor and one supporting in the lower back (see Fig. 160)—to give stable support so that the receiver can concentrate on our pressure.

Another standard posture is kneeling on all fours (see Figs. 247, 318). In this position it is important that our back be naturally straight and again we move from the hips. Our knees are usually a few inches from the body. The further back they are, the stronger the pressure we can apply.

Other standard positions also include the principle of support. That is, where possible we support the receiver with our own body. This support enables the receiver to relax and concentrate on our touch without the need to make compromising adjustments to uncomfortable postures. For example in doing the shoulders in a sitting position, our feet follow the shape of the buttocks and our knees offer support within the shoulder blade area (see Fig. 174).

Another useful posture is what we shall term half or semi-kneeling, similar to genuflection. In this position we integrate our movement by leaning the outside leg on our arm: here, pressure actually comes in a circle from the supporting hand, through the body to the hand giving shiatsu (see Fig. 191).

• *The Supporting Hand*

Once we assume a comfortable posture we apply the supporting hand. Usually support is with a palm, free of tension, that follows the contours of the receiver's body. However we can also use thumb, elbow, or palms and knee together for support. Sometimes the support comes from the opposite direction of the hand giving shiatsu (see Figs. 153, 191, 245). In his case the pressure is coming in a circle from the supporting hand to the hand giving shiatsu. In other words we lean forward with the giving hand and simultaneously lean back with the supporting one. In shiatsu there is no pushing or pulling.

We can perform some tests that show the importance of the supporting hand:

(i) Sit in seiza opposite your partner and apply pressure with your right thumb anywhere on the inside middle arm. Without letting up, apply the same amount of pressure with the left thumb, just above the right. If the receiver is concentrating, he or she should notice that the first way felt sharper and indeed that pressure with support was more comfortable. With support we can apply stronger and deeper pressure without any additional discomfort.

(ii) If we hold a toy slinky with our hands close together, we will notice that it will move quickly and rhythmically. However as we move our hands apart, the slinky's movement will begin to falter and at a certain point collapse. Similarly, in giving shiatsu it is wise that our supporting hand remain close to the moving one. The precise distance apart will depend on the type of pressure we are giving and the condition that we are treating.

• *The Moving Hand*

The following are the standard ways of giving Zen Shiatsu:

(1) General palm pressure
(2) Heel of palm pressure
(3) Clasping pressure
(4) Thumb pressure
(5) Fingertip pressure
(6) Elbow pressure
(7) Knee pressure

(1) *General Palm Pressure*

General or whole of palm pressure employs an open palm that follows the contours of the receiver's body. Pressure is even, from the heel of the palm to the tips of the fingers (Fig. 129). General palm is the most commonly used type of pressure in Zen Shiatsu and is usually applied to an area before other techniques such as thumb or elbow pressure. It is the most soothing and relaxing form, accustoming the body to our touch before applying deeper or stronger pressure. It is also the most sensitive way to feel for a response. For these reasons it is perhaps the best technique for those beginning to learn shiatsu.

Fig. 129

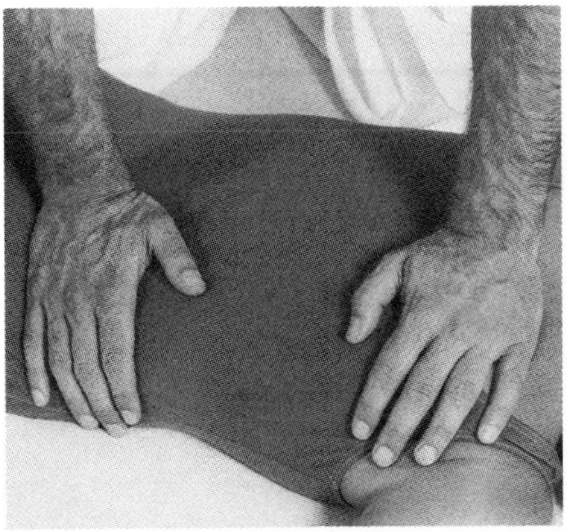

(2) *Heel of Palm Pressure*

Heel of palm simply focuses pressure within this area of the hand. It is deeper than general palm pressure and can be quite strong. The fingers do not necessarily touch the body, and once again the entire palm is free of tension (see Fig. 256). With general palm pressure we cover a whole area, for example the side of the upper leg with 3 to 4 placements of pressure. With heel of palm pressure we would focus on just one meridian in that area.

When giving either general or heel of palm pressure to an arm or leg, the supporting hand rests above or over a joint (see Figs. 213 and 274). The most common postures for these two kinds of pressure are seiza on toes and kneeling on all fours. The most common form of support is an open palm.

(3) *Clasping or Squeezing Pressure*
Clasping pressure is excellent for the arms, especially on aged, frail or thin people. In the supine position we can also use clasping pressure on the lower legs. Clasping comes not from the fingertips but from even contraction of the whole palm, similar to gentle squeezing (Fig. 130, left hand).

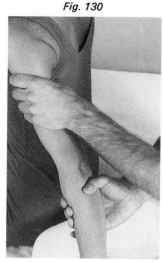
Fig. 130

(4) *Thumb Pressure*
In traditional shiatsu, thumb pressure is the most commonly used technique. The most comfortable postures are variations on seiza, kneeling on all fours, and kneeling on one knee with one foot on the floor (see Figs. 131, 154, and 243). The most often used forms of support are with palm or thumb (see Figs. 131 and 133).

When we apply pressure we use neither the padding of the thumb nor the tip, but the area in-between. The thumb should not be bent at the joint, but rather

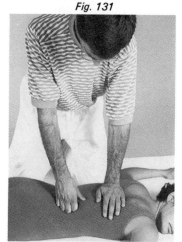
Fig. 131

should follow one naturally straight line flowing along the arm to the fingertip (Fig. 132).

There are two popular forms of thumb pressure:

(a) *Using the fingers splayed for support.* In this method the splayed fingers act like shock absorbers for the pressure focused in the thumb. The best support is the same form with the left

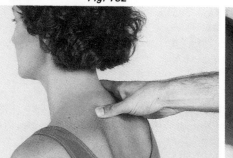
Fig. 132
Fig. 133

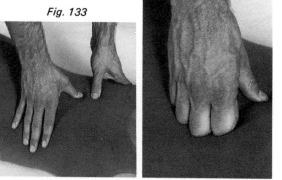
Fig. 134

hand (Fig. 133). In general, both thumbs apply pressure to points on the same meridian.

(b) *Making a fist.* The second phalange of the fingers follows the contours of the body and supports the pressure focused in the thumb (Fig. 134). The best form of support with this technique is an open palm (see Fig. 131).

Another method which Masunaga used in the sitting position employed the second phalange of the index finger with the thumb. This technique covers more area as the pressure is even between the thumb and finger joint. The thumb and finger can be together or apart. What is important is that the whole second phalange of the finger rests on the body (Fig. 135).

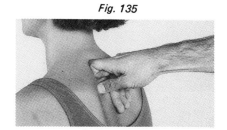

Fig. 135

Thumb pressure can be deep but it is a little sharp and lacks the power of elbow pressure. It can also be tiring for the practitioner. When possible, the most effective method is to apply pressure along a line of no more than 6 inches or so. Then move the supporting hand down to the last point of pressure and continue on, for example Figs. 258 and 259.

(5) *Fingertip Pressure*

Fingertip pressure is effective over the chest in the sitting position or around the shoulder joint in the side position (see Fig. 174). Pressure is given with support by the thumb on the shoulder or arm and simply leaning your body forward: the pressure comes from your whole body through your fingertips, not solely from the fingertips.

(6) *Elbow Pressure*

Since elbow pressure can be very strong, it is best to master the preceding techniques first. However, after general palm pressure elbow pressure is the most commonly used technique in Zen Shiatsu.

There are definite advantages in the use of elbow pressure. It is easier on the giver and covers more area more quickly. The pressure is stronger and yet it is more comfortable than some of the other techniques mentioned. Further, with practice one can develop as much sensitivity to the receiver's response as with the other methods. We feel for relaxation in the receiver's muscles: it will prompt us to release then reapply pressure in order for our elbow to feel correctly placed.

There are a number of postures especially appropriate for elbow shiatsu. These include seiza on toes, kneeling on all fours, and seiza with one leg pointed directly in front, the other at an angle of 45 degrees away or more. The further we extend our body away from the receiver the more we lean, hence the stronger our potential pressure. Fig. 137 is a milder version of Fig. 136 which demonstrates this principle. Sometimes we kneel on the knee closest to the receiver's body and place our other foot on the floor (see Fig. 248).

Fig. 136

Fig. 137

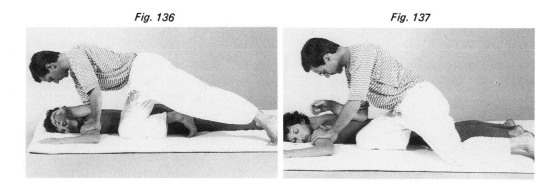

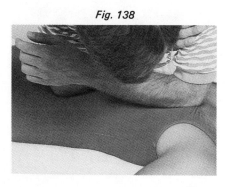

Fig. 138

The most common form of support is with the palm (see Fig. 250), however we can use our elbow instead (Fig. 138). Support can be at a distance, as when we give shiatsu beside the spine in the prone position, or close by when working over a limited area.

The hand of the arm can be open or closed. If closed make a loosely clenched fist, which contracts just slightly with the application of pressure. When applying elbow pressure, always begin with a broad, flat angle; to intensify, raise your arm gradually. The best area of the elbow to apply pressure with, even when broad and flat, is toward the area below the elbow. Although it may sometimes appear otherwise in the photographs in this book, this is indeed how pressure is being applied (Fig. 139-1). Pressure can be applied with the upper arm as well. In this technique lean forward to apply the elbow, then lean back with your whole body, drawing the elbow toward you (Fig. 139-2).

With the elbow, it is best to apply pressure across the muscle, which means the lower arm will constantly vary its direction as you move from one point to the next.

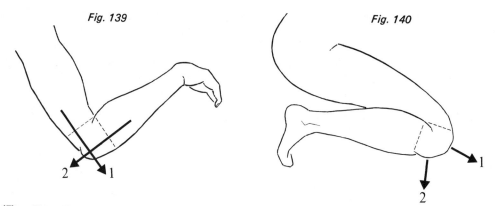

Fig. 139

Fig. 140

(7) *Knee Pressure*

Knee pressure is commonly used on the arms and legs, especially in supine and prone positions. Since knee pressure can be very strong, it is important that it be administered correctly.

Usually after giving general palm pressure we apply support with both hands. In the posture of seiza on toes, move your body forward and let the knee giving shiatsu rest on the beginning point (see Fig. 263). Get comfortable. Then raise your body to a height in accordance with the amount of pressure you wish to apply (see Fig. 264).

We can give pressure with the front of our knee (Fig. 140-1) or with the part connecting with the lower leg (Fig. 140-2). To apply the former method we simply move forward; to apply the latter technique we move downward.

Surprisingly, knee pressure can be more effective if both knees are employed. However this technique requires more skill than using one knee alone. Place the supporting hands on the body then the supporting knee above the knee (Figs. 141 and 142) or elbow joint (Fig. 143), resting comfortably. With all support systems stable, apply pressure with the moving knee.

Both knees can also be applied to give stationary pressure. In this case, knees are usually together. This technique is especially useful when the meridian is kyo (Figs. 144 through 146).

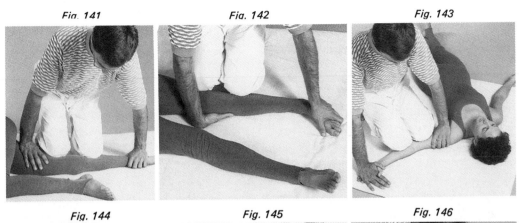

Fig. 141   Fig. 142   Fig. 143

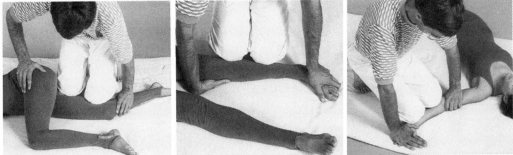

Fig. 144   Fig. 145   Fig. 146

3. Vertical Pressure

Visualize a cross-section of a limb as a circle. Shiatsu pressure is dominated by heaven's force, a force moving toward the center of the limb from all directions. In other words, that force would appear as vertical at any point on the surface. To be in harmony with this force our pressure is always vertical to the surface of the body receiving shiatsu.

4. Natural Leaning Pressure

Shiatsu is natural leaning pressure. Natural pressure is heaven's force, or gravity going vertically downward. It is the vertical application of the hands to the body in a relaxed state. Leaning pressure is earth's force, it is the horizontal movement of our body from one hand to the other which makes the deep application of pressure possible. In other words, with natural leaning pressure we harmonize heaven's and earth's forces within ourselves at the point of pressure.

Further, if we follow through with this principle our weight should be in our hands, since heaven's force is moving downward. This situation will indeed be the case if we are relaxed. In addition, we move our consciousness into our hands at the point of pressure, uniting mind and body by simply concentrating on what we are doing.

5. Keeping the Tanden as Center, Apply Shiatsu by Moving Your Whole Body

Masunaga used to say that hara equalled intention, while hips equalled behavior. That is, our intentions manifest into behavior through our hips. The tanden lies some three finger-widths below the navel. It is the energy center of the whole body, the center common to all people. Keeping the tanden as center as you change positions involves moving the whole body.

If we imagine energy bifurcating at the tanden into two lines ending in our hands, then we can visualize our whole body as a lever. To experience this for yourself extend your arms horizontally and turn from the hips slightly to one side. This motion will automatically extend one arm and draw back the other. It can be contrasted with moving only from the wrists. In the latter case the arms move but the body does not; the giver loses connection with his or her own center and the two points of pressure will feel as two distinct points. However, by moving from the tanden the two points will feel as one. We can compare this action with the functioning of screwdrivers. We can take out a screw with either a short or long screwdriver. Both can do the job. However, it can be done more easily, with less effort, by using the longer tool. In like manner, both a four cylinder and V8 powered car can travel at fast speeds, but the latter will do it with greater ease and comfort.

By moving from our tanden, it is easier on the giver and more comfortable for the receiver, even though the pressure may be deeper and stronger.

6. Apply Pressure Slowly in the Beginning and Follow Through

If one car towing another takes off too quickly a rope connecting the two would snap. However, if the same auto takes off slowly, it can build up momentum and both cars can travel quite rapidly.

By applying pressure slowly in the beginning, we can sense the amount of pressure comfortable for the receiver. While our pressure may be deep and strong, we always remain well within the receiver's threshold of pain. If we exceed this limit, the receiver's body will close up to our pressure. Indications of this effect can show in the most subtle of reactions at various places throughout the receiver's body.

Further, with each application we visualize applying pressure even before touching the body and visualize following through after maximum pressure is applied. We could liken this approach to a tennis player who begins the swing before hitting the ball and continues the movement after hitting.

7. Don't Make Waves

In some schools of shiatsu, pressure is applied to a point and then released by taking the thumbs off the body and moving to the next point. This approach is similar to Dō-In which tends to stimulate the body into activity, while Zen Shiatsu tends to promote relaxation.

Thus in Zen Shiatsu we apply pressure to a point by leaning in on the hand applying pressure and release by moving our body weight back onto the supporting hand. Still maintaining contact with the receiver's body, we slide our hand to the next point and once more lean in to apply stationary pressure. The distance between points of pressure is fairly constant. However, the tempo and depth to which we apply pressure are coordinated with the response that we sense from the receiver's body. Overall, we establish a rhythm, keeping a natural flow of one movement leading into the next.

The receiver should breathe normally, although their respiration rate will be largely regulated by the timing of our pressure. The giver should also breathe normally, exhaling upon applying pressure, inhaling while moving on to the next point.

8. The Pressure of Both Hands Equals One

We can observe this principle within the symbol of yin and yang: the Tai Chi Tu. That is, the more pressure we apply with one hand, the less proportionately is given with the other. Thus we subtly and constantly shift our weight from one hand to the other as we apply pressure.

9. Maximum Comfortable Stretch

In the morning soon after arising, we are likely to stretch before beginning with the day's activities. Simple stretching promotes the flow of ki along the meridians. In our practice we employ this principle where possible, stretching a meridian before giving shiatsu. Stretching also has the effect, in some cases, of drawing a meridian toward the surface, making it easier to treat.

We may take the leg meridian stretches as examples. Each stretch is actually two simultaneous stretches. First, with the supporting hand over the hara, the stretch is downward at the knee. It is also away from the hara along a line of the meridian you are working on, extending into infinity (see Figs. 320 and 324).

Another important point regarding stretching relates to support. When we are stretching against a joint, the joint needs to be well supported in a way counter to the stretch. This principle can be seen in arm meridian stretches (see Fig. 172). Here the stretch is upward and backward simultaneously and the shoulder joint is well supported by pressure coming from the opposite direction. The receiver's body is supported by our hara and upper leg.

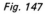

Fig. 147

In the case of wrist stretches it is important that the support with the index finger and thumb be right over the joint (Fig. 147). In this example we first stretch the palm upward against our support; then to intensify the stretch we draw the arm slightly downward at the wrist.

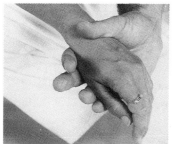

10. Constantly Adjust Your Pressure According to the Condition of the Receiver's Body

When we drive a car our feet are constantly on either the brake or accelerator as we increase our speed on clear roads and slow down for the corners. In our shiatsu we establish a basic rhythm suitable for each individual receiver. However within that overall rhythm we will need to constantly adjust the depth, intensity, and general quality of our pressure as we note changes in the response. In this way we maintain oneness with the receiver.

We will notice in the following chapter such phrases as "with the right palm stationary, give left thumb pressure across the left shoulder in 5 to 6 places." These "5 to 6 places" represent points to which we apply stationary pressure. They are usually along a line and only some, if any, are recognized tsubos. On average it would take less than 5 to 6 seconds to complete this line of pressure. The general tempo at which we apply pressure is about the same as a normal rate of counting from 1 to 6 or a little faster.

However, we adjust the tempo as well as strength and depth of pressure more individually. Shiatsu can be deep and strong but it should be comfortable and well within the limits of a person's threshold of pain or discomfort. Basically, shiatsu should be an enjoyable experience.

Let us now consider the variations on what we might call standard pressure. First we need to consider the connection between kyo and jitsu. As we have seen in Chapters 1 and 2, the focus of Zen Shiatsu is in strengthening a weakness rather than maximizing a strength. We establish balance by attracting energy to a kyo area from a jitsu area. The first tenet of Zen Shiatsu is to "treat kyo first." Thus we first treat the weaker side of the body or the most underactive meridian. While the general tempo, strength, and depth of pressure will depend upon the receiver's overall condition, we make variations on this according to the condition of each meridian.

● *Kyo Meridians*

Kyo meridians fall into two basic categories: yin kyo and yang kyo. Each manifests as a different body condition and should be treated differently.

(1) *Yin kyo*

Since this is a yang condition the receiver may appear strong. Consequently one may think that he or she can take strong pressure when more yin, that is, a soft approach, is actually needed. In this condition the receiver has ample energy to resist strong pressure; consequently sharp or quickly applied pressure to an area will elicit muscular resistance there. Upon the release of pressure however, the flesh will be slow to resume its original shape. This is due to the lack of yin, which normally causes energy to move to the surface. The flesh in this condition lacks tone or resilience.

We can treat this condition in the following manner:

(i) Following general palm pressure, apply firm but gentle support not too distant from the hand which will move from point to point.

(ii) Apply heel of palm or broad flat elbow pressure slowly and gently until you feel the area softening; at that time you can slowly apply even deeper and stronger pressure. We thus hold at each point for at least a few seconds, sometimes even longer. An indication that the area is softening is the feeling that our pressure no longer sits properly. The muscles have relaxed and a different angle of pressure is now appropriate. Thus we gently release pressure and immediately reapply, continuing with the same procedure until we feel the area has relaxed to its maximum. We then move to the next point on that meridian.

(2) *Yang kyo*

(i) Apply firm but gentle pressure with the stationary supporting hand, in close proximity to the hand which moves from point to point. This support will instill confidence in receivers that they will not be hurt.

(ii) Since the meridian is deeper, we need a sharper angle of pressure. We may use thumb, fingertip or elbow, applied at a slightly acute angle. If we can first stretch the meridian, as is the case with the meridians in the legs (Chapter 7, section 33) it would be quite helpful.

(iii) Apply general palm pressure to the area. Now imagine applying pressure to a still surface of liquid. We wish to apply pressure without disturbing the surface any more than is possible. This means that we need to apply pressure very slowly and gently. We begin with a broad angle of pressure that gradually gets sharper once we sense the receiver's response.

As we discussed earlier in Chapter 1, our different kinds of shiatsu pressure can be considered as a "language of touch." We can compare this language with actual verbal communication in this particular case. The broad angle can be likened to general conversation while sharper pressure could be seen as equivalent to questioning that focuses on the receiver's problem. Slow and gentle pressure is analogous to the slow and gentle nature of the conversation. At the slightest sign of resistance, indicated by muscular contraction or tension anywhere throughout the body, we stop and hold our pressure at that depth—in conversation our questioning or probing is beginning to provoke resistance. We wait until such signs of tension subside and then continue to apply deeper pressure—akin to becoming more involved in discussion with the person's problem. We may have to stop and wait two or three times before we actually connect with the meridian—we wait in conversation until the person is relaxed or feels comfortable enough to open up to our question. If we feel a deep hardness we have reached the body's last line of resistance for defending this weakness— we have now been told the real cause of the problem.

In your shiatsu approach with caution; gently hold your pressure until you feel the hardness softening, then move to the next point on that meridian.

● *Jitsu Meridians*
Jitsu meridians fall into two basic categories: yang jitsu and yin jitsu. Again, each materializes in a different body condition and should be treated differently.

(1) *Yang jitsu*
There are two ways we can treat this meridian. We can make an analogy of each of these shiatsu methods with two different approaches to counselling that one might employ. The first way, which requires the least discomfort, is to find some attractive activity for a person to pour their energy into. With shiatsu, the corresponding treatment would locate the kyo meridian and employ various techniques to draw energy away from the area of excess to the area of deficiency. This approach is the one Masunaga recommended.

In the second approach, we would clearly indicate to the person that we are a friend and that we wish to help. With this relationship established we would then tell them of the necessity for change and continue to remind and encourage them to do so. The more we gain confidence and attention, the more emphatic and stronger will be possible our manner of expression. However this approach can develop into a kind of nagging, that no one really enjoys, but it may work. This way, less than ideal, represents in shiatsu work directly on the jitsu meridian.

Since yang jitsu may represent a very stagnated condition, it is still likely to need stimulation even if we choose the method of attracting excess to kyo. We can illustrate this condition with two metaphorical situations.

First, we can imagine a dog tied to his kennel. Obviously he wants to move and barks at every passing object. Even though he has plenty of energy, sooner or later he gets bored and falls asleep. While asleep another dog passes by. Unless this passing dog makes a sound the tied-up dog will sleep through the experience.

In the second, we can imagine ourselves caught in an elevator. One's immediate reaction is to bang on the walls and call out for assistance. If, over a considerable period of time no help arrives we may fall asleep. It may be a light sleep and even the faintest sound may cause us to awaken, but some stimulus is needed to once more arouse us into action.

Like these situations yang jitsu may represent a condition where energy is asleep. There is plenty of energy but it needs to be stimulated into action. In a wider sense yang jitsu may indicate a person with plenty of energy who is in a rut, in the wrong job for example, yet unable, for one reason or another to make a change in their life.

Let us see how we can apply shiatsu directly to a yang jitsu meridian.

Since it is a full condition some element of pain or discomfort may be involved in the application of pressure. It is analogous to the pain or discomfort we may face when we are forced to make changes in our life that we resist, even though we realize they are good for us.

(i)   Apply the supporting hand to the body.
(ii) Following general palm pressure, apply appropriate forms of pressure: heel of palm pressure or a broad, flat elbow pressure.
(iii) Since the predominant force, yang, is moving in the same direction as our shiatsu we may be able to apply pressure to a certain depth before causing discomfort—as one would squeeze and take up any slack in a loosely filled laundry bag until feeling its density. Once we know this depth we apply pressure to that level: this shiatsu is analagous to a conversation where we are attempting to get a person's attention, at first slowly and gently. Slow and gentle pressure in the beginning of shiatsu is equivalent to establishing a friendship. Then in our shiatsu from one point to the next our pressure is light and brisk: it is analogous to light and casual conversation when first meeting someone, finding out their interests. Our shiatsu is also repeated: along a meridian we repeat our application of pressure at least once. These repetitions are equivalent to verbal reminders. With each repetition of shiatsu, the pressure can become a little stronger and deeper, equivalent to a stronger and more forceful message.

This approach in shiatsu should cause an area to soften and make your efforts to attract the yang excess to a kyo area more effective.

(2) *Yin jitsu*

Since our pressure is going in the opposite direction to the predominant force of yin, the surface is likely to be tender and it is very easy to cause pain or discomfort by applying strong pressure. As this condition is very active it needs little pressure to move the energy. Since yin is in excess, direction and grounding are needed. These qualities are supplied through locating the most kyo meridian and applying holding pressure to a point there, attracting energy from the yin jitsu meridian.

We can also work directly on the yin jitsu meridian, in the following manner:

(i)   Apply the supporting hand to the body.
(ii) Following general palm pressure select a broad kind of pressure: heel of palm or a broad, flat elbow pressure.
(iii) From one point to the next, apply light and brisk pressure. Probably only one repetition of pressure will be necessary.

● *Working on Both Kyo and Jitsu Areas Simultaneously*

There are two basic ways we can work on kyo and jitsu areas simultaneously. In one method both hands are stationary; in the other one hand is stationary while the other hand moves.

(1) *Both hands stationary*
    In a relaxed state, place the left palm, thumb or finger, over the jitsu area. Pressure should be light, just enough to take up any slack. The other hand slowly applies at a sharp angle, deep holding pressure to the kyo area or point. If the diagnosis is correct and the technique applied properly, then the stiffness you feel in the jitsu area will naturally subside. This method is especially effective over the hara in supine position and on the back in the prone position.

(2) *One hand stationary, the other moving*
    In this technique you apply deep holding pressure to a point on a kyo meridian, usually with your thumb. The other hand applies brisk, light, repetitious pressure along the jitsu meridian. The latter pressure activates the energy along the jitsu meridian. The stationary pressure acts as a beacon showing where the excess energy should move to. This technique is effective when you work on the neck in the side position or the upper back in the prone position (see Figs. 191 and 232). In both examples the stationary hand is shown giving support. To effect this technique, this supporting hand's thumb applies stationary pressure to a point on the kyo meridian passing through that area.

Chapter 7

The Zen Shiatsu Form

I have entitled this chapter "The Zen Shiatsu Form" since the way Zen Shiatsu is practiced is indeed a form. At Masunaga's clinic in Tokyo, whatever the receiver's problem, all practitioners follow the same basic procedure in giving shiatsu. Within that overall form however, each would make variations for the following reasons:

1.   A practitioner may begin a sequence on the opposite side to that presented in this text. This decision would depend on the diagnosis.
2.   Some practitioners would concentrate on certain meridians only, skipping those they feel do not need treatment. To be effective this approach demands a great deal of diagnostic understanding.
3.   Practitioners select a style or approach to this form suitable to their own physique and to what they deem suitable for each particular receiver. For example, where one practitioner may use elbow, another uses knee. Where elbow is suitable for one receiver, on another the same practitioner may choose to use knee.

I too have developed my own approach, faithful to the spirit and principles of Zen Shiatsu. For example, I like to use heel of palm pressure more often than is practiced at Masunaga's clinic. It is I feel, a particularly useful technique, especially for those whose body is hard, dense, or very tight. Also, it is an excellent technique for beginners. It is easier to sense the receiver's response than when using elbow or knee and consequently safer.

Due to space limitations certain parts of the Zen Shiatsu form have been deleted. The most noticeable deletion is a way to treat the arms in the side position. While it provides an excellent method of treating the arms, there are other, better ways which I have presented in this chapter. With these exceptions, this chapter provides a faithful representation of Zen Shiatsu as it is practiced at Masunaga's center in Tokyo.

The photographic material emphasizes two important aspects:

1.   The sequential aspect of this form
I have endeavored to show how movements are fluid and natural, one movement flowing into the next. In this way a practitioner can create a sense of peace and relaxation for the receiver.
2.   The positioning and posture of the giver
There is a tendency for students to want to know where to press without paying due attention to the way of applying pressure.

This latter aspect depends upon the giver's positioning and posture. Since it is often overlooked, I have decided to emphasize this point. However, emphasizing positioning and posture creates problems in showing where to press. As much as possible I have tried to explain where to press in the accompanying text. However, at some point or other one will need to gain a copy of Masunaga's meridian chart and some text on point location. Recommended books and sources for them are listed in the bibliography.

Masunaga developed a unique theory on the constellation of meridians. In his approach, all twelve meridians pass through the hands and arms. He discovered these, he said, by using his own intuition. As one becomes more familiar with the body through practicing shiatsu, one can confirm for oneself the existence of these meridians. However since this matter is quite complex, Masunaga's meridians in the arms will not be addressed, nor some in the neck. But the techniques to treat these meridians are presented, so those students keen to do so can explore for themselves. Masunaga did not consider the direction of pressure application important. It appears that he was more concerned with creating a flow in the giver's movements. In this respect, with few exceptions, I have followed Masunaga's approach, as opposed to the more conventional view that has the giver applying pressure in the same direction as the flow of the meridian.

Allow me to finish this introduction with some advice on how to use this material:

- Begin with the premise that you want to give an enjoyable massage. If receivers do not like your shiatsu, then they have already closed up on you, despite your technical skill and theoretical understanding, and it will be doubly difficult for your shiatsu to be effective.
- In the beginning, do not be too concerned with the precise location of meridians or tsubos. Pay more attention to the way your hand or thumb molds to the contours of the receiver's body and to your posture and positioning.
- Begin with the safer and more sensitive techniques. First go through the entire form from start to finish using only thumb or palm pressure. Only when you have mastered those techniques should you move on to elbow or knee pressure. In this way there is more opportunity to develop sensitivity to each receiver's condition and response, consequently less chance of causing harm.
- Try to develop fluid, natural flowing movements.
- If you feel that this form is too long (it should take about ninety minutes) then first eliminate sequences from the side position.
- If you find some of the postures uncomfortable, try some of the exercises in Chapter 5. Simply by practicing shiatsu though, your body will gradually adjust.

Sitting Position

1. Preparation and Diagnosis

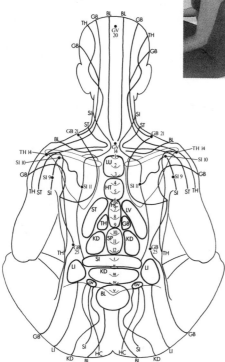

Fig. 148

The receiver sits comfortably, cross-legged or with legs outstretched. Sit seiza behind the receiver at natural arm's length. Place your right palm between the shoulder blades, close your eyes, and harmonize your breathing with the receiver's (Fig. 148).

Open your eyes and bring both hands to the shoulders. Gently feel in 2 to 3 places along the shoulders, then down the arms to the elbows in the same way (Fig. 149).

Slide your hands back, placing thumbs on each side of the first thoracic vertebra (Fig. 150). Gently slide your palms down the sides of the spine, main-

Fig. 149

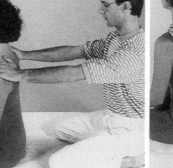

Fig. 150

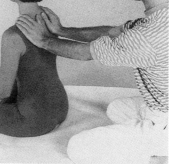

Fig. 152

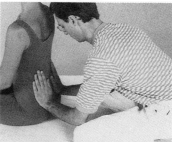

Fig. 151

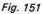

taining full palm contact with the back until reaching the iliac crest (Fig. 151).

Beginning in this position, the receiver can concentrate solely on touch, and the giver, by observation and touch, can begin to evaluate the receiver's condition (Fig. 152).

We are mainly looking for subtle changes in the quality of the flesh. Meridians intersect which can make evaluation difficult. We therefore follow lines. We look for some kind of regularity along a line (a meridian), passing beyond the point of intersection.

1. Check the general way of sitting. If the receiver slumps, from what level? This posture could indicate to us, through our knowledge of diagnostic areas along the spine, trouble in associated organs.
2. Check the level of the shoulders. Decide which shoulder is normal. If the other is higher it suggests a jitsu condition in one or more internal organs on that side: if lower, a kyo condition.
3. When a spine curves, the concave side of the curve represents the jitsu side: convex represents the kyo side.
4. We can consider the effects of diet as outlined in Chapter 2.
5. We can utilize our understanding of kyo and jitsu in the following areas;

• *Check*

LU. Rounded shoulders, distortions around the spine surrounding T_1, T_2, and T_3

L.I. The hips for flabbiness, softness or fullness. Pain or discomfort above the iliac crest. A slumping posture with no structure (kyo).

ST. The area below the left shoulder blade

SP/P. The area surrounding T_{10}, T_{11}, and T_{12}

HT. Very rounded back. Area surrounding T_4, T_5, T_6.

S.I. Area at base of neck, area within shoulder blades surrounding S.I.11, area surrounding L_1 and L_2

BL. Sacrum area: when this is flatter than the buttocks it suggests a kyo condition. Slumping from the lower back also suggests BL. kyo. When the muscles each side of the spine are very pronounced, it suggests BL. jitsu.

KD. Area beside L_3 and L_4. Area over the lower rib cage each side of the spine.

H.C. Area surrounding T_7, T_8, T_9

T.H. Area on the left side of T_8, T_9 and tense shoulders (as if you feel cold)

GB. Area to the right of T_9, T_{10}. Area around sides of shoulder blades. Discomfort below the base of the skull on each side of the spine.

LV. Area below right shoulder blade

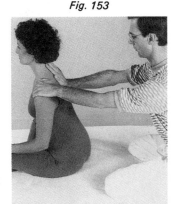

Fig. 153

2. Upper Back

(a) *Over the spine and beside the spine (BL.m)*
Place your left hand on the left shoulder. Come up onto your toes if necessary. With your right palm parallel with and over the spine at T_2, lean forward and apply general palm pressure in 2 to 3 places, moving down the spine to a point level with the base of the shoulder blades (Fig. 153).

On a line approximately 1 1/2 thumb-widths to the left of the midline of the spine, lean forward from your lower back and apply either of the following techniques:

(i) *Thumb pressure*—in 6 to 7 places from T_2 to T_8 (Fig. 154). Repeat.

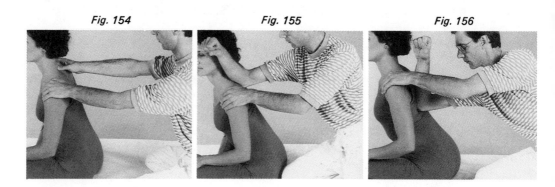

Fig. 154   Fig. 155   Fig. 156

(ii)   *Elbow pressure*—in 3 to 4 places from T_2 to T_8 (Figs. 155 and 156). Repeat. With elbow pressure bring your right knee more forward and your left knee more to the outside. Your right fist should be pointing at an angle of between "10 and 11 o'clock."

Full body coordination necessitates stretching back on the left shoulder, focusing and intensifying the pressure applied with the right thumb or elbow. In addition, while we may begin on our toes, most likely we will finish with the backs of our feet on the futon, adjusting our position so that we always maintain vertical contact with the point of pressure.

Repeat thumb pressure or elbow pressure, in mirror image on the right side.

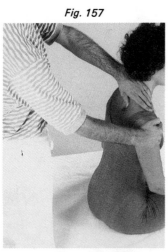

Fig. 157

(b)   *Around and beside the shoulder blades (GB.m)*

We can apply either thumb pressure or elbow pressure around the shoulder blades. Apply either in the following way:

(i)   *Thumb pressure*

Assume a kneeling posture, facing slightly toward the receiver's right side. Slide your right hand onto the arm just below the shoulder. Place your left thumb beside, but not too close to, the upper part of the right shoulder blade. Leaning forward, apply pressure, moving your body downward and to the right to consistently maintain vertical pressure as you give shiatsu around the shoulder blade (Fig. 157). Apply pressure in 5 to 6 places toward the base of the shoulder blades (Fig. 158). Repeat.

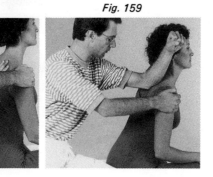

Fig. 158   Fig. 159

(ii)   *Elbow pressure*

Sit seiza facing slightly toward the receiver's right side and slide your right hand onto the arm just below the shoulder. Come onto your toes if necessary. Apply pressure as above in 4 to 5 places (Fig. 159), in the beginning with the angle of the fist in a nearly vertical position. Repeat.

As above, continually adjust your body position to maintain vertical pressure, and coordinate the simultaneous stretching back and leaning forward motions of your arms and hands by full coordination of your body. Repeat step (b), (i) or (ii) in mirror image on the other side.

3. Arms

We can give palm and thumb pressure, or elbow pressure to the arms. The former is easier for beginners and better when the receiver is thin or frail or when there is a great difference in height between giver and receiver. When well executed, elbow pressure is quicker to do and the pressure is stronger yet comfortable. Elbow pressure is also less taxing on the giver.

Clasping and thumb pressure

Sit seiza on toes, with your right knee facing the receiver's spine and the left knee at a 45 degree angle. Support the receiver's back by placing your right knee in the small of the back, just to the left of the spine.

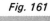
Fig. 160

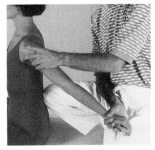

Keeping your back naturally straight, take the left wrist between your right thumb and index finger and rest your elbow on your lap. With your left palm on the upper arm just below the shoulder, apply gentle clasping pressure in 3 places down the upper arm (Fig. 160). Then support the arm just below the elbow.

Give clasping pressure with your right hand down the inside of the receiver's upper arm in 3 places, then return to support at the wrist with right thumb and index finger. With your left palm, give gentle squeezing pressure to the underside of the upper arm, in 3 places. On the upper side, from the elbow apply thumb pressure down the center of the lower arm along the T.H.m in 6 to 7 places (Fig. 161). Repeat. In this position we can also give shiatsu to the L.I.m and S.I.m. With your left hand holding the fingers, turn the palm face up. Giving support in this way, apply thumb shiatsu from the elbow down the center of the lower arm along the H.C.m in 6 to 7 places (Fig. 162).

Fig. 161

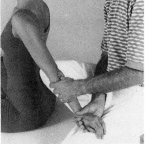

Repeat. In this position we can also give shiatsu along the HT.m and LU.m.

Fig. 162   *Fig. 163*

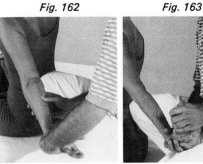

Return the palm face down and again support firmly at the wrist with your right thumb and index finger. With the receiver's fingers in your left palm, gently stretch the fingers backward (Fig. 163). To increase the stretch, keep the receiver's elbow straight and lower the arm slightly.

Then, let the fingers drop and place your left palm over the back of the hand, still

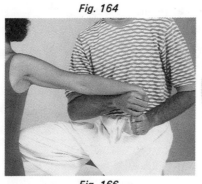

Fig. 164

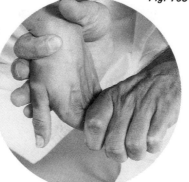

Fig. 165

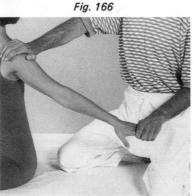

Fig. 166

supporting firmly at the wrist as before. Gently stretch the wrist (Fig. 164). To increase the stretch, keep the elbow straight and gently raise the arm slightly.

Release the stretch, and with the same support at the wrist, take the fingers and rotate the hand twice in each direction. Finish by pressing down on the back of the fingers (Fig. 165). Holding the fingers in your left hand, place your right hand on the left shoulder (Fig. 166). Come into a kneeling posture with your right leg supporting the left side of the receiver's back. As you change your position let the arm drop to the side in preparation for doing the arm meridian stretches.

Elbow pressure

Standing on the left side and slightly behind, place your right foot beside the left hip and your right knee in the armpit. Support the arm at the wrist in your left hand, with the middle finger behind the wrist, palm facing down.

Holding the wrist just above your left knee, come into a mild squat, keeping your back straight. Gently stretch the arm by moving your left leg away from the receiver's body. If your legs are too long for the receiver's torso, move the right foot back slightly. If your legs are too short, raise the right heel.

By simply leaning your upper body forward, from T.H.14, give shiatsu to the T.H.m down the upper arm to the elbow, in 3 to 4 places (Fig. 167). Repeat.

Then, from L.I.15 give shiatsu to the L.I.m in the same way. Repeat.

Turn the palm over and hold as though shaking hands. With the left elbow resting just above your left knee, give shiatsu to the LU.m from the shoulder toward the elbow, in 3 places

Fig. 167   Fig. 168

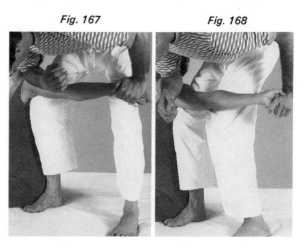

(Fig. 168). Repeat.

Raise the arm slightly on your upper left leg. Leaning still further forward, repeat as above to the H.C.m; followed by thumb pressure to H.C.3 in the hollow of the elbow, 3 times.

Continue along the H.C.m from H.C.3 to the wrist, H.C.7, in 3 to 4 places. Repeat. In this movement your left leg moves outward as your elbow also moves outward, acting as support. Tilt the palm up slightly to reveal the LU. m. From the elbow to the wrist, give elbow shiatsu to the LU.m, in 3 to 4 places (Fig. 169). Repeat.

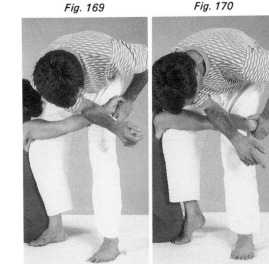

Fig. 169   Fig. 170

Fig. 171

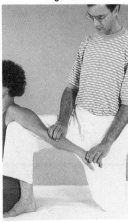

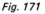

Turn the palm over, supporting at the wrist with your left thumb and index finger. With your left knee again just below the elbow, give shiatsu as above to the T.H.m, from the elbow, finishing at T.H.4 on the wrist (Fig. 170).

Tilt the hand upward slightly and in the same manner give shiatsu to the S.I.m.

Maintaining the support under the armpit, come down into a half kneeling posture. With your left index finger, give pressure to L.I.4 between the index finger and thumb.

Place the fingers of your right hand on the L.I.m beside and on L.I.11 by the crease in the elbow. With these fingers, give pressure down the L.I.m in 4 to 5 places (Fig. 171). Repeat.

Support the wrist with clasping pressure from your right index finger and thumb (this time with thumb below) and prepare to perform the wrist stretches and rotations as in the previous section under "palm and thumb" pressure (see Figs. 163 through 166).

Fig. 172   Fig. 173

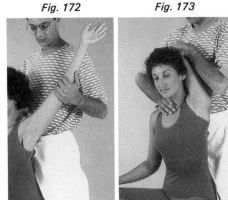

4. Arm Meridian Stretches

Come into a kneeling posture, with your right upper leg supporting the left side of the receiver's back. Place your right hand on the receiver's left shoulder, directly in front of your hara. Pick the arm up under the elbow with your left hand. Stretch upward and toward yourself simultaneously, at an angle of 10 o'clock, stretching the LU.m (Fig. 172).

Hold for a few moments, release the

stretch, and follow through in a circular movement to the side.

Continuing to hold at the elbow, raise the arm again, to a vertical angle of 12 o'clock, stretching the H.C.m. Release as before and once again bring the receiver's arm into a vertical stretch.

At the point of maximum stretch, move your supporting right hand to the right side of the neck. Bend the arm at the elbow, allowing the hand to drop behind the head. Supporting and pressing slightly forward with your hara in the back, gently stretch the arm behind the head, stretching the HT.m in the upper arm (Fig. 173).

Guide the arm to rest by the side.

Repeat steps *3*, (i) or (ii) and *4* in mirror image on the right arm.

5. Chest

• *Finger and thumb pressure*

Come into a standing posture behind the receiver. Place your feet beside the buttocks with your knees supporting in the shoulder blade area. Visualizing the shoulders as a pivot, place your thumbs on the shoulders and your fingertips on the chest. Lean forward and extend your fingertips downward as far as possible.

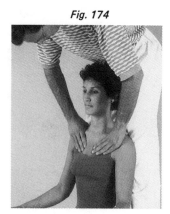

Fig. 174

Along a line from inside to outside, give shiatsu across the chest with your fingertips in 4 places along the H.C.m (Fig. 174). Repeat.

Raise your fingertips some 2 thumb-widths and repeat again as above to the HT.m. Repeat.

Locate the midpoint on the clavicle between the neck and arm. With your middle fingers 1 to 2 thumb-widths below this point, give pressure to LU.1, 3 times. Come up vertically on a line through this point to just below the clavicle and repeat the same to LU.2.

With the index and middle fingers, give pressure in 4 places across the pectoral muscles around the front of the shoulders (LV.m). Repeat.

6. Shoulders

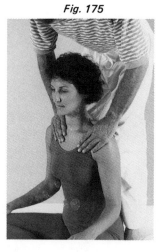

Fig. 175

Techniques employing either thumb pressure or elbow pressure are effective for shiatsu across the shoulders.

• *Thumb pressure*

Bringing the receiver's body forward slightly by gently pressing your knees into the shoulder blades, place your thumbs on either side of the spine, with your fingers resting on the chest. With the right palm stationary, give thumb shiatsu across the left shoulder, in 5 to 6 places (Fig. 175). Repeat. Repeat in mirror image over the right shoulder. Give shiatsu on 2 or more lines, depending on which meridians you wish to treat.

• *Elbow pressure*

Elbow shiatsu to the shoulders can be very strong yet

very relaxing if applied correctly. In the same posture as above, begin by giving palm pressure across the shoulders, in 3 places each side. Then rest your right hand on the right shoulder beside the neck and move your body to the right slightly. With your left arm, give broad elbow pressure across the left shoulder to the arm, in 3 places (Fig. 176). Repeat.

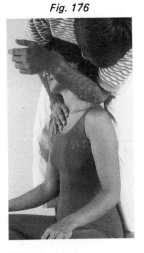

Fig. 176

Repeat in mirror image across the right shoulder.

The location of your pressure depends upon which meridian you wish to treat. Again, you apply pressure by simply leaning, varying the angle and direction of pressure according to which part of the shoulder you are treating.

The area of the shoulders beside the neck relates to the intestines, especially the S.I.m. This area is often very hard, usually reflecting a stagnated condition of the intestines. Elbow pressure incorrectly applied here can easily cause pain. Conversely, properly applied elbow pressure can be very effective. So that the elbow does not slip off the muscle, we can apply pressure here in a slightly different way.

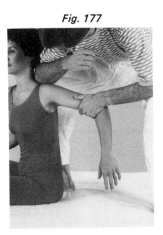

Fig. 177

Beginning on the left side first, change your position to a squat. Your right leg supports the back on the right side, parallel with the spine. The left leg is extended back slightly. Take the left arm, just above the elbow, in your left hand and raise it slightly, so that your left elbow rests above your left knee. This movement will relieve tension in the left shoulder beside the neck. By leaning your body in toward the neck, you can apply a very focused angle of pressure.

Stretch back slightly with your left hand. At the same time apply pressure with your right elbow to this area beside T_1 (Fig. 177). Hold momentarily. Repeat at least twice. Repeat, in mirror image, on the right shoulder.

7. Back

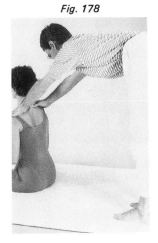

Fig. 178

Change to a standing posture with your knees giving support in the shoulder blades. Place your thumbs on either side of T_1 and take one step backward. Leaning forward while keeping your back straight, apply alternate thumb pressure on either side of the spine (Fig. 178), walking down it with your thumbs, in 6 to 7 places on each side. Do not let the fingers leave the shoulders.

8. Neck Rotation and Stretch

Sit seiza, on toes with your left leg parallel with and beside the receiver's upper left leg. Raise your right upper leg to

Fig. 179

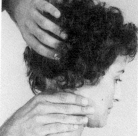

be horizontal with the floor, resting in the lower back area. Place the V-area between the thumb and index finger of your right hand over the area just below the base of the skull (Fig. 179). Place your left hand over the receiver's forehead, above the eyebrows.

Draw the head back onto your right hand and rotate, first counterclockwise twice, then clockwise twice.

Adjust your pressure slightly so that your upper right leg is parallel with the floor, and your right inner thigh is

Fig. 180

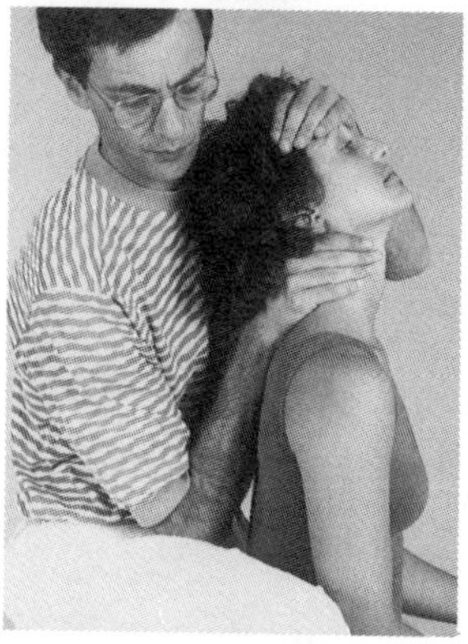

Fig. 181

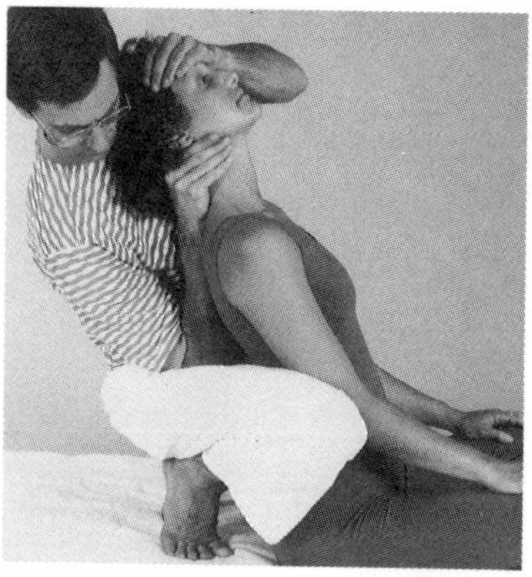

Fig. 182

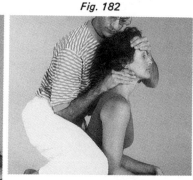

in line with the receiver's spine. Your right arm rests parallel with and over the spine. Remind the receiver to relax completely.

Draw the receiver's forehead backward, taking out any slack (Fig. 180). Together, lean backward until your elbow reaches your lap. Then lean further backward a fraction, stretching the neck upward in a line vertical with the spine (Fig. 181). Hold for a few seconds. To release the stretch, simply lean forward together (Fig. 182).

9. Stretching Both Arms Together

Fig. 184

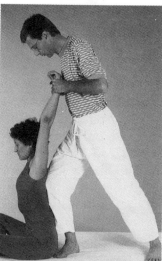

Stand up with your right foot turned inward and the outer part of the lower right leg parallel with and supporting the spine. Your left leg extends straight back with your left foot also turned inward. Bending forward from the lower back, come up onto the toes of the left foot and pick the arms up at the elbows (Fig. 183).

Fig. 183

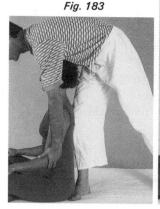

Slide your hands to the wrists, with your middle fingers supporting on the underside of the wrists and your thumbs just below the receiver's index fingers on the back of the hand. Raising your upper body, bring the receiver's hands to your chest. Now using your whole body as a lever, lift the arms vertically by raising your upper body further (Fig. 184).

Leaning back, shift your weight onto your left foot and stretch the arms vertically (Fig. 185). At the point of maximum stretch bend the

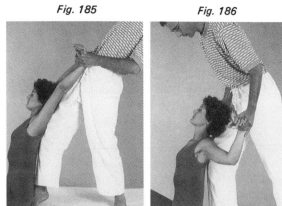

Fig. 185   Fig. 186

Fig. 187 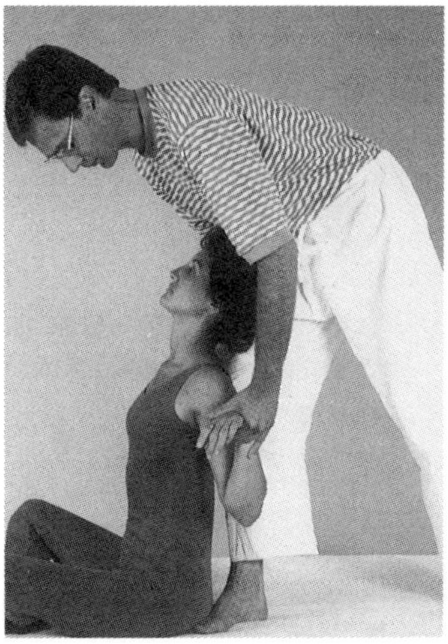   Fig. 188 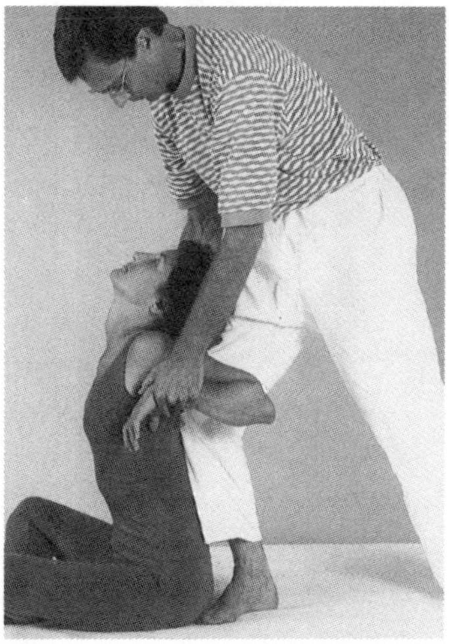   Fig. 189

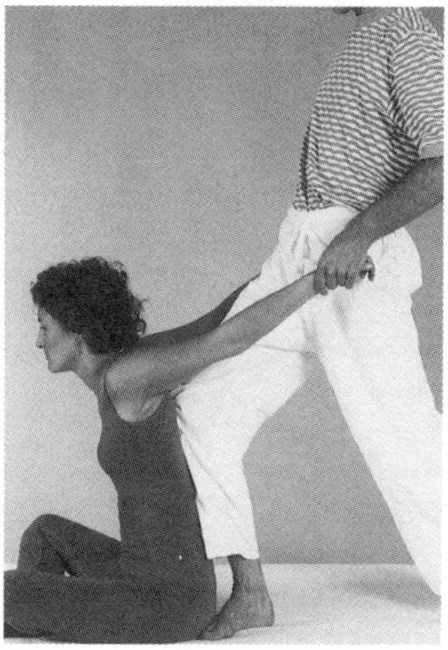

wrists forward at a 90 degree angle. Move the arms out to the side and in a downward direction with the receiver's lower arms moving perpendicularly toward the floor (Fig. 186). In this way the stretch will open up the chest.

Keep coming down until the elbows touch the sides (Fig. 187) and repeat the stretch again. The second time, after the elbows touch the sides, bring the wrists up into the armpit area, raising the shoulders upward (Fig. 188). Make sure to maintain back support with your lower right leg. Hold this stretch for a few moments and then cover the back of the receiver's hands with your palms.

Holding the stretch, with your right knee in the receiver's back, stretch the arms backward and slightly upward with palms down (Fig. 189). Hold the arms at the wrists with thumb and index fingers. Hold the stretch for a few seconds, then place the arms gently in the receiver's lap.

Come forward and again support the receiver's back by resting your knees in the shoulder blades. Take the upper arms in your hands and gently raise and release the shoulders 2 to 3 times to check that the shoulders are relaxed. Then come forward to the receiver's left side with your left hand giving support on the side of the neck. With your right hand pointing downward, finish with a gentle rubdown along the spine, 3 times or so.

Side Position

10. Preparation

Generally we begin with the receiver lying on the right side, which is more restful for the heart. The receiver's head rests on a small pillow with the right arm extended forward away from the body. The right leg is slightly bent at the knees while the left leg rests across at a 90 degree angle. Make sure both knees are resting comfortably on the futon. The lower part of the left arm rests on the hip or behind it.

Fig. 190

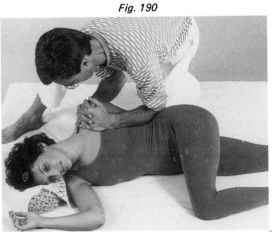

11. Neck

Assume a half-kneeling posture with your left knee beside the lower back. Interlace your fingers and gently stretch the shoulder toward you (Fig. 190). The angle of the stretch should be parallel with the floor. Holding the stretch with your left hand, move your body forward a few inches. Support your right elbow with your right knee and place your 4 fingers on the back of the neck.

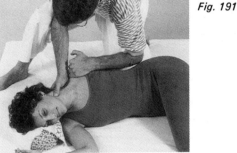

Fig. 191

With your right thumb, give shiatsu to the ST.m immediately in front of the sternocleidomastoid muscle, in 4 places toward the clavicle (Fig. 191). Repeat.

Returning to the beginning position, rotate your hand to the right 1 thumb-width and give thumb pressure to the L.I.m along the sternocleidomastoid muscle; in 4 places. Repeat.

Return to the previous beginning point and rotate to a point on the anterior border of the same muscle. Toward a point 2 thumb-widths to the left of the midline at T_1 (S.I.15), give shiatsu along the S.I.m, in 5 to 6 places. Repeat.

Return to the last beginning point and rotate your hand some 2 thumb-widths to the right and give shiatsu to the GB.m in a downward direction toward the shoulder; in 4 to 5 places. Repeat.

Rotate back still further, 1 thumb-width, and as above give shiatsu to the T.H.m.

When treating each meridian, we not only stretch the shoulder but also move it into a different position to maximize the stretch.

Maintaining the stretch on the shoulder with the left hand, give thumb pressure, as above, across the base of the skull, from behind the ear to the spine in approximately 5 places. Repeat. The angle of pressure is in an opposite direction to the angle of the stretch held on the shoulder. Repeat.

12. Face and Head

The right thumb gives support gently just behind the ear, while the left thumb gives shiatsu along the cheekbone from S.I.19 toward the nose (S.I.18), in 3 to 4 places (Fig. 192).

From a point, T.H.21, just above S.I.19, give thumb shiatsu toward the outer tip of the eyebrow, T.H.23, in 4 to 5 places.

| Fig. 192 | Fig. 193 | Fig. 194 | Fig. 195 |

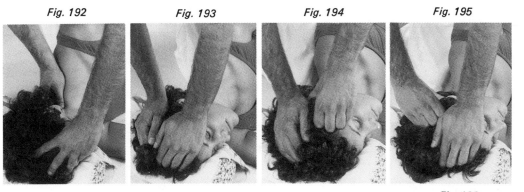

Fig. 196

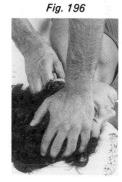

Place both palms on the side of the head and by leaning, gently apply pressure (Fig. 193). Upon releasing pressure, with the left hand remaining stationary, the right hand moves downward applying pressure to a second area, behind the ear. Repeat. The right hand supports as in Fig. 193 while the second phalanges of the fingers of the left hand give shiatsu to the temple area going toward the cheekbone, in 2 places (Fig. 194). Repeat.

The left hand supports on the temple area while with the right hand we give shiatsu as above, on an inside line around the ear, in 3 to 4 places (Fig. 195). Repeat. Follow with the same kind of pressure on an outside line.

Finish by giving shiatsu in the same way as above, across the base of the skull from ear to spine, in 3 to 4 places (Fig. 196). Repeat.

• *Elbow pressure to neck*

Just below the base of the skull, tension and stiffness often arise. This is most often related to stagnation along the GB.m. Elbow pressure here can be very effective.

Fig. 197

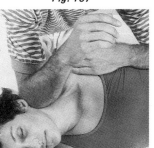

Sit seiza with knees wide apart, facing the receiver's neck. Lean forward and with your left hand gently stretch the shoulder in the direction of the feet. With your right elbow, beginning just behind the ear and just below the base of the skull, apply light but firm pressure (Fig. 197). Follow the contours of the neck and apply pressure in 3 to 4 places toward the spine. Repeat at least once. With each repetition, as the stiffness subsides, apply deeper pressure.

To be effective, leave a space between the base of the skull and the place where you apply pressure.

240

13. Left Shoulder

Assume a half kneeling posture, with your left
upper leg by the receiver's back and your
right leg extended away. Your right knee supports your right shoulder as your right hand
rests on the shoulder, stretching downward. By
leaning forward, apply elbow pressure at the
base of the neck beside C_7 and T_1 (Fig. 198).
Repeat twice.

Support the shoulder with your left hand
and gently stretch downward. Lean in with your
body, in a slightly counterclockwise motion and
apply thumb pressure from beside T_1 on an
outside line toward the arm; in 4 to 5 places
(Fig. 199). Repeat. Follow with similar pressure
along a line across the top of the shoulder.

14. Around the Left Shoulder Blade —
GB.m and Left Side of Spine — BL.m

In the same half-kneeling posture, move your
body a few inches toward the feet. Thread your
left supporting hand around the shoulder and
armpit. Press the shoulder blade away from
you and assume a lower body angle. With the
same knee support on your right elbow as
above, place your right thumb on a point
beside the upper part of the shoulder blade
(Fig. 200). Remember to leave a space between
the shoulder blade and the line to which you
apply pressure.

Lean in, and in a downward direction give
thumb shiatsu around and toward the base of
the shoulder blade in 5 to 6 places. Repeat.

Maintaining the same support system, give
thumb shiatsu down the left side of the spine
(BL.m) from beside T_2 to T_8 in 7 to 8 places,
sliding your left knee a few inches down as
you proceed (Fig. 201). Repeat.

The supporting hand moves to the hara and
you continue down the BL.m to the iliac crest;
in 7 to 8 places (Fig. 202). Repeat.

15. Hips

For the remainder of the side position, all
movements are toward the feet.

Fig. 198

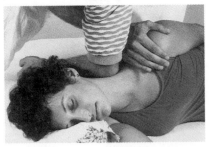

Fig. 199

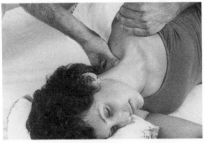

Fig. 200

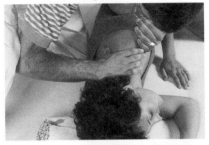

Fig. 201

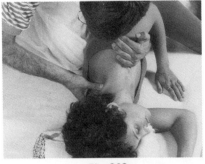

Fig. 202

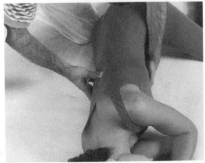

Fig. 203

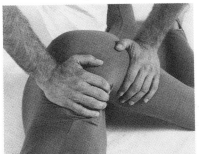

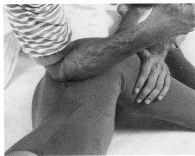
Fig. 204

Move your body further down toward the feet. Assume a half-kneeling posture and place your left supporting hand on the upper leg. With your right hand give general palm pressure on an inside line beside the sacrum in 2 places, followed by the same on an outside line over the hip (Fig. 203). Then apply either heel of palm pressure or elbow pressure along these same lines.

   (i) *Heel of palm pressure*
      Apply deeper and more focused pressure by using the heel of the right palm.

  (ii) *Elbow pressure*
      To apply elbow pressure, come into a kneeling posture with knees apart. As this area of the body is usually more solid, elbow pressure can be especially effective. However, it is important to remember to vary the direction, angle, and intensity of pressure according to the different contours of the body in this area (Fig. 204).

16. Left Leg

Maintaining the same posture, with knees slightly wider apart, place your left supporting hand below the left knee. With your right elbow, give shiatsu to the hip area in 1 to 2 places (Fig. 205).

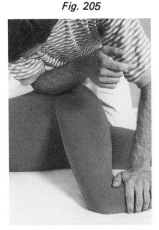
Fig. 205

(1) *T.H.m*
    The T.H.m runs along a line midway between the front of the leg and the outer side. Give general palm pressure in 3 places (Fig. 206). Follow with heel of palm pressure or elbow pressure, in 3 to 4 places (Fig. 207). Repeat.

(2) *GB.m*
    The GB.m runs down the outer side of the leg, approximately in alignment with the outer seam of a pair of trousers. Slide the left supporting hand down toward the ankle and apply general palm pressure down the side of the leg toward the knee, in 3

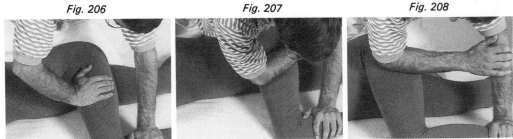
Fig. 206   Fig. 207   Fig. 208

to 4 places. Follow with heel of palm pressure or elbow pressure (Fig. 208), in 3 to 4 places. Repeat.

(3) *L.I.m*
Change position. Assume

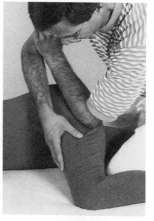
Fig. 209

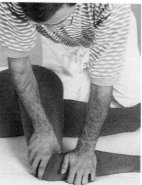
Fig. 210

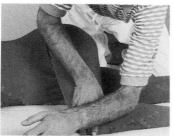
Fig. 211

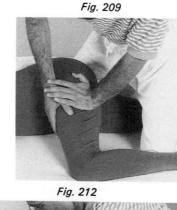
Fig. 212

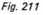
Fig. 213

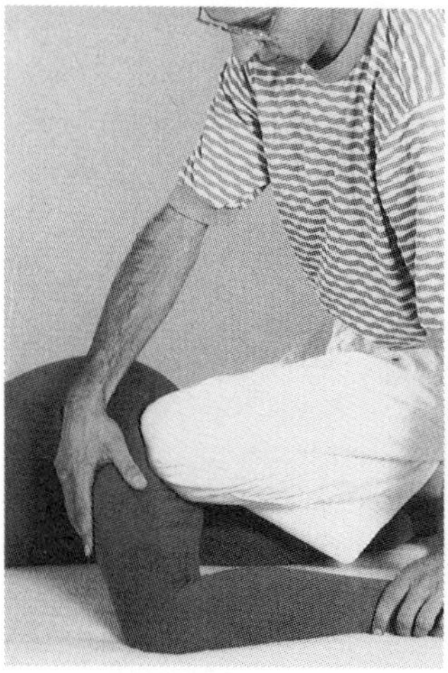

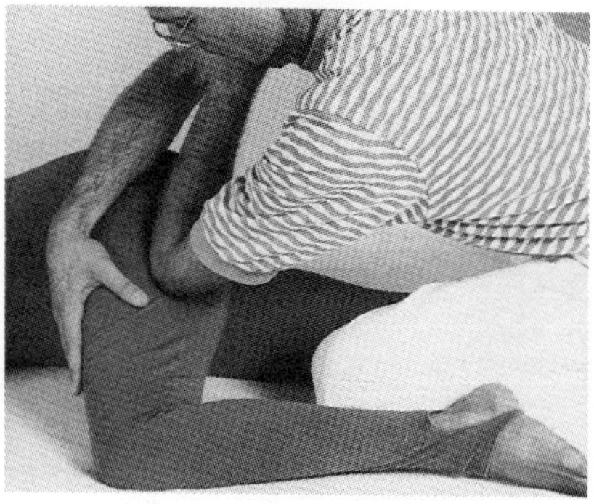

seiza posture on your toes facing the upper half of the left leg. Place your right hand over the upper part of the T.H.m. The L.I.m flows just below the vastus lateralis muscle, some 3 to 4 thumb-widths below the GB.m. With your left palm give general palm pressure, in 3 to 4 places (Fig. 209). Follow with heel of palm pressure or elbow pressure, in 4 to 5 places. Repeat. When applying elbow pressure the right hand moves along, parallel with the elbow giving support as you move down the leg (Fig. 210). Knee pressure is also very effective and is applied in a similar manner to elbow pressure (Fig. 211).

(4) *KD.m*
The KD.m runs parallel with and some 2 thumb-widths below the L.I.m. With a lower body angle give elbow pressure as applied to the L.I.m, only at a sightly sharper angle (Fig. 212). Step back, and kneel behind the right leg. Place your right supporting hand above the left knee. Give general palm pressure down the side of the lower leg in 4 to 5 places.

Fig. 214

(5) *GB.m*
In the lower leg, the GB.m continues its course down the outside bony region of the leg, which is approximately in alignment with the outside seam of a pair of trousers. Begin applying pressure from GB.34, which is just below a bony extension (the head of the fibula), moving toward the outside of the ankle. Apply heel of palm pressure, in 4 to 5 places (Fig. 213). Repeat.

Fig. 215

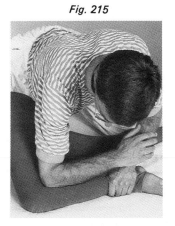

Or apply elbow pressure, in 4 to 5 places
(Fig. 214). Repeat.

(6) *L.I.m*

The L.I.m runs parallel with and some 2 thumb-widths posterior to the GB.m, beside the fibula. Apply heel of palm pressure, in 5 to 6 places. Repeat. Or apply elbow pressure. Use your right elbow to cover the upper half in 3 places (Fig. 215). Repeat. Use the left elbow for the lower half, to the ankle, in 3 to 4 places (Fig. 216). Repeat.

17. Right Leg

Step back and assume a kneeling posture, facing the upper half of the inside leg. Place your left supporting hand below the knee. With your right hand give general palm pressure in 2 to 3 places, toward the knee.

Heel of palm, elbow, and knee pressure can all be very effective here. Keep in mind that the area above the knee along the LV.m is very sensitive on most people, so be careful.

Fig. 216

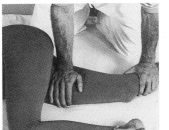

Fig. 217

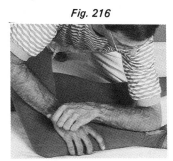

Fig. 218

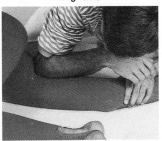

(1) *LV.m*

The LV.m flows on a line some 2 1/2 inches inside of the front of the upper leg, toward the inside of the knee.

Place your left supporting hand below the knee. Apply one of the following techniques:
  (i) Heel of palm pressure, in 3 to 4 places (Fig. 217). Repeat.
  (ii) Elbow pressure as above (Fig. 218).
  (iii) Left knee pressure, in 2 places. The right hand supports on the right hip.

(2) *HT.m*

Running parallel with the LV.m, but some 2 to 3 thumb-widths closer to you, lies the HT.m. Apply pressure as above, to the HT.m.

(3) *BL.m*

From the point BL.50, some 3 to 4 thumb-widths closer to you than the HT.m and just below the buttocks, the BL.m flows to the point BL.54, the centerpoint behind the knee.

Knee pressure is most effective here. Place your left supporting hand below the knee and your right hand on the hip. Using your left knee, apply pressure toward the receiver's knee, in 3 to 4 places (Fig. 219). Repeat.

For the lower half of the inside leg, change positions. Kneeling, face the lower leg and place

Fig. 219　　　　　　　Fig. 220　　　　　　　Fig. 221

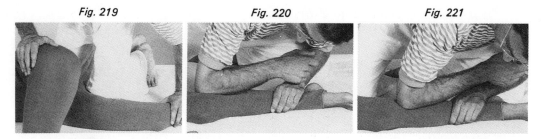

your right supporting hand above the right knee. Give general palm pressure to the lower leg in 3 to 4 places. The left hand now gives support below the calf muscle.

Fig. 222

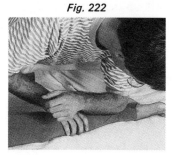

(4) *KD.m*

From KD.10, beside the knee, to KD.9, at the base of the calf muscle and a little more than 1 inch from the tibia, apply pressure with your right elbow, in 3 to 4 places (Fig. 220). Repeat.

(5) *LV.m*

From LV.8, also beside the knee, along a line on the inside of the calf muscle to LV.6, halfway down the lower leg, apply pressure as to the KD.m in 3 to 4 places.

(6) *SP.m*

From SP.9, on the head of the tibia, apply elbow shiatsu halfway down the lower leg, beside the tibia in 3 to 4 places (Fig. 221). Repeat.

Your right hand now rests on the calf muscle. With your left elbow give shiatsu to the SP.m in the lower half of the inside leg to a point just anterior to the ankle, in 3 to 4 places (Fig. 222). Repeat.

18. Right Foot

Either thumb or knee pressure can be effective on the sole of the foot.

(i) *Thumb pressure*

Change to a half-kneeling posture, with your left hand supporting the foot. Imagine 3 lines on the foot: inside, center, and outside. From the balls of the foot to the heel, give thumb pressure in 5 to 6 places along each line and repeat.

Finish with thumb pressure to KD.1, which is in the center just below the balls of the foot (Fig. 223). Repeat 3 times.

(ii) *Knee pressure*

Sit in seiza facing the receiver's head. Your right hand clasps above and

Fig. 223　　　　　　　　Fig. 224

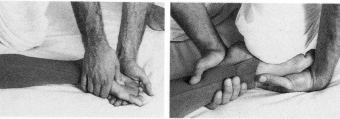

around the ankle and your left hand supports over the top of the foot. With your left knee lean in, and apply pressure to the sole of the foot—in 1 or 2 places (Fig. 224).

Repeat 2 to 3 times.

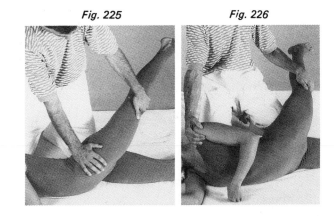

Fig. 225   Fig. 226

19. Side Stretch

Upon finishing shiatsu to the foot, rest the outside leg on the inside leg. Change to a seiza posture, facing the receiver's back. Lift the top leg at the knee with your left hand, while at the same time pressing the hip forward with your right (Fig. 225).

On your toes, place your left knee in the left buttock. Press the upper back forward slightly and place your right knee below the shoulder blade. Place your right hand around the left shoulder with your middle finger resting in the armpit (Fig. 226).

Lean back and stretch the knee and shoulder toward you. Hold for a few moments, then relax and finish with a gentle rubdown to the spine in a half-kneeling posture. Repeat steps *11* through *19* in mirror image on the receiver's right side.

Prone Position

20. Preparation

The receiver lies on the stomach with arms by the sides, palms up, the head to whichever side is more comfortable. A large thin pillow can be placed under the stomach for additional comfort; it will also help to relieve discomfort in those with stiff necks.

Sit seiza, above the head, facing the feet, and observe which side of the back is more relaxed: this side is the one we begin on. For practice, with the exception of the upper back, we begin on the right side.

21. Upper Back

Come into a kneeling position and place your right palm parallel with and over the spine, in line with the base of the shoulder blades. Place your left palm over your right.

Fig. 227   Fig. 228   Fig. 229

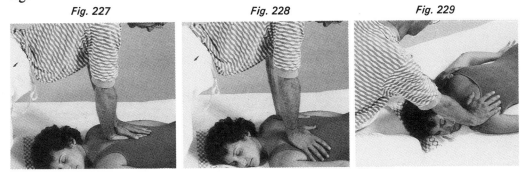

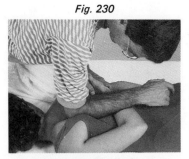

Fig. 230

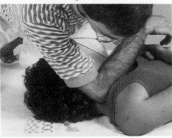

Fig. 231

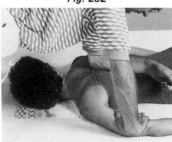

Fig. 232

Lean forward and apply pressure (Fig. 227). Then release by shifting your weight back. In the same manner apply pressure in 2 more places over the spine, moving toward the neck.

Place each palm over the base of the corresponding shoulder blade. Lean forward, apply pressure (Fig. 228), then release. In the same manner apply pressure in 4 to 5 more places, moving toward and onto the shoulders. From the third place of pressure begin to stretch the shoulders down and away from you, keeping in mind to change your body angle to maintain vertical pressure (Fig. 229).

- *Elbow pressure*
  a. *Around and beside the left shoulder blade*
     In a kneeling position, take the receiver's left hand in your left hand as though shaking hands and gently stretch toward you. This movement has the effect of elevating the shoulder blade away from the body. Move your position to the right side of the receiver's head.

     With your right fist pointing toward the right hand, apply pressure beside but not too close to the shoulder blade (Fig. 230). Moving toward and onto the shoulders, apply pressure to the G.B.m, in 5 to 6 places. Repeat. Keep in mind that with each application of pressure it is necessary to change your body position

slightly to maintain vertical pressure (Fig. 231). Release.

b. *Left side of spine*
   Change to a kneeling posture above the left side of the receiver's head and place your right hand above the left elbow. With your

Fig. 233

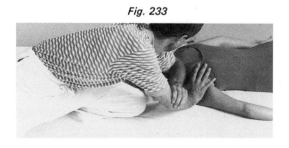

left hand facing toward the receiver's left hand, lean in and apply pressure along the left side of the spine from a point level with the base of the shoulder blades (Fig. 232).

Apply pressure toward the neck in 3 to 4 more places. Repeat.

c. *Left shoulder*
   Change position. Assume a lower body angle with your right hand resting on the upper arm, closer to the shoulder. Apply pressure at a sharper angle beside T_1 (Fig. 233): one place, 3 times.

   With points of pressure closely spaced, apply pressure across the shoulder in 3 to 4 places. Repeat.

Note: On many people the upper back is very tight and stiff. This condition may require more shiatsu than usual. You may have to apply pressure along the same line a number of times before you feel the area yielding.

Repeat movements (a), (b), and (c) in mirror image on the right side, then continue onto the lower right arm.

22. Lower Right Arm

Sitting seiza, face the lower right arm at right angles. Come into a kneeling position and place your right hand above the elbow. Give general palm pressure down the arm in 3 to 4 places, then proceed with shiatsu to the following meridians:

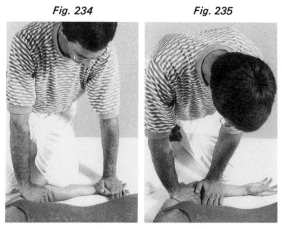

Fig. 234   Fig. 235

(1) *HT.m*

The HT.m flows from the inside of the elbow (HT.3) toward the little finger side of the wrist (HT.7). Apply either of the following:

(i) Heel of palm pressure with your left hand; in 3 to 4 places. Repeat.

(ii) Knee pressure with your left knee. Your left hand supports by resting on the right palm; 3 to 4 places (Fig. 234). Repeat.

(2) *H.C.m*

The H.C.m follows a center line from the elbow (H.C.3) to the wrist (H.C.7). It is easier to treat the H.C.m by moving the arm toward the receiver's shoulder a few inches.

From elbow to wrist, apply pressure as above with either:

(i) Heel of palm pressure (Fig. 235)

(ii) Knee pressure

23. Right Hand

Change to a half-kneeling posture facing in the direction of the feet, with your left hand, palm up, under the receiver's hand for support.

Apply thumb pressure to the following points 3 times each, holding for a few moments with each application of pressure.

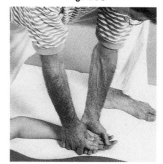

Fig. 236

LU.7, LU.8, LU.9 just above the wrist at the base of the thumb

LU.10 on the fleshy area below the thumb

H.C.7 on a midline almost on the crease of the wrist

H.C.8 in the center of the palm (Fig. 236)

Shift support to the right hand and with the left thumb apply pressure to the following points:

H.T.7 just above the crease of the wrist on the side of the little finger

H.T.8 midway between the wrist and the base of the little finger

248

Change position, gently moving the arm in the opposite direction to above the head. Sit seiza facing the lower right arm. Come into a kneeling position and place your right hand over the receiver's right hand. Give general palm pressure to the lower arm in the direction of the elbow in 3 places.

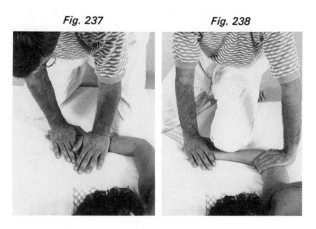

Fig. 237   Fig. 238

(1) *L.I.m*

The L.I.m follows an inside line from a point beside the thumb side of the wrist (L.I.5) toward a point beside the end of the crease in the elbow (L.I.11). Apply either:

(i) Heel of palm pressure with your left hand from the wrist, in 3 to 4 places (Fig. 237). Repeat.

(ii) Knee pressure with your left knee, in 3 to 4 places. Repeat. Your left hand supports above the elbow.

(2) *T.H.m*

From a midpoint on the wrist (T.H.4) along a central line to the elbow, give shiatsu as above to the T.H.m (Fig. 238).

(3) *S.I.m*

Along an outside line, from the wrist (S.I.6) to the elbow, give shiatsu as above to the S.I.m.

Change position. Face the upper arm, in seiza posture, on your toes. Your left hand supports on the shoulder while your left thumb supports your right thumb, which applies pressure to S.I.9 just below the armpit. Repeat 3 times.

24. Right Side Shoulder Blade Area, Rib Cage and Lower Back Area

Change to a half-kneeling position and give shiatsu to S.I.11 in the center of the shoulder blade, 3 times, by either of the following techniques:

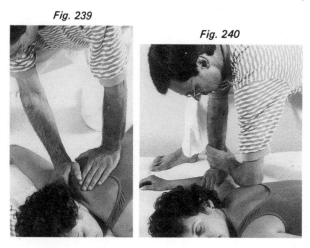

Fig. 239

Fig. 240

(i) *Heel of palm pressure*
The left hand supports around the shoulder blade while you apply pressure with your right hand (Fig. 239).

(ii) *Elbow pressure*
Place your right hand over the elbow. Your left hand clasps your right wrist. Your right knee rests on your right arm. Lean in to apply pressure (Fig. 240).

In the same posture, move your

body position toward the waist some 6 inches. Place
your left hand in the lower back area, left side, for
support. With your right palm, give general palm pressure across the rib cage toward the lower back area
in 3 to 4 places (Fig. 241). Heel of palm pressure can
be applied in like manner. By changing to a kneeling
posture we can also apply elbow pressure along the
same line, in 3 to 4 places (Fig. 242).

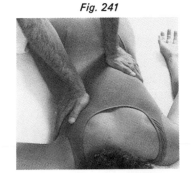

Fig. 241

Beside the lumbar vertebrae measure out 2 thumb-
widths. Apply shiatsu by either of the
following techniques:

Fig. 242   Fig. 243

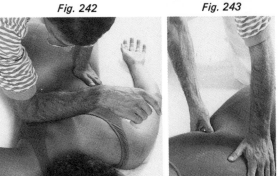

(i) *Thumb pressure*
   Your supporting hand is
   on the left side of the spine.
   From L_1 to L_4 apply pres-
   sure in 4 places (Fig. 243).
   Repeat.

(ii) *Elbow pressure*
   Elbow pressure is especially
   effective here. When applying pressure it is important
   to maintain a low body
   angle.

Fig. 244

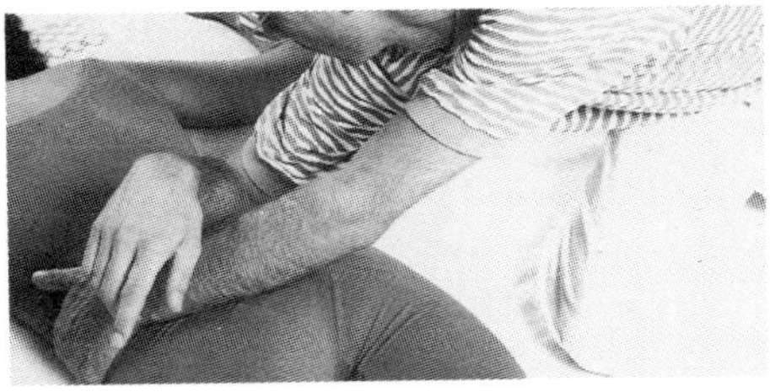

Beside T_{12} (KD.), L_1
and L_2 (S.I.), sit seiza facing the hips, and
place your left hand around the waist
(Fig. 244). With an angle of pressure more
acute than usual, lean in and beside each
area apply pressure and hold for a few
seconds. Repeat at least once or until you
feel the area responding to your shiatsu.

In mirror image, change your position. Sit
seiza facing the head, right hand over the left side at the waist. Apply pressure as
above beside L_3 and L_4 (KD.) (Fig. 245) and toward L_5 (BL.), then beside and along
the iliac crest (L.I.) in the same manner as above. Sometimes the area corresponding
to the L.I.m is very tight. In this case raise the right leg along the futon (Fig. 246).

Repeat steps *22* to *24* (Figs. 234 through 246) in mirror image on the left side.

25. Beside the Spine

Kneel on the receiver's left side some 6 to 9 inches away, further back if you wish to
apply stronger pressure. Place your right palm parallel with and over the upper spine,
the left palm on your right, the left finger and thumb lightly clasped around the
right wrist. By leaning, apply pressure (Fig. 247). Release, then apply again in 5 to
6 more places toward and onto the coccyx, sliding from 1 point to the next. Repeat.

General palm pressure, heel of palm pressure, thumb pressure, and elbow pressure

Fig. 245

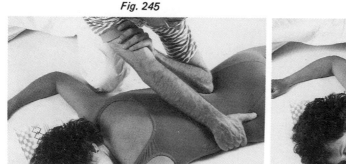

Fig. 246

Fig. 247

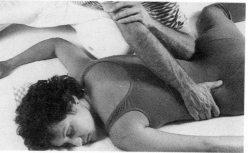

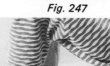

can all be very effective over the back. General palm pressure helps to induce relaxation. Heel of palm pressure is deep and soothing but not as strong or sharp as elbow pressure. Thumb pressure is generally sharper, less powerful than elbow and especially effective over limited areas. Elbow pressure is the most widely practiced technique in Zen Shiatsu.

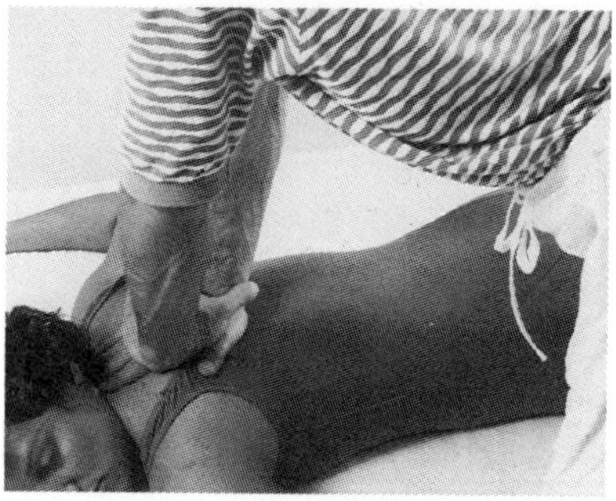

(i) *Elbow pressure*

Place your left hand over the left shoulder. Begin on the more relaxed side. For our practice begin on the left side. Assume a half-kneeling posture, with your left foot beyond the receiver's head and your right knee about 6 inches away from the receiver's body, in line with the middle back area. The left knee rests on your left elbow. Apply pressure from T_4 to L_4, in 5 to 6 places (Figs. 248 and 249). Your arm is pointed at an angle of between 10 and 11 o'clock and your point of pressure is approximately one and a half thumb-widths away from the midline, but aiming toward the spine. Repeat at least once. Then, to give shiatsu along the right side of the spine, assume a kneeling posture, with your knees apart. The angle of pressure is such that your arm is pointed between 1 and 2 o'clock. Continue as on the left side from T_4 to L_4 (Figs. 250 and 251). Repeat at least once.

Fig. 248

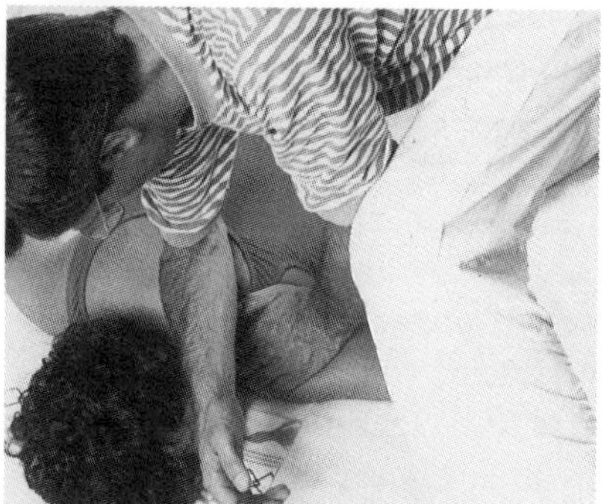

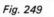

Fig. 249

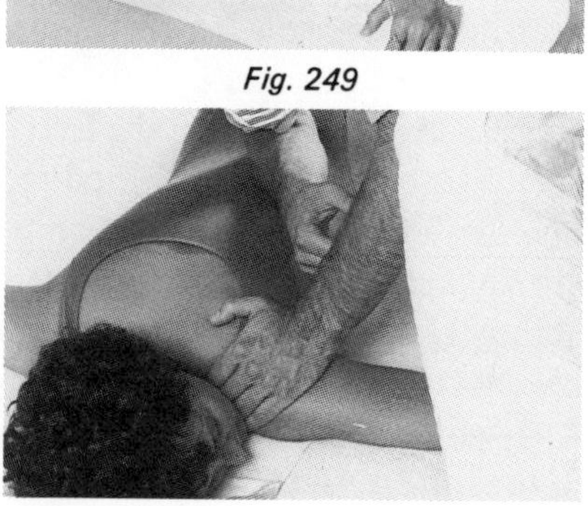

Fig. 250

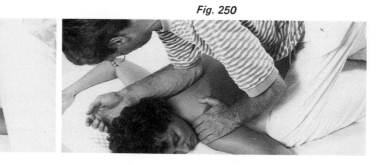

Keep in mind that you may have to move your whole body slightly as you move down the spine. The first sequence of pressure should not be too strong; if appropriate gradually build up with each following sequence of pressure. Also, without going to extremes, the further you move away from the body the stronger your pressure can be. (Refer to Chapter 6.)

When working within a small area, assume a different posture.

Sit seiza with your left knee extended some 45 degrees away. Place your left supporting hand in close proximity to the area to which you wish to give shiatsu. Begin with a flat

Fig. 251

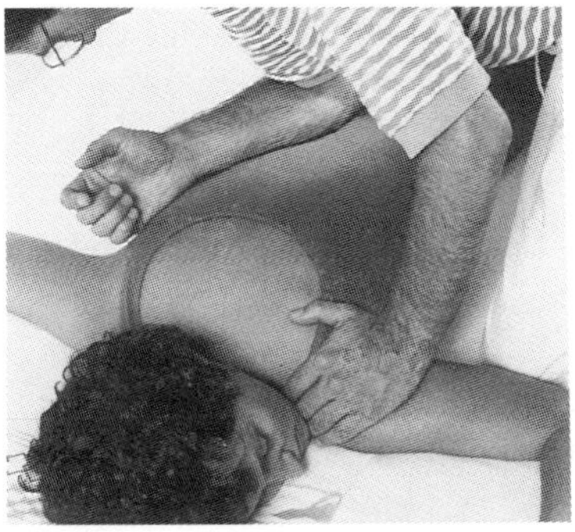

Fig. 252   *Fig. 253*

Fig. 254   *Fig. 255*

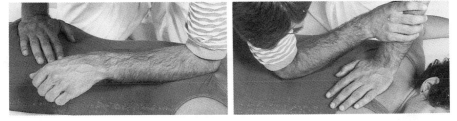

broad angle of pressure (Fig. 252). Upon further applications you can slowly raise your arm slightly, increasing the intensity of pressure (Fig. 253).

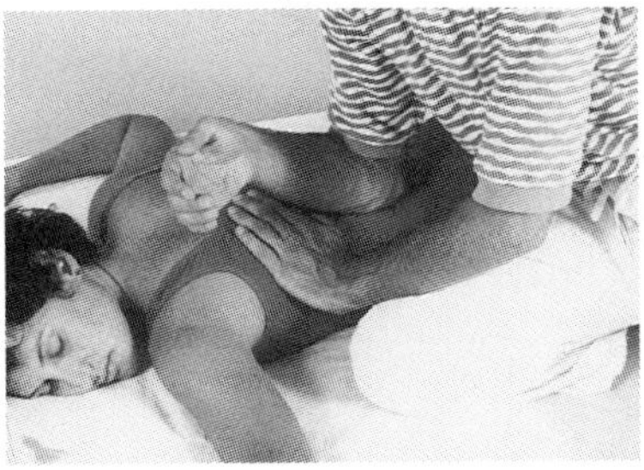

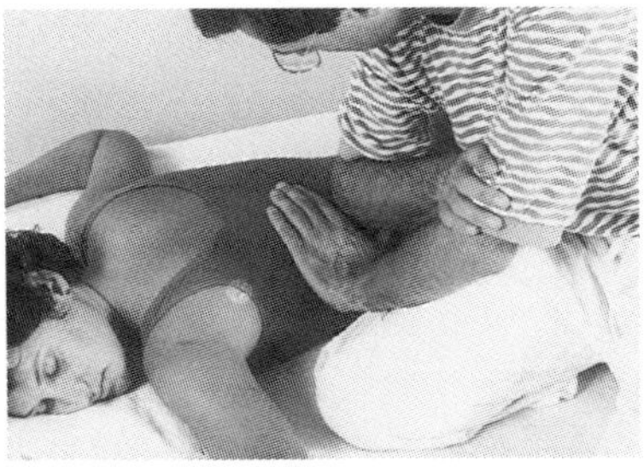

To give elbow shiatsu to the second BL.m, change to a kneeling position facing the back, in preparation for working on the right side, if you are kneeling on the left. (If kneeling on the right side, prepare to work on the left.) Use your left elbow to apply pressure to the upper half of the back (Fig. 254) and your right for the lower (Fig. 255). In each case the supporting hand rests in the opposite area and you proceed toward the hips.

With your left elbow you can give shiatsu to the areas relating to the liver and gallbladder: with your right elbow apply pressure to that area related to the right kidney (Fig. 255).

Working from the receiver's right side place your supporting hand in the lower back area, left side, and give shiatsu with your right elbow to areas relating to the stomach and triple heater; then place your right hand between the spine and shoulder blade, and with your left elbow give shiatsu to the area relating to the left kidney.

(ii) *Heel of palm pressure*
Heel of palm pressure can be most effective when you are working in a kneeling position facing the body, to apply pressure down the BL.m on the opposite side from the side you are kneeling on. Use

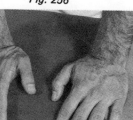
Fig. 256

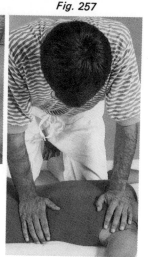
Fig. 257

your left hand for the upper and right for the lower, with the supporting hand resting comfortably in the opposite area.

In this example, the left hand remains stationary between the shoulder blade and spine, while the right heel of palm gives shiatsu down the BL.m (Figs. 256 and 257). Repeat these steps in mirror image on the opposite side.

(iii) *Thumb pressure*

Thumb pressure is most effective when focusing on a small area. Begin on the left side. In a half-kneeling position with your left knee resting against your left arm begin with the left thumb placed above the right. On the left side, the left thumb remains stationary while the right thumb gives shiatsu along a line of

Fig. 260

Fig. 258   Fig. 259

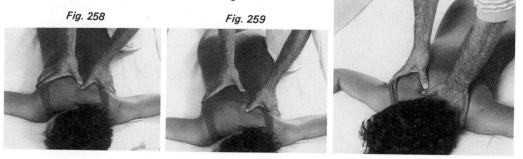

some 4 to 6 inches, in 4 to 6 places (Figs. 258 and 259). For thumb shiatsu along the right side of the spine, assume a kneeling posture and clasp your left hand around the left shoulder, with your left thumb resting on the right side of the spine. Apply pressure with your right thumb from a point immediately below the left, in 4 to 6 places (Fig. 260). When using thumb pressure you will most probably have to repeat your pressure a number of times to be effective.

Next, return to the left side and from the last point of pressure, once more progress down the spine in 4 to 6 places, then the right side again, and so on.

26. Hips

All movements from here are toward the feet. From the waist down we begin shiatsu on the side which is more relaxed: for practice, the right side. Begin in a half-kneeling posture on the receiver's right side and place your left supporting hand over the sacrum. Imagine a line some 2 inches, and another 5 inches, lateral to the sacrum and somewhat parallel with the spine.

(i) *General palm pressure*

From top to bottom on the inside line beside the sacrum, apply palm pressure in 2 places (Fig. 261). Repeat in the same way on the outside line. With your right hand resting on the last point of pressure, give general palm pressure with your left hand to the upper leg, along an inside line toward the knee, in 2 to 3 places (Fig. 262). Now continue with your right hand, toward the knee with general palm pres-

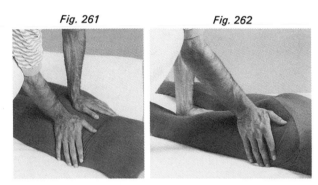

Fig. 261   Fig. 262

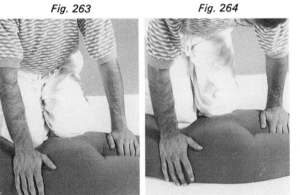

Fig. 263   Fig. 264

sure on an outside line in 2 to 3 places.

(ii) *Heel of palm pressure*

Over the buttocks for stronger, deeper pressure, apply shiatsu as above with the heel of palm, in 2 to 3 places along each line. Repeat.

(iii) *Knee pressure*

Change position. Face the hips in a squatting position and place your left hand on the upper leg and your right hand in the lower back area, left side. Your right knee gently rests in the lower back area, right side, while your left knee rests on the inside line (Fig. 263). When comfortable, come up into a kneeling position and give shiatsu along the inside line, in 2 places (Fig. 264). Repeat. Follow with knee shiatsu on the outside line in 2 places. Repeat.

27. Upper Leg

Change position. In a kneeling posture, face the receiver's upper leg. From the buttocks to just above the back of the knee we work along 3 lines: the BL.m on a center line, the LU.m a little to the outside of the center line, and the KD.m on an outside line. Along each line apply heel of palm pressure, with your right hand, in 3 to 4 places. Repeat. Or apply knee pressure, with your left knee. Your right hand rests on the sacrum. Again, in 3 to 4 places. Repeat.

(i) *Heel of palm pressure*

(1) *BL.m*

As though holding a suitcase, pick up the foot and draw the leg toward

254

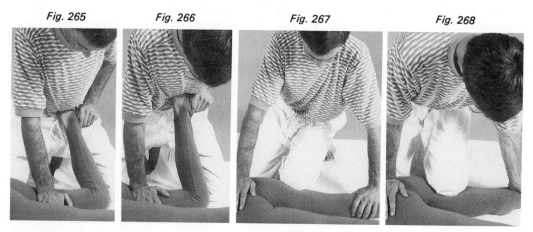

Fig. 265   Fig. 266   Fig. 267   Fig. 268

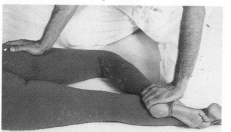

Fig. 269

you, resting it in your lower left abdominal area. While leaning in, apply pressure (Fig. 265).

(2) *LU.m*

Move the foot away from you so that the lower leg is perpendicular to the floor and resting in the left side of your abdomen. While leaning in slightly apply pressure (Fig. 266).

(3) *KD.m*

In seiza, with knees apart, move the foot away from you, making it easier to treat an outside line.

(ii) *Knee pressure*

For knee pressure a different approach is more appropriate. Place your right palm over the sacrum and your left palm over the right knee.

(1) *BL.m*

Turn your left palm in reverse and gently stretch the leg toward you and downward. Apply shiatsu along a center line with your left knee, in 3 to 4 places (Fig. 267).

(2) *LU.m*

Focus the stretch downward toward the foot. Give shiatsu down a line just to the outside of the center line as above.

(3) *KD.m*

Turn your left palm around, facing away from you. Gently stretch the leg away from you and downward slightly. Give shiatsu with your left knee to the KD.m, in 3 to 4 places (Fig. 268).

(4) *L.I.m*

Place the right foot above the left ankle, which is supported by your left hand. Change to seiza posture with legs wide apart on each side of the knee.

(i) *General palm pressure*

With your right hand, apply pressure beside the iliotibial ligament toward the knee, in 4 to 5 places (Fig. 269). Then apply either heel of palm or elbow pressure.

(ii) *Heel of palm pressure*
Apply pressure as above, using the heel of the right palm. Come up on your toes if necessary.

(iii) *Elbow pressure*
Elbow pressure can be most effective but it is stronger and sharper. Along the same line, with your elbow almost at right angles to the muscle, apply pressure, in 5 to 6 places (Fig. 270). Repeat.

(5) *GB.m*
Move the right leg so that the right root rests comfortably just above the left knee, supported and held in place by your left hand. From hip to knee, along an outside line, give general palm pressure, in 3 to 4 places. Follow with either heel of palm pressure or elbow pressure in 3 to 4 places (Fig. 271). Repeat. The angle of elbow pressure should be at a diagonal across the muscle, with either seiza, or seiza on toes posture.

Fig. 270

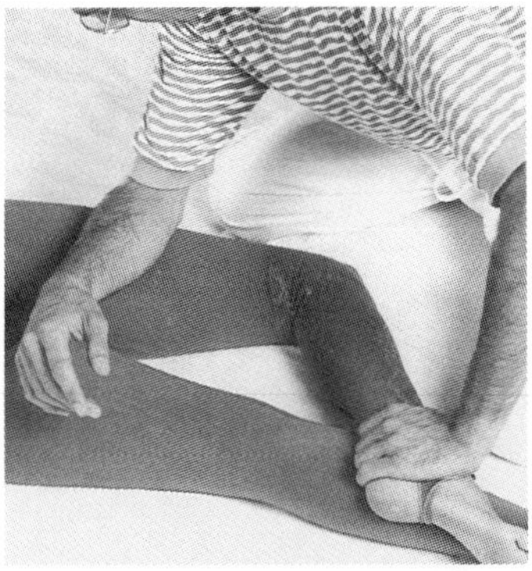

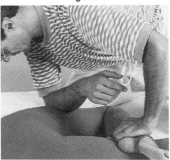

Fig. 271

28. Lower Right Leg

GB.m
Turn your position to face your left hand, sitting seiza on your toes with knees apart. From knee to ankle apply the following techniques:

(i) *General palm pressure*—in 3 to 4 places, followed by either:

(ii) *Heel of palm pressure*—in 3 to 4 places

(iii) *Elbow pressure* across the muscle from GB.34 in 4 to 5 places (Fig. 272)

Facing the lower leg, come into seiza on toes posture and place your left hand around the right heel, so that the sole of the right foot is resting on your lower arm. With your right hand give general palm pressure to the lower leg, toward the ankle, in 3 to 4 places.

Fig. 272

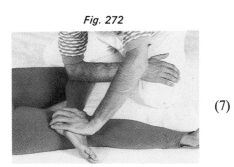

(7) *T.H.m*
The T.H.m flows midway between the GB.m and the front of the leg. Along the T.H.m we can apply either heel of palm pressure or knee pressure.

(i) *Heel of palm pressure*
Apply heel of palm pressure with your right hand from knee to ankle, in 4 to 5 places. Repeat. As you apply pressure with your right hand, stretch the Achilles tendon and draw the foot toward you, thus increasing the pressure of your shiatsu.

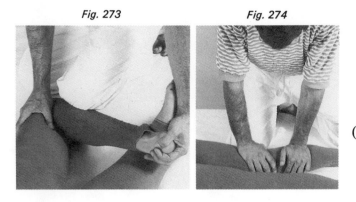

Fig. 273   Fig. 274

(ii) *Knee pressure*
Apply left knee pressure, in 3 to 4 places as above (Fig. 273). Repeat. Your right hand rests over the right knee.

(8) *ST.m*
Apply knee pressure as to the T.H.m, along a line just beside the tibia, from ST.36 to the ankle.

(9) *BL.m*
Return the leg to its normal position. In a kneeling posture, face the lower leg and place your right hand above the knee. With your left hand, give general palm pressure from just below the knee to the heel, in 3 to 4 places (Fig. 274). Rest your left hand over the Achilles tendon. Follow with either heel of palm pressure with the right palm or elbow pressure. The BL.m over the calf muscle is often tight and painful to the touch. While knee pressure can be applied here it may be a little too strong. Heel of palm pressure applied slowly is safe, deep and soothing. Elbow pressure is stronger and sharper, yet the giver has more control, and more sensitivity to the receiver's reaction than with knee pressure.

(i) *Heel of palm pressure*
From just below the knee toward BL.57 at the base of the calf muscle, apply pressure in 2 to 3 places. Repeat. This area may require a number of repetitions of pressure before you feel a positive response.

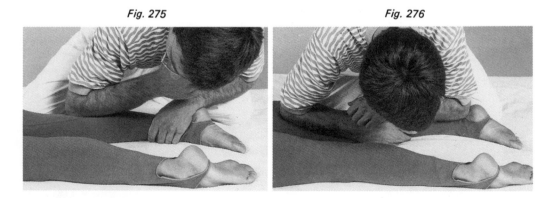

Fig. 275   Fig. 276

(ii) *Elbow pressure*
Facing the lower leg, in seiza with knees wide apart, brace your left elbow on your left knee. Place your left hand around the right ankle and gently stretch the leg downward, and hold the stretch. With your right elbow, apply pressure from the knee down the BL.m, in 2 to 3 places to BL.57 (Fig. 275). Place your right hand under the middle of the lower leg. With your left elbow, give shiatsu to the inside of the lower half of the lower leg toward the ankle, in 2 to 3 places (Fig. 276).

29. Sole of Right Foot

Shiatsu can be given with either thumb or elbow pressure.

(i) *Thumb pressure*

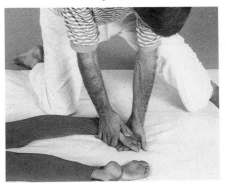

Fig. 277

Assume a semi-kneeling posture, facing the right foot. Place your left hand under the right foot, with your left knee resting on your left arm. With your right thumb, give shiatsu to KD.1, 3 times, holding momentarily each time (Fig. 277). In the same manner, pressure can be applied to various lines along the foot: inside, center, and outside, for example, in 5 to 6 places along each line.

Fig. 278

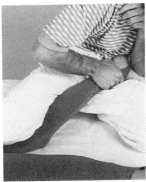

(ii) *Elbow pressure*

Change to seiza posture on toes, with your right knee resting just above the back of the receiver's right knee. The top of the receiver's right foot rests on your left lap. Grasp just above the ankle with your right hand. Gently stretch the leg away, simultaneously pressing at the knee with your right knee. While gently applying pressure with your right knee, apply counter pressure to KD.1 on the sole of the foot with your left elbow (Fig. 278). Repeat twice. In the same manner, pressure can be applied to various points on the foot

30. Joint Stretches

Change to a seiza posture facing the receiver's head, with the knee between your knees and lower leg at a perpendicular angle to the floor. With the fingertips of both hands give simultaneous pressure along a center line running along the sole of the foot (Fig. 279). Your thumbs support at the base of the toes.

Fig. 279

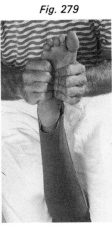

Fig. 280

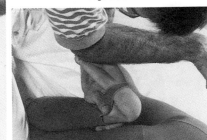

Support over the balls of the foot with your left index finger and thumb, and briskly rub the toes backward and forward a few times.

Place your left hand just above the ankle. With your right hand holding the foot, rotate it in each direction 2 to 3 times.

Fig. 281

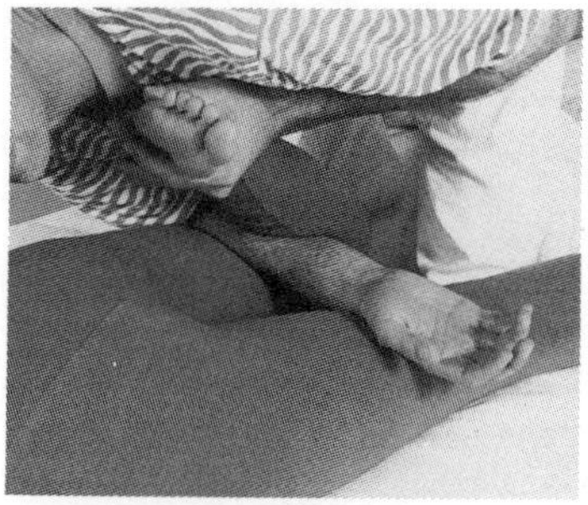

Fig. 282

Fig. 283

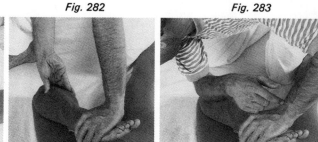

Fig. 284

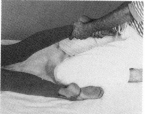

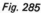

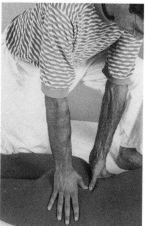

Fig. 285

Fig. 286

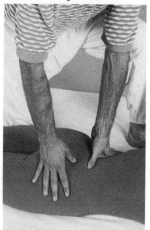

Bring the lower leg to a vertical position. Place your right elbow on the ball of the foot and lean forward, thereby stretching the Achilles tendon. Intensify the stretch by moving the leg toward the buttocks (Fig. 280). Hold briefly, then release.

Place the top of the foot on your chest, supported by your left hand. Place your right elbow behind the knee. Slowly lean forward and press the leg toward the buttocks, gently stretching the knee joint (Fig. 281). Hold briefly then release. Repeat. Take your elbow away and press the sole of the foot toward and if flexible enough, onto the buttocks. Hold and change to a half-kneeling posture. With your right thumb give shiatsu to the ST.m from ST.36 to ST.40, in 3 to 4 places (Fig. 282). Repeat.

Elbow pressure can also be applied here, instead. Place the left palm over the back of the right foot. While holding the stretch, apply pressure over ST.36, then toward and to ST.40, in 3 to 4 places (Fig. 283). Repeat.

Bring the leg back into its natural position. Sitting seiza, hold the leg with your left hand above the ankle and your right hand on the top of the foot. Leaning back, gently stretch the leg 2 to 3 times (Fig. 284). Allow the leg to rest, with toes pointed inward.

Repeat steps *26* through *30*, mirror image on the left leg with the following exception. Begin the left side sequence with thumb pressure on each side on the sacrum, in 3 to 4 places, beginning on the right side (Figs. 285 and 286).

31. *Both Legs Together*

(1) *The feet*

There are two main ways to give shiatsu to the feet: standing or kneeling.

(i) *Standing*

This method is best if the receiver has reasonably

Fig. 287

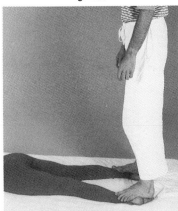

flexible ankles. Place your right foot inward at right angles, on the sole of the right foot. Then, turn your foot outward so that the toes and ball of your foot rest above the heel. Repeat these steps on the left foot.

Fig. 288

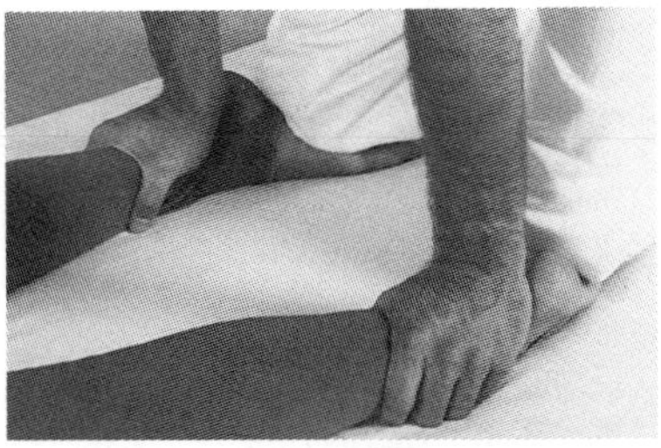

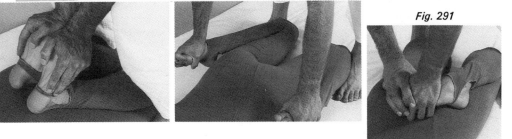

In a relaxed and centered state, gently shift your weight from one foot to the other, for 15 to 30 seconds, stretching the ankles as well as applying pressure to the feet (Fig. 287).

Fig. 289   Fig. 290   Fig. 291

(ii) *Kneeling*

Place your hands for support just above the heels. Assume a kneeling posture by placing your knees on the soles of the feet. Again, shift your weight from one knee to the other, gently giving knee pressure to each foot alternately (Fig. 288). While holding with your knees on the soles of the feet, lean forward and apply palm pressure from knees to heels, in 3 to 4 places, simultaneously. Repeat.

(2) *Stretches*

Lift both feet and bring them slightly toward the buttocks. With your feet beside the outsides of the knees, place the heels of your palms over the toes, and stretch them toward the floor. Intensify the stretch by moving both heels toward the buttocks. Hold briefly, then release (Fig. 289).

Fig. 292

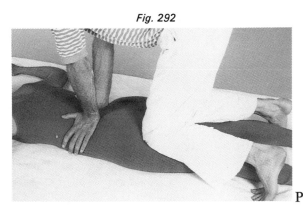

Straightaway, reverse the position of the feet so that the soles are facing the floor. Lean forward, and gently press the feet toward the floor (Fig. 290). Hold briefly, then, placing the sole of one foot on top of the other, press both feet together toward the sacrum (Fig. 291). Repeat, with the other foot on top. Let both legs rest naturally with toes turned inward. Place your hands on the receiver's

Fig. 293 Fig. 294 Fig. 295

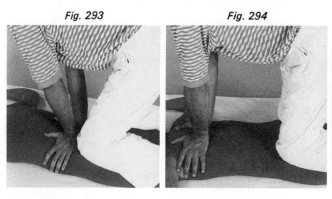

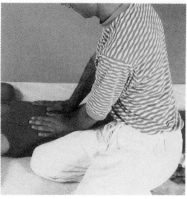

waist. Come into a kneeling position with your toes in proximity to the outside of the receiver's calves.

Apply knee pressure to both legs simultaneously, from the buttocks to just above the knees, in 2 to 3 places (Fig. 292). Repeat.

Place your knees on the buttocks just below the iliac crest. In the same manner as above, give shiatsu in 2 to 3 places and repeat (Fig. 293). Holding, with your knees on the buttocks, place your palms between the shoulder blades. Lean forward and give palm pressure simultaneously down both sides of the spine in 4 to 5 places (Fig. 294).

Fig. 296

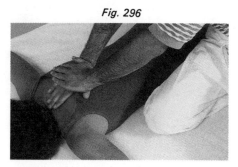

Change to a kneeling position on the left side and repeat thumb pressure or elbow pressure down each side of the spine at least twice. At this time the back should be much more relaxed, and once again, you can treat those areas of kyo and jitsu.

Finish by giving gentle forward-backward motion pressure with your palms in the lower back area 2 to 3 times, followed by the same to the middle back area (Fig. 295).

Around the shoulder blade area, give a rotating kind of palm pressure with "inside to outside" circles, 2 to 3 times. Place your left palm over your right and give a gentle but brisk rubdown to the spine 2 to 3 times (Fig. 296).

Supine Position

32. Hara Diagnosis

Sit seiza on the receivers' right side, parallel with their body. Place your right palm over the center of the hara and hold lightly for a few seconds (Fig. 298). Apply light pressure to the 4 other sections of the hara: to the receiver's right side, upper hara, left side, lower hara, and once more to the center. In this way, feeling for hot or cold, tightness, stiffness, weakness and flaccid muscles, the giver can gain an overall feeling of the receiver's condition.

Raise the heel of your right palm and place your left palm horizontally over the lower hara.

1. *HT.* With the fingers of the right hand, apply pressure at a 45 degree angle to the heart diagnosis area, just below the sternum (Fig. 299).
2. *H.C.* In the same manner, at a more vertical angle, apply pressure to an area midway between the navel and sternum (Fig. 300).
3. *GB.* With index and middle fingers, apply pressure at a perpendicular angle toward the rib cage on the receiver's upper right side (Fig. 301).
4. *LV.* Employing index and middle fingers, with the palm at an oblique angle, apply pressure under the middle area of the rib cage on the right side (Fig. 302).
5. *LU. right side.* In the same manner as above but at a more vertical angle, apply pressure under the lower part of the rib cage on the receiver's right side (Fig. 303).
6. *LU. left side.* Apply shiatsu with your right hand under the lower rib cage, left side (Fig. 304).
7. *ST.* Apply pressure perpendicular to and under the rib cage, on the receiver's upper left side (Fig. 305).

Fig. 297

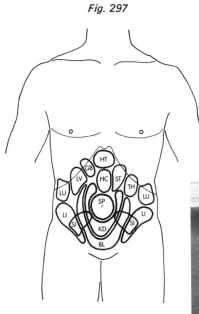

Fig. 298

Fig. 299

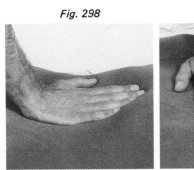

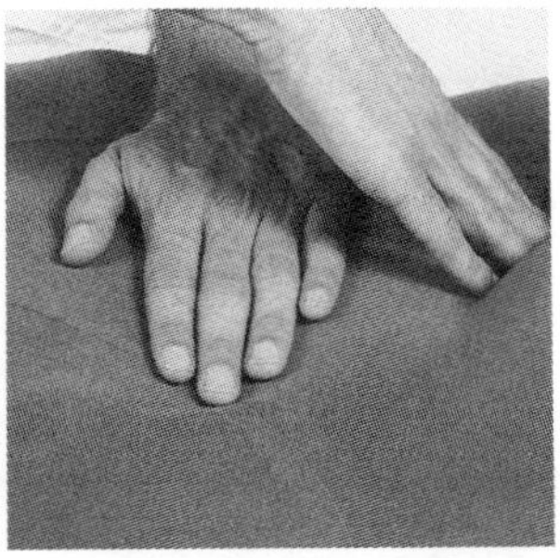

Fig. 300

Fig. 301

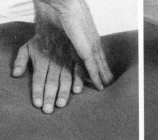

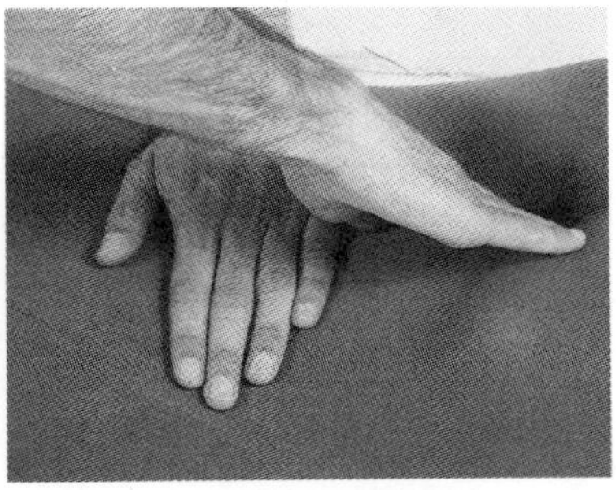

Fig. 302   *Fig. 303*   *Fig. 304*   *Fig. 305*

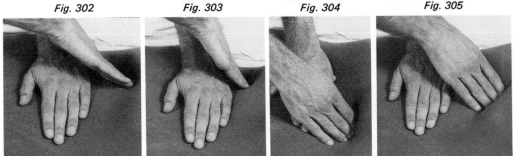

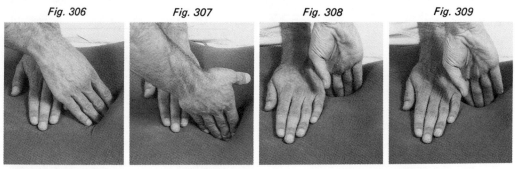

Fig. 306   Fig. 307   Fig. 308   Fig. 309

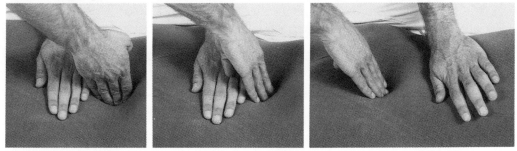

Fig. 310   Fig. 311   Fig. 312

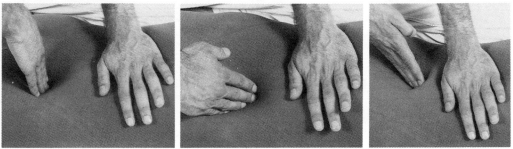

Fig. 313   Fig. 314   Fig. 315

8. *T.H.* In like manner, as above, give shiatsu to the area between lung and stomach areas on the left side (Fig. 306).

9. *BL. left side.* Immediately below the triple heater area, to an area almost level with the navel, apply vertical pressure (Fig. 307).

10. *BL. right side.* Give shiatsu to the same area on the opposite side (Fig. 308).

11. *KD. right side.* Slide your right hand to within 1 inch of the central vertical line. Apply vertical pressure (Fig. 309).

12. *KD. left side.* Turn your hand around and apply pressure to the same line on the left side (Fig. 310).

13. *SP.* Apply almost vertical pressure with 3 fingers around the navel area (Fig. 311).

14. *KD. lower.* Place your left hand over the upper hara for support. With your right hand at a fairly sharp angle, give shiatsu to an area 2 inches below the navel (Fig. 312).

15. *BL. lower.* To an area 2 inches below the KD. area, apply pressure as above, at an even more vertical angle (Fig. 313).

16. *S.I. left side.* From a point 2 inches below the hip bone, at an angle directed toward the navel, give shiatsu at a diagonal across the lower hara (Fig. 314).

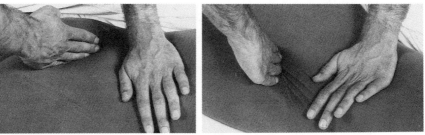

Fig. 316   Fig. 317

17. *S.I. right side.* Give shiatsu as above, on the right side in mirror image (Fig. 315).
18. *L.I. right side.* With your right hand parallel with and over the groin, apply pressure (Fig. 316).
19. *L.I. left side.* In the same area as above, on the left side, apply shiatsu (Fig. 317).
20. Repeat steps *1* through *19*.
21. Select the areas which are most jitsu. Let us assume that there are three such areas. This time apply pressure to one area with one hand and to another with the other. Give gentle alternate pressure to test for the most jitsu area. Now compare in the same manner this area with the remaining jitsu area and decide which is the most jitsu area.
22. Repeat the above process to the most kyo areas.
23. Apply very light pressure over the jitsu area, just enough to take up any slack. Apply deep holding pressure over the kyo area. If we have chosen the two areas of greatest opposite distortion then the stiffness in the jitsu area will subside. The change may be subtle so we have to judge carefully. If the jitsu area does not change try the same technique with each of the kyo areas.
24. If you still cannot find the correct pair, check the meridians in the legs.
25. Once a decision is made, these meridians and their partners are the two pairs of opposites we will pay special attention to throughout the final part of the treatment. In actual clinical practice at Masunaga's clinic, hara diagnosis was carried out three times during a massage: at the beginning, at this point in the treatment, and at the end.

33. Legs

All movements are toward the feet. With one exception, the left hand should remain on the hara at all times. We usually apply general palm pressure to an area first, followed by heel of palm, thumb, elbow or knee pressure. We work mostly from the receiver's right side.

(a) Choosing the leg to which we first give shiatsu
General practice is to treat the whole of one leg at a time. Sit seiza facing the receiver, at his or her feet. To choose which leg is first, bring the legs to a 90 degree angle and open them. Observe which leg opens more. That is the leg which is more relaxed or flexible, the leg we begin on. If this is not obvious, then in a kneeling position apply gentle pressure at the knees. For practice we begin on the left leg.

(b) Upper left leg

In the following sequence the leg is moved into different positions. The purpose is to stretch the meridian related to each position, bringing it close to the surface, making it easier for treatment. For some people such positions may cause discomfort in which case a cushion may be placed underneath the knee.

Kneel on the receiver's right side, facing the upper leg. Place your left hand over the hara.

Fig. 318

Fig. 319

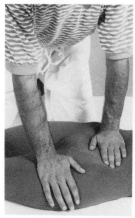
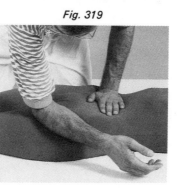

(1) *ST.m*

The ST.m runs along the front of the leg, approximately 1 inch lateral to a center line in the upper leg and continues toward the lateral side of the kneecap. Give general palm pressure to the upper leg in 3 places toward the knee (Fig. 318), followed by either:

(i) Heel of palm pressure
(ii) Elbow pressure (Fig. 319). In 3 to 4 places, toward the knee. Repeat.

(2) *SP.m*

Change the position of the leg so that the toes of the left foot are in line with the right heel. Give general palm pressure in 3 places to the inside of the upper leg, in 3 places to the lower leg, and once on the arch of the foot. The SP.m in this position runs approximately 1 1/4 to 1 1/2 inches from the lateral side of the leg toward the knee. Gently stretch the SP.m by applying pressure at the knee with your right hand (Fig. 320). Follow by applying either:

(i) Heel of palm pressure
(ii) Elbow pressure (Fig. 321). In 3 to 4 places, toward and onto the knee. Repeat.

Fig. 320

Fig. 321

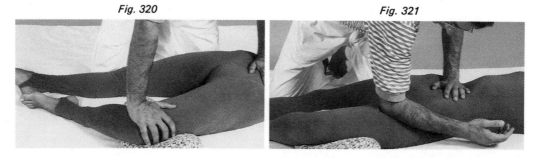

(3) *S.I.m*

Move the heel of the left foot in line with the right knee. Change your position so that your right knee rests just below the left ankle, preventing the leg from moving. In this position the S.I.m runs on a midline in the upper leg. Gently stretch the S.I.m by applying pressure at the knee with your right hand. Apply either:

Fig. 322

Fig. 323

Fig. 324

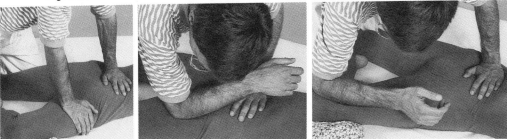

Fig. 325

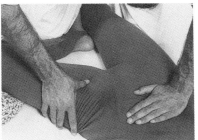

Fig. 326

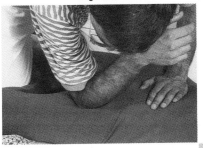

(i)   Heel of palm pressure, in 3 to 4 places (Fig. 322)

(ii) Thumb pressure in 6 to 7 places

(iii) Elbow pressure in 3 to 4 places, toward and onto the knee (Figs. 323 and 324). Repeat.

In this same position apply thumb pressure to the HT.m, which lies approximately 3 thumb-widths below the gracilis muscle, in 4 to 5 places. Repeat.

(4) *H.C.m*

Move the arch of the left foot in line with the right knee and gently stretch the H.C.m by applying pressure at the knee. The H.C.m in this position travels just above and behind the gracilis muscle. Apply either:

Fig. 327

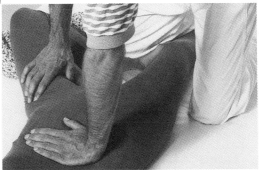

(i)   Thumb pressure in 5 to 6 places (Fig. 325)

(ii) Elbow pressure in 3 to 4 places (Fig. 326). Repeat.
The angle of pressure should be aiming toward the inside of the gracilis muscle.

(5) *LV.m*

Move the ball of the left foot in line with the right knee and gently stretch the LV.m by applying pressure at the knee. The LV.m follows a line just below the gracilis muscle. Apply either:

(i)   Thumb pressure in 5 to 6 places (Fig. 327)

(ii) Knee pressure with your right knee, in 2 to 3 places (Fig. 328). Repeat. Your

Fig. 328

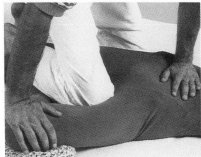

right hand gives support at the knee. Knee pressure can then be applied to the H.C.m (Fig. 329).

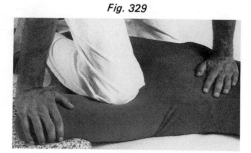
Fig. 329

(6) *T.H.m*

Move the big toe of the left foot in line with the right ankle and gently stretch the left leg across the right leg. Secure the leg in position with the lower inside of your right thigh, and support the knee with the left side of your abdomen.

Your crotch should not touch the receiver's body. Make sure to counterbalance the stretch with firm but gentle pressure on the hara.

Along a line midway between the front and outer side of the leg give general palm pressure (Fig. 330), in 3 to 4 places toward the knee followed by either:

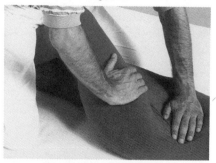
Fig. 330

(i) Heel of palm pressure
(ii) Elbow pressure (Fig. 331). In 3 to 4 places toward the knee. Repeat.

(7) *GB.m*

Move the arch of the left foot in line with the right knee; stretch the left leg across the right and secure the lower leg with the inside of your lower right thigh. Tuck the left knee below the left side of your rib cage. Along an outside line (approximately placed on the outside seam of a pair of trousers), apply general palm pressure, in 3 to 4 places toward the knee, followed by either:

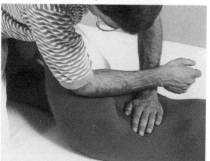
Fig. 331

(i) Heel of palm pressure
(ii) Elbow pressure in 3 to 4 places toward and onto the knee (Fig. 332). Repeat.

(8) *L.I.m*

Take the left knee in your right hand and stretch toward the right shoulder. Along a line at the edge of the iliotibial ligament apply general palm pressure, followed by either:

(i) Heel of palm pressure, in 3 to 4 places
(ii) Elbow pressure in 3 to 4 places, toward the knee (Fig. 333)

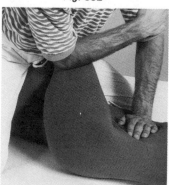
Fig. 332

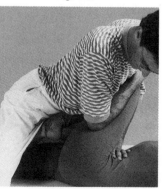
Fig. 333

(iii) Knee pressure in 2 to 3 places. Repeat. Move your body to the receiver's left side, and place your right hand on the hara. In seiza posture on your toes, while holding the stretch, take the left knee in your left hand and draw the

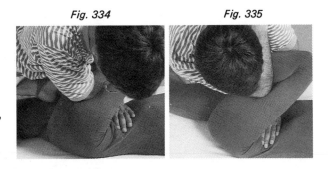

Fig. 334   Fig. 335

leg onto your right knee. Hold, release, then apply pressure in 2 more places toward the knee. Repeat. Fig. 358 shows a mirror image of this move.

(9) *KD.m*

Take the left knee in your right hand and stretch toward the right side of the face. The KD.m flows parallel with the LI.m some 2 to 3 thumb-widths toward the back of the leg. Apply either:

(i) Elbow pressure in 3 to 4 places toward the knee (Fig. 334)

(ii) Knee pressure in 2 to 3 places. Repeat.

Knee pressure is applied in the same manner as pressure to the L.I.m, only this time use your left knee.

(10) *LU.m*

Take the left knee in your right hand and stretch toward the nose. Along a line a little to the outside of the center of the back of the leg apply elbow pressure at a fairly acute angle in 2 to 3 places toward the knee (Fig. 335). Repeat.

(11) *BL.m*

Take the left knee in your right hand and stretch toward the left side of the face. Standing on the receiver's left side, squat slightly and place your left knee on a point some 2 thumb-widths inside of the LU.m. Place your right hand over the left on the hara. Lean forward and apply pressure to this one point, 2 to 3 times (Fig. 336). Change position.

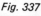

Fig. 336

(12) *ST., m*

Kneeling on the receiver's left side facing the upper left leg, place your right hand on the knee. With your left hand, grasp the arch of the left foot, and bring the lower leg underneath but slightly to the outside of the upper leg.

With your right hand over the hara, apply pressure at the knee with your left hand, stretching the ST.m (Fig. 337). For many people this stretch is painful and it is advisable to stretch the leg only as far as it is comfortable.

If the knee can rest on the futon you can apply either:

(i) Heel of palm pressure with your left

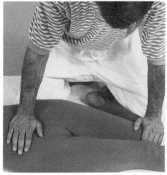

Fig. 337

palm in 3 to 4 places (Fig. 338)

(ii) Knee pressure with your left knee in 3 to 4 places (Fig. 339). Repeat. Your left hand placed over the left knee gives support.

(c) Lower leg

Return the leg to its natural position. In a kneeling position, face the lower leg. Place your right hand, bent at the wrist, under the left knee for support.

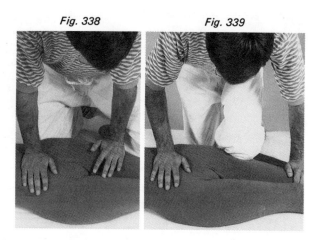

Fig. 338   Fig. 339

The ST.m in this position follows a line on the lateral side of the tibia.

Following general palm pressure apply either:

(i) Heel of palm pressure in 3 to 4 places

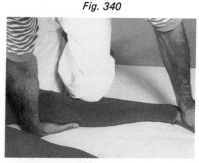

Fig. 340

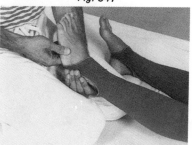

Fig. 341

(ii) Knee pressure in 3 to 4 places (Fig. 340). Repeat.

With knee pressure your left hand rests on the top of the left foot. It simultaneously stretches the foot toward the floor and inward. In the same manner, pressure can be applied to the T.H.m some 2 thumb-widths lateral to the ST.m.

(d) Left foot

Facing the receiver, change to seiza at the base of the feet. Hold the heel in your right hand and give clasping pressure with your left palm from behind the knee and along the back of the leg, in 3 places then once on the arch of the foot with the right hand.

Consider the little toe the outside and the big toe as the inside. Imagine 6 points, 4 at the outside of the base of each of the smaller

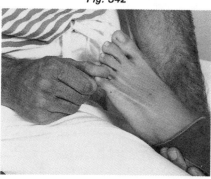

Fig. 342

toes, 1 at the base of each side of the big toe. Hold the heel in your left hand. From ankle to toes, apply thumb pressure along each of 6 lines in 4 to 5 places. Begin along the BL.m (outside line) and finish along the inside line (SP.m) (Fig. 341). Repeat to each line.

Beginning with the little toe, give pinching pressure to each toe with your index

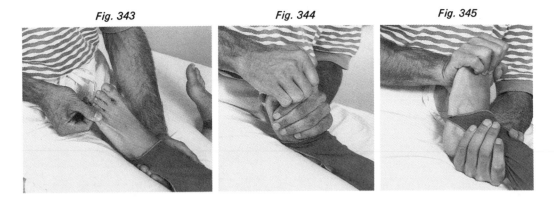

Fig. 343   Fig. 344   Fig. 345

finger and thumb, first on the outside in 2 places, then on the top and bottom in 2 places, stretching each toe toward you as you apply pressure (Figs. 342 and 343).

Supporting with the left hand over the top of the foot, grasp all toes between the heel of your palm and fingertips, stretch the toes toward the receiver and then gently toward you (Fig. 344). Your fingertips should rest on the foot, not on the toes. Then rotate the toes twice in each direction.

(e) **Stretching the left ankle joint**

Give support just above the ankle with your left hand. With your right hand over the top of the foot, gently stretch toward you, then grasp the toes with your right hand and rotate the ankle twice in each direction (Fig. 345). Now stretch the foot toward you again and then toward the receiver.

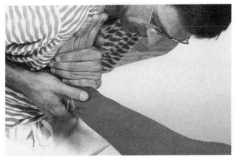

Fig. 346

In this last move, holding the heel in your right hand, place the sole of the foot in the center of your chest with your left hand over the top of the foot, and lean forward in a downward direction (Fig. 346).

Fig. 347

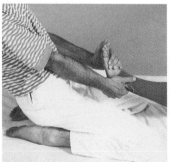

Fig. 348

This movement will stretch the Achilles tendon and muscles along the back of the leg. In making the stretch it is most important to lean downward. If you push the leg toward the receiver it could cause misalignment in the hips.

Now stretch the whole leg toward you (Fig. 347). Interlace your fingers and hold the receiver's foot between your hands. Gently rock the body forward and backward (Fig. 348).

270

(f) Stretching the hip joint

Change to a kneeling position. Take the left knee in your hands. Then gently place your left knee above the right knee. Ask the receiver to breathe in. Upon exhalation, gently press the knee toward the chest (Fig. 349). Repeat.

The angle of the stretch should be along the line of the kyo meridian as explained in (8) to (11). For a general stretch point the knee toward the nose.

Fig. 349

Fig. 350

Fig. 351

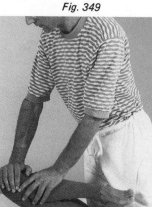
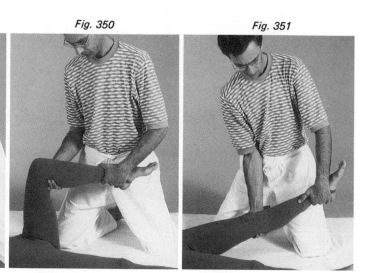

Fig. 352

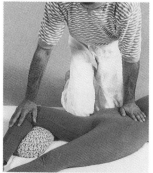

(g) Hip rotation

In a kneeling position hold the left ankle in your left hand and the left knee in your right hand (Fig. 350). Making a large arc, rotate 3 times in either direction, clockwise first if the kyo meridian is on the outside. Still holding the ankle with the left hand support the knee with your right hand. Briskly extend the leg in the direction of the feet 3 times (Fig. 351). Then bring the leg to its normal position.

(h) Right leg

Shiatsu to the right leg should be done in mirror image with the following exceptions:

(i)   Maintain support over the hara with the left hand while still working from the right side.

(ii) *ST.m.* You may find it easier to use your right knee instead of your right elbow. The right hand gives support over the knee.

(iii) *SP.m.* Again, knee pressure with your right knee may be easier (Fig. 352).

(iv) *S.I.m.* Positioning is different: in seiza, with your knees on either side of the knee (Fig. 353).

Fig. 353

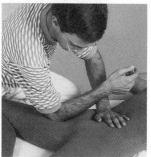

(v)   *H.C.m.* Almost the same body position as for S.I.m; elbow pressure is probably easiest, with pressure going inward toward the gracilis muscle (Fig. 354).

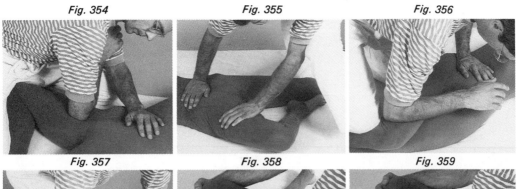

Fig. 354 Fig. 355 Fig. 356

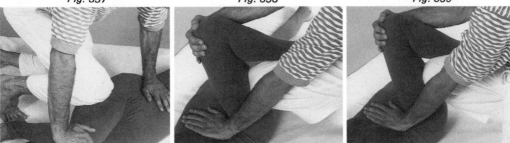

Fig. 357 Fig. 358 Fig. 359

(vi) *LV.m.* For the LV.m only, use your right hand for support. With your left knee resting against your left elbow, apply left hand thumb pressure (Fig. 355).

(vii) *T.H.m.* Place your left knee under the buttocks for support and your right knee below the receiver's right knee (Fig. 356).

(viii) *G.B.m.* Place your left knee further under the buttocks but this time give support at the knee with your right hand and apply knee pressure (Fig. 357).

(ix) *L.I.m.* Place your left hand over the hara. Stretch the right knee toward the left shoulder and hold. Then sit seiza on your toes, knees apart. Place your right hand over the knee and your left knee over the L.I.m, at the base of the buttocks (Fig. 358). Lean forward sightly with your left knee. Then draw the leg onto the left knee. In this manner, apply pressure toward the knee in 2 to 3 places. Repeat.

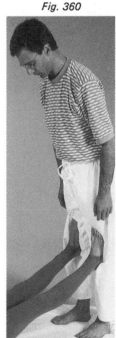

Fig. 360

(x) *KD.m.* Place your left hand over the hara. Stretch the right knee toward the left side of the face and hold. Sit seiza on your toes, knees apart. Place your right hand over the knee and your right knee on the KD.m, just below the buttocks (Fig. 359). Lean forward with your right knee and stretch the leg back onto the knee with your right hand. Apply pressure along the KD.m, in 3 to 4 places, moving toward the knee.

(xi) When giving shiatsu to the feet you may find it easier to apply pressure with your right thumb in the same manner as on the left foot.

(i) Both legs simultaneously
Stand up and place both the receiver's feet on your knees (Fig. 360). Lean forward and pick the legs up at

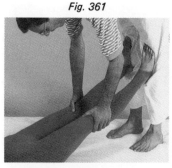

Fig. 361

Fig. 362

Fig. 363

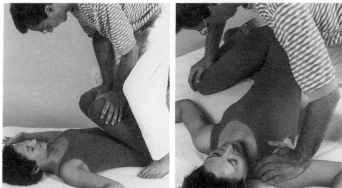

Fig. 364

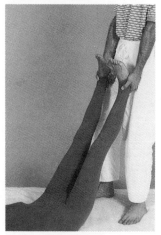

the knees (Fig. 361). Walk in until both knees are by the chest, but keep the sacrum on the floor as much as possible. Press gently to see which leg is more flexible (Fig. 362). If the right leg is more flexible, draw the left leg forward slightly, place your left hand on the right shoulder and stretch the right leg to the left side with your right hand (Fig. 363).

The right shoulder should not rise from the floor and you should not force the stretch. Make the stretch in the direction of the kyo meridian. Repeat on the other side; right hand on left shoulder, left hand on knee. Bring the knees back to the chest as in Fig. 362, and you should now find them closer to the chest, indicating more flexibility in the lower back area.

Supporting the legs with your legs as in Fig. 362, rotate the hips in small circles, two times each way. Grasp the ankles and stretch the legs vertically (Fig. 364). Holding the stretch gently shake the legs while bringing them to the floor. With the legs a few inches from the floor, gently and briskly move the legs sideways, causing the body to "wriggle" sideways throughout (Fig. 365).

Fig. 365

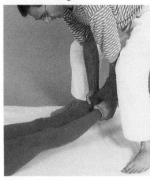

34. Arms

Fig. 366

Sit seiza a few inches above the head, facing the receiver's feet.

(a) **Selecting on which arm to begin shiatsu**
Observe which shoulder is more elevated from the floor. If this is not obvious, assume a kneeling position and place your hands on the shoulders. Leaning forward, apply gentle pressure (Fig. 366). The more relaxed side is

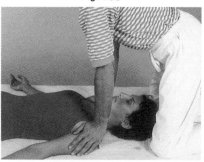

Fig. 367

Fig. 368

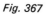

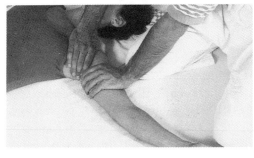

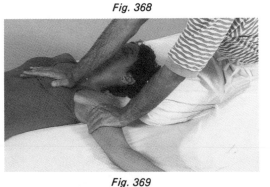

Fig. 369

the one we begin on: for practice, the left arm.

(b) Left arm

The arm with palm up should be placed at right angles to the body. Support at the shoulder with your right hand and give general palm pressure with your left hand down the arm, in 4 to 5 places (Fig. 367).

(1) *LU.m*

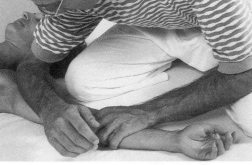

Fig. 370

Give support with your left hand on the upper arm by the armpit. Gently apply heel of palm pressure to LU.1 in the chest area 3 times (Fig. 368).

Support on the shoulder with your right hand. Apply either:

(i) Heel of palm pressure toward LU.5 at the outside crease in the elbow in 3 places. Repeat. Support below the elbow with your left hand.

(ii) Elbow pressure. Sit seiza with legs apart. Brace your left elbow with your left knee. With your left hand clasping below the left elbow, very gently stretch the arm away from the body. From the shoulder to the elbow, apply elbow pressue in 2 to 3 places (Fig. 369). Slide your left supporting hand onto the left hand as though shaking hands while still maintaining a gentle stretch. By leaning in with your right elbow apply a counter-stretch as well as pressure, from the left elbow toward a point midway down the lower arm, in 2 to 3 places (Fig. 370). Repeat.

Sit seiza on toes. Support with your right hand over the left elbow. With your left elbow, apply pressure from a point midway down the lower arm, toward and onto the wrist in 2 to 3 places (Fig. 371).

Fig. 371

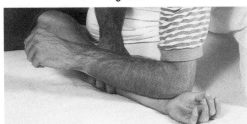

(2) *L.I.m*

Turn the palm over and support with your right hand on the shoulder. With your left hand give general palm pressure toward the hand in 5 to 6 places. Then apply either:

(i) Heel of palm pressure. With your left hand supporting below the elbow, apply right heel of palm pressure toward the elbow in 2 or 3 places. Repeat.

(ii) Elbow pressure. Sit seiza, with knees apart, your left elbow braced on your left knee. With the left hand clasping below the left elbow, gently stretch away from the shoulder. With your right elbow apply a counter-stretch as well as pressure to the L.I.m, from the shoulder toward the elbow, in 2 to 3 places (Fig. 372). Repeat.

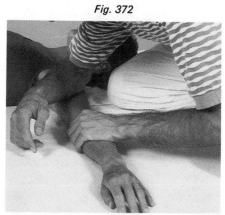

Fig. 372

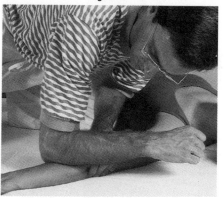

Fig. 373

Change position. Face the lower arm from the opposite side, seiza on toes, knees apart. Give support above the elbow with your left hand.

The L.I.m runs from L.I.11, at the crease in the elbow, to the thumb side of the nail of the index finger. Apply either:

(i) Heel of palm pressure with your right hand toward the thumb side of the wrist in 3 to 4 places. Repeat.

(ii) Elbow pressure. With your right elbow, give shiatsu from L.I.11 toward L.I.5, by the crease of the wrist, thumb side, in 3 to 4 places (Fig. 373). Repeat.

(3) *H.C.m*

Turn the palm over and raise the angle of the arm 45 degrees.

The H.C.m follows a central line from armpit to wrist. On the upper arm apply in 3 to 4 places either:

Fig. 374

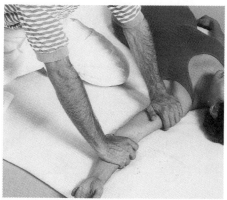

(i) Heel of palm pressure. Support below the elbow with your right hand and apply pressure with your left heel of palm (Fig. 374). Repeat.

(ii) Elbow pressure. Sit seiza, knees apart, with your right elbow braced on your right knee. Clasp the arm below the elbow, and gently stretch the arm away from the shoulder. With your

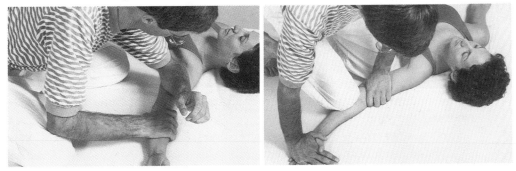

Fig. 375   Fig. 376

left elbow, from the receiver's armpit toward the elbow, apply elbow pressure in 2 to 3 places (Fig. 375). Repeat. Sit seiza on toes. Your left hand gives

Fig. 377

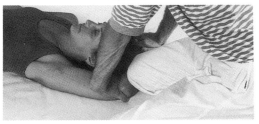

Fig. 378

support above the elbow, and your right hand gives support over the palm. Apply right knee pressure from the elbow toward the wrist in 3 to 4 places (Fig. 376). Repeat.

(4) *HT.m*

Sit seiza on toes, knees apart, facing the upper arm, which is now pointing above the head. Support above the elbow with your right hand. With your left elbow, from armpit to elbow, apply elbow pressure in 3 to 4 places (Fig. 377). Repeat. Extend the arm behind the receiver's head. Sit seiza, facing the upper arm. Your left hand gives support above the elbow, and your right hand rests over the receiver's left hand. With your right knee, from elbow to wrist, give shiatsu in 3 to 4 places. Repeat (Fig. 378).

Fig. 379

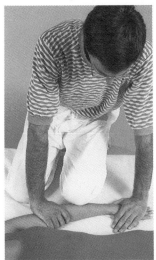

Change the position of the arm so that it rests by the side, palm down. Kneel, facing the lower arm. Give support above the elbow with your right hand. Apply left hand general palm pressure along the lower arm in 3 places.

(5) *T.H.m*

The T.H.m follows a central line toward the wrist. Apply heel of palm pressure or knee pressure in 3 to 4 places (Fig. 379). Repeat. For knee pressure, your left hand rests over the palm.

(6) *S.I.m*

The S.I.m follows an outside line from the elbow to the little finger side of the wrist (S.I.6). Apply pressure to the S.I.m, as above with the T.H.m.

(c) **Left hand**

Stand up, place your right foot lightly over the receiver's upper arm and interlace your little fingers between the little finger and ring finger, and the thumb and index finger. Apply pressure downward and slightly forward, opening and stretching the palm.

Apply shiatsu with your thumbs along 3 lines: outside, center and inside, in 2 to 3 places each line (Fig. 380).

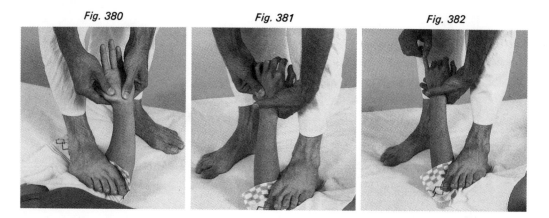

Fig. 380   Fig. 381   Fig. 382

Change position. Stand on the opposite side of the arm, facing the face. Place your left foot over the arm just above the elbow. Support the arm at the wrist with your left hand. With your right thumb, apply shiatsu along 3 lines between the knuckles (Fig. 381); followed with shiatsu using the left thumb to L.I.4, between the index finger and thumb.

(d) **Fingers**

Maintain support at the wrist with your left hand. Take the little finger between index finger and thumb and give shiatsu to the sides toward the nail in 2 to 3 places (Fig. 382). The last point is most important, so give shiatsu to that point 3 times.

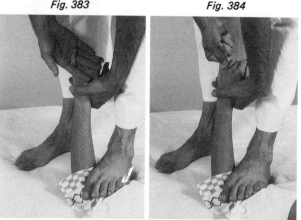

Fig. 383   Fig. 384

Then, give shiatsu to the top and bottom of the finger in 3 places, stretching it as you apply pressure. Finish by stretching the finger away from the hand (Figs. 383 and 384). Repeat on the other 3 fingers.

Apply shiatsu to the thumb in like manner with your left hand, while supporting with your right. With left hand supporting the wrist between your thumb and index finger, interlace your fingers between the receiver's finger and thumb, and gently stretch downward and slightly toward you (Fig. 385). Raise the arm off the futon and gently shake (Fig. 386).

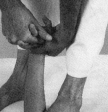

Fig. 385

(e) Shoulder joint

Place your left hand over the shoulder, and with your right hand hold the arm at the wrist with your fingers over the back of the wrist and your thumb in the center of the palm, and the arm above the receiver's head (Fig. 387). Make 3 clockwise rotations, sliding the upper arm along the futon on the downward move until the receiver's elbow touches the side (Figs. 387 through 390). Then beginning with the arm just above a line perpendicular to the body, begin a downward and outward movement stretching away from the shoulder (Fig. 391). (N.B., the hand over the receiver's hand is facing in the opposite direction to the hand over the shoulder.) This will cause the shoulder to rise. Holding the shoulder firmly while performing this move will help to stretch and loosen it.

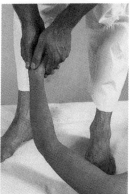

Fig. 386

After holding this position for a few moments, move the wrist in toward the armpit (Fig. 392). From here, making a circular motion, slide the arm at the wrist

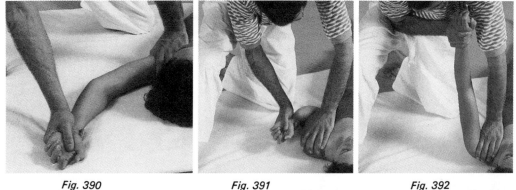

Fig. 387   Fig. 388   Fig. 389

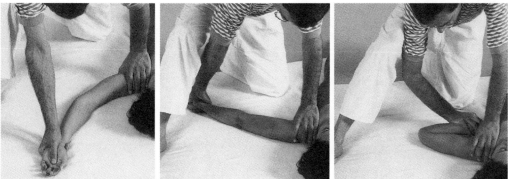

Fig. 390   Fig. 391   Fig. 392

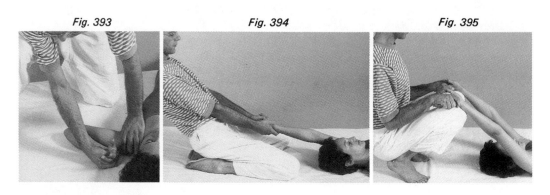

Fig. 393   Fig. 394   Fig. 395

over the shoulder to a position just above it (Fig. 393).
Repeat these moves at least twice.

Change position to seiza above the receiver's head. Hold as though shaking the receiver's left hand with your left hand and place your right hand over the wrist. Gently stretch the arm toward you at a low angle from the floor (Fig. 394). Hold momentarily, then lay the arm by the side. Repeat step *34* (b) through (e) mirror image on the right arm.

(f)   Both arms

In a squatting position, take both hands in yours as though shaking hands. Lean back so that the wrists are resting on your knees. By leaning back further, take up any slack and stretch both arms (Fig. 395).

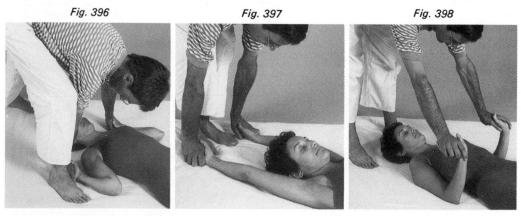

Fig. 396   Fig. 397   Fig. 398

Fig. 399

Stand up, bring both arms forward, elbows by the side and rest the upper arms on the floor (Fig. 396). With brisk but gentle movement draw the arms toward you (Fig. 397). Repeat.

Standing and using your whole body, stretch one arm upward, then the other. Repeat to each side twice. Bring the arms forward, with elbows on the floor and upper arms vertical to the floor. With your palms on the receiver's palms, gently stretch the wrists (Fig. 398).

Finish by resting the arms by the sides (Fig. 399).

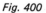
Fig. 400

35. Neck

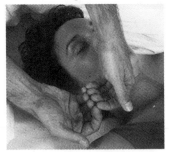

Fig. 401

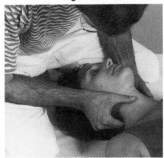

Sit seiza, knees apart, above the receiver's head. With the 4 fingertips of each hand, give deep but gentle shiatsu to each side of the spine, from neck to base of skull, in 4 to 5 places (Figs. 400 and 401). Repeat.

Place the receiver's head in your left palm and tilt slightly toward the left. With your 4 fingers resting over the back of the neck, give thumb shiatsu to ST. and L.I. meridians on the right side of the neck, in 3 places to each line, from clavicle to jaw (Fig. 402). Repeat this move, mirror image on the left side.

Supporting the head with both hands, rotate it to both left side and right (Fig. 403). Come back to center,

Fig. 402

Fig. 403

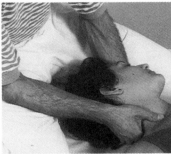
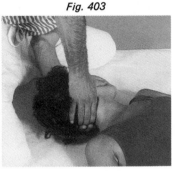

Fig. 404

Fig. 405

Fig. 406

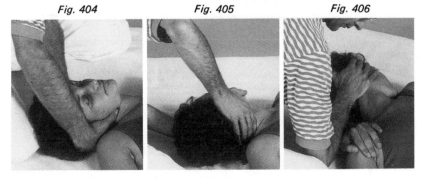

then, bend the head to the right side and left (Fig. 404). Return to center. Combine both moves by bending to the right side, then rotating to the left, and very gently stretch to the point of maximum comfort in the stretch (Fig. 405). Repeat in mirror image on the other side. In this position, we may create a stable but intense stretch. Move to the right side slightly, with knees apart. With the receiver's head in the position created by the previous stretch, place your right palm over the base of the skull and your left palm over the right shoulder. (Your left arm should be under your right arm.) Place your elbows inside your knees. Squeeze your knees together slightly, causing your elbows to contract inward and your palms to move away from each other (Fig. 406). In this stretch the right hand hardly moves at all, while the left moves downward, creating the stretch on the neck. Repeat this step on the other side.

Fig. 407 Fig. 408

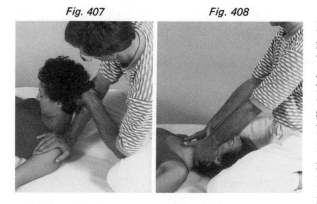

Sit seiza above the receiver's head, knees apart. Support the receiver's head in your left hand. With your right arm resting under your left hand, and your right hand resting on the receiver's left shoulder, ask the receiver to breathe in. While the receiver exhales, stretch the head upward by raising your right arm (Fig. 407). Hold momentarily. Repeat, mirror image, on the other side.

To finish off, place your left palm over the back of the neck, with your right palm over your left. Gently stretch toward you in a wavelike motion a few times (Fig. 408). On the last stretch, continue to the point where the receiver's feet show signs of moving upward.

36. Face

Sit seiza above the head, knees apart.
- (i) Place your thumbs between the eyebrows and give shiatsu toward the hairline, in 4 to 5 places (Fig. 409).
- (ii) From a central point, just below the hairline give shiatsu across the forehead to the ear, in 5 to 6 places (Fig. 410). Repeat on 2 more horizontal lines, moving down toward the eyebrows.
- (iii) With your index fingers between eyelid and eyebrow gently stretch toward you (Fig. 411).
- (iv) Give shiatsu beside the bridge of the nose with your index fingers (Fig. 412).
- (v) Give shiatsu to the outside corner of the eyes, with your thumbs (Fig. 413). Be very careful.

Fig. 409 Fig. 410

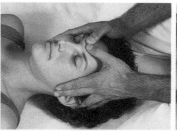
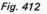
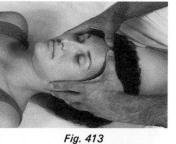

Fig. 411 Fig. 412 Fig. 413

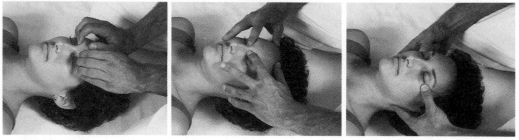

281

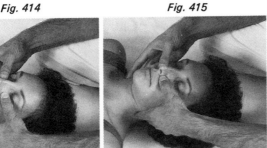

Fig. 414   Fig. 415

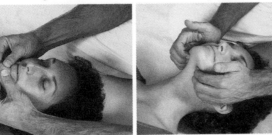

Fig. 416   Fig. 417

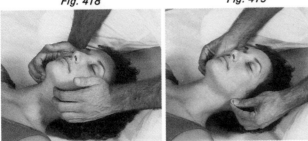

Fig. 418   Fig. 419

(vi) Give shiatsu with your thumbs below the eyes, from the nose extending outward (Fig. 414).

(vii) Give shiatsu to points beside the nostrils (Fig. 415).

(viii) Give shiatsu to the area above the upper lip, from center to outside.

(ix) Give shiatsu to the area below the lower lip, from the chin, along the jawbone to the ears (Fig. 416).

(x) Give shiatsu beneath the jaw by stretching with the fingers toward you (Fig. 417).

(xi) With the heels of the palms, apply pressure to the temple region (Fig. 418).

(xii) With thumb and index finger, apply gentle pinching pressure from the earlobes around the ridges of the ears (Fig. 419).

Fig. 420

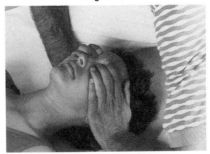

Fig. 421

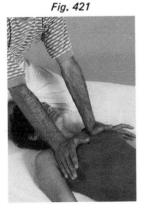

(xiii) Finish with gentle relaxation to the eyes. Place the fingertips over them and hold momentarily (Fig. 420). Check first that the receiver is not wearing contact lenses.

37. Chest

Still sitting seiza above the head, place the heels of the palms over LU.1 (Fig. 421). Gently apply alternate pressure with each palm, twice or more, holding momentarily each time.

Fig. 422

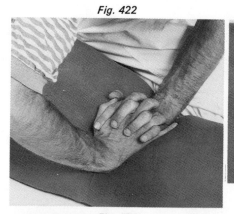

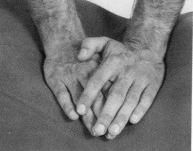
Fig. 423

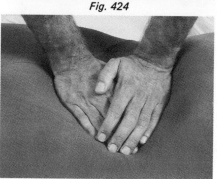
Fig. 424

38. Hara

Sit seiza, facing the receiver on the right side. Once more give hara diagnosis and finish with hara massage. There are 2 techniques for possible experimentation:

(i) Interlace the fingers and place horizontally over the hara. With the heels of the palms, in an undulating motion, press side to side in rhythmic, horizontal motions (Fig. 422).

(ii) Sit seiza, facing the receiver. Place your right palm on the lower hara, and your left palm over your right hand on the upper hara. With the heels of your palms, massage the right side by leaning forward (Fig. 423). With your fingertips, massage the left side by drawing backward (Fig. 424). Repeat in undulating motions from 5 to 10 times on each side. Finish with stationary pressure over the central hara area for 30 seconds or more.

Suggest that the receiver rest for a few minutes before getting up.

Additional Techniques

There are some techniques that I use less often but they can be useful from time to time.

1. Sitting position

(i) *Thumb pressure beside the spine, from base of shoulder blades to iliac crest*
Assume a half-kneeling posture. Place your left hand over the receiver's hara and your right knee over your right elbow. Apply thumb pressure in 6 to 8 places, down the left side. Then move your body over a few inches and repeat on the right side (Fig. 425).

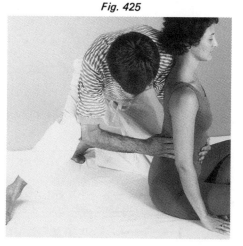
Fig. 425

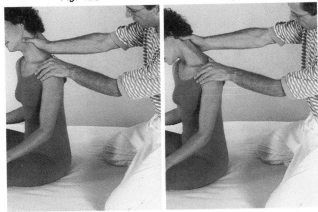

Fig. 426   Fig. 427

(ii) *Thumb shiatsu to the neck*
Place your left hand on
the left shoulder for support. Direct the neck at
an angle that stretches
the meridian you wish to
treat. Place your four
fingers over the back of
the neck for support and
apply thumb pressure
down the side of the
neck in 3 to 4 places.
Repeat (Fig. 426—ST.m,
Fig. 427—GB.m). Repeat
mirror image on the opposite side.

2. **Side position**
   (i) *Elbow shiatsu to the shoulder*
   Sit beyond the receiver's head
   and facing the feet, seiza with
   knees apart. Place your left hand
   on the shoulder and lean forward to stretch it. With your
   right elbow, from neck to arm,
   apply pressure in 3 to 4 places
   (Fig. 428). Repeat.

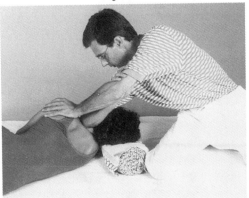

Fig. 428

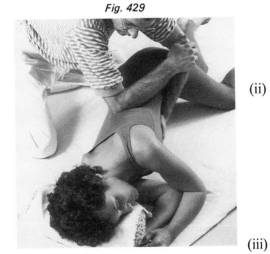

Fig. 429

(ii) *Elbow shiatsu beside the spine, lower back*
Seiza with knees apart. Place your
left hand over the hara for support.
With your right elbow, following the
contours of the receiver's body, apply
shiatsu on the left side of the spine, over
the middle back region, toward the
sacrum in 3 to 4 places (Fig. 429).
Repeat.

(iii) *Side stretch*
Following the general side stretch (see
Figs. 225 and 226), keep your left knee on the left buttock but place your
right knee on the floor. Against your left knee, stretch the receiver's left
shoulder away from you and the left leg toward you in a downward direction,
gently stretching the body along one line (Fig. 430). Then reverse the stretch.
Draw the shoulder toward you and stretch the hip away from you. Do not

overstretch: perform gently. The upper left leg is approximately 90 degrees to the torso and your left elbow is resting in your hara (Fig. 431).

3. Prone position

(i) *HT. and LV. meridians*

Place your left hand over the sacrum to give support. Pick up the foot as though holding a suitcase and extend it away from you. With your left knee, apply pres-

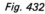

Fig. 430

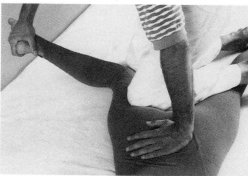

sure to the HT.m in 2 to 3 places and then, by extending the foot further away from you, to the LV.m in the same manner (Fig. 432).

(ii) *Manipulating the spine*

Place your left hand over the sacrum. Place your right hand

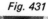

Fig. 431

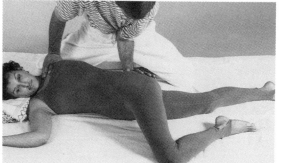

over the right knee. Maintaining firm but gentle pressure over the sacrum, raise the receiver's right knee by leaning your body to the left, thus creating a gentle stretch in the lower spine (Fig. 433). Repeat on the left leg. Draw the leg up from the outside this time (Fig. 434).

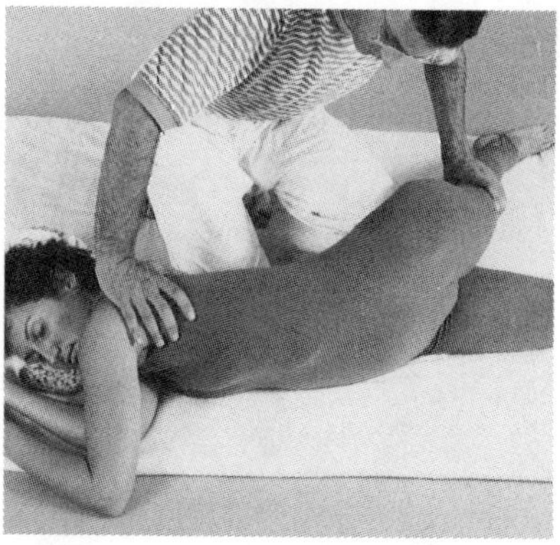

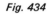

Fig. 432

Fig. 433

Fig. 434

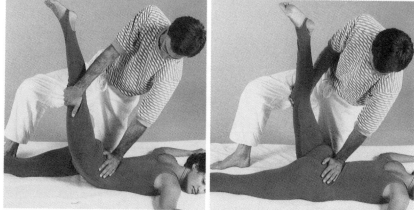

End Notes

Chapter 1

[1] Daisetsu Teitaro Suzuki, *The Awakening of Zen* (Boulder: Prajna Press, 1980), 27.

[2] Henri Wei, *The Guiding Light of Lao Tsu* (Wheaton, Illinois: Quest The Theosophical Publishing House, 1982), 160.

[3] D. T. Suzuki, *Studies in Zen* (New York: Delta Books, 1955), 153.

[4] Nahum Stiskin, *The Looking Glass God* (Brookline, Mass.: Autumn Press, 1972). Refer to pages 27–33 for a detailed explanation of the logarithmic spiral.

[5] Koichi Tohei, *Ki in Daily Life* (Tokyo: Ki no Kenkyukai, 1978), 20.

[6] Wei, op cit, 160.

[7] Frederick Franck, *The Buddha Eye: An Anthology of the Kyoto School* (New York: The Crossroad Publishing Company, 1982,) 92.

[8] Wei, op cit, 188.

[9] Noel Perrin, *Giving Up the Gun: Japan's Reversion to the Sword* (Boulder: Shambhala, 1980).

Chapter 2

[1] Lama Anagarika Govinda, *The Inner Structure of the I Ching: The Book of Transformations* (Tokyo and New York: Weatherhill, 1981), 158.

[2] John Blofeld, *Taoism: The Road to Immortality* (Boston: Shambhala, 1978), 93.

[3] Wei, op. cit, 160.

[4] Taoist Master N., Hua-Ching, *Tao: The Subtle Universal Law and the Integral Way of Life* (Calif.: The Shrine of the Eternal Breath of Tao, 1979), 27.
Lama Anagarika Govinda, op cit, 57.
Mme. Dr. M. Hashimoto, *Japanese Acupuncture* (New York: Liveright, 1966), 18–19.
Michio Kushi, *How to See Your Health: The Book of Oriental Diagnosis* (Tokyo and New York: Japan Publications, Inc., 1980), 21.
Ilza Veith, *The Yellow Emperor's Classic of Internal Medicine* (Berkeley, Los Angeles, and London: University of California Press, 1972), 21.

[5] Stephan D. R. Feuchtwang, *An Anthropological Analysis of Chinese Geomancy* (Vientiane, Laos: Editions Vithagna, 1974), 42.

[6] Lama Anagarika Govinda, op. cit, 161.

[7] Michio Kushi, *The Book of Macrobiotics: The Universal Way of Health, Happiness and Peace* (Tokyo and New York: Japan Publications, Inc., 1986), 31.

[8] Da Liu, *The Tao and Chinese Culture* (New York: Schocken Books, 1979), 114.

Chapter 3

[1] Hung Ying-Ming, *The Roots of Wisdom: Saikontan*, trans., William Scott Wilson (Tokyo and New York: Kodansha International Ltd., 1985), 9.

[2] Michio and Aveline Kushi, with Alex Jack, *Macrobiotic Diet* (Tokyo and New York: Japan Publications, Inc., 1985).

[3] Seibin and Teruko Arasaki, *Vegetables from the Sea: To Help You Look and Feel Better* (Tokyo and New York: Japan Publications, Inc., 1983). Please refer to this book for an in-depth study of sea vegetables.

Chapter 4

The Liver and Gallbladder Meridians:

[1] Gia-Fu Feng and Jane English, *Chuang Tsu: Inner Chapters* (New York: Vintage Books, 1974), 95.

[2] General References
Ted J. Kaptchuk, *The Web That Has No Weaver: Understanding Chinese Medicine* (New York: Congdon & Weed, 1983), 59–62.
Felix Mann, *The Meridians of Acupuncture* (London: William Heinemann Medical Books, Ltd., 1964), 101–108.
John O'Connor and Dan Bensky, *Acupuncture: A Comprehensive Text*. Shanghai College of Traditional Medicine (Seattle: Eastland Press, 1981), 12.
Yoshiaki Omura, *Acupuncture Medicine: Its Historical and Clinical Background* (Tokyo and New York: Japan Publications, Inc., 1982), 28.

[3] Omura, 1982, 28.

[4] O'Connor and Bensky, 1981, 12.

[5] Ibid, 12.

[6] Kaptchuk, 1983, 59.

[7] O'Connor and Bensky, 1981, 12.

[8] General References
Omura, 1982, 107–110.
An Outline of Chinese Acupuncture, The Academy of Traditional Chinese Medicine (Peking: Foreign Language Press, 1975), 184–191.

[9] Shizuto Masunaga with Stephen Brown, *Zen Imagery Exercises: Meridian Exercises for Wholesome Living* (Tokyo and New York: Japan Publications, Inc., 1987), 72–74.

[10] Masunaga, 1987, 203.

[11] Shizuto Masunaga with Wataru Ohashi and the Shiatsu Education Center of America, *Zen Shiatsu: How to Harmonize Yin and Yang for Better Health* (Tokyo and New York: Japan Publications, Inc., 1977), 47.

[12] Masunaga, 1987, 203–204.

[13] General References
Rudolph Ballentine M.D., *Diet and Nutrition: A Holistic Approach* (Honesdale, Pennsylvania: The Himalayan International Institute, 1982), 325–331.
The Illustrated Encyclopedia of the Human Body (New York: Exeter Books, 1984), 110–111.
The Rand McNally Atlas of the Body (Chicago, San Francisco and New York: Rand McNally & Company, 1980), 46–47.

[14] Ballentine, 1982, 327.

[15] *Atlas of the Body*, 1980, 46.

[16] General References
Rob Allanson, *The Liver Bodyhealth: A Guide to Keeping Your Body Well* (Boston: East West Books, 1985), 35–37.
The Columbia University College of Physicians and Surgeons, *Complete Home Medical Guide* (New York: Crown Publishers, Inc., 1985), 518–520.
Michio Kushi, *Natural Healing through Macrobiotics* (Tokyo and New York: Japan Publications, Inc., 1978), 88–89.

[17] *The Complete Home Medical Guide*, 1985, 520.
Allanson, 1985, 37.

[18] *The Complete Home Medical Guide*, 1985, 519.

[19] *The Complete Home Medical Guide*, 1985, 518.
Kushi, 1978, 89.

[20] *The Complete Home Medical Guide*, 1985, 519.
Allanson, 1985, 37.

[21] Omura, 1982, 28.

[22] Mann, 1964, 95.

[23] Ibid, 95.

[24] Ibid, 95.

[25] Omura, 1982, 100–106.
An Outline of Chinese Acupuncture, 1975, 172–184.

[26] Masunaga, 1987, 72–73.

[27] Ibid, 202–203.

[28] Masunaga, 1977, 47.

[29] Masunaga, 1987, 203.

[30] General References
The Illustrated Encyclopedia of the Human Body, (New York: Exeter, 1984), 108, 110.
Edwin B. Steen/Ashley Montagu, *Anatomy and Physiology* vol. 1 (New York, Hagerstown, San Francisco, and London: Barnes and Noble Books, 1959), 164–165, 187, 192.
Rob Allanson, *The Gallbladder Bodyhealth: A Guide to Keeping Your Body Well* (Boston: East West Books, 1985), 55–58.

[31] *The Human Body*, 1984, 108, 110.
Complete Home Medical Guide, 1985, 520, 521.
Allanson, 1985, 57.

[32] *The Human Body*, 1984, 110.

[33] Michio Kushi, *How to See Your Health*, 1980.
Bill Tims, *The Liver Bodyhealth: A Guide to Keeping Your Body Well* (Boston: East West Books, 1985), 39–41.

[34] Michio Kushi and Alex Jack, *The Cancer Prevention Diet* (New York: St. Martin's Press, 1983), 231–234.

The Heart and Small Intestine, Heart Constrictor and Triple Heater Meridians:

[1] General References
Katchuk, 1983, 54–55.
Mann, 1964, 54–57.
Omura, 1982, 28.

[2] Omura, 1982, 28.

[3] Huai-Chin Nan, trans., Wen Kuan Chu Ph.D., *Tao and Longevity: Mind-Body Transformation* (York Beach, Maine: Samuel Weiser, Inc., 1984), 106.

[4] Kaptchuk, 1983, 54.

[5] General References
Omura, 1982, 70–74.
An Outline of Chinese Acupuncture, 1975, 127–131.

[6] Masunaga, 66–68.

[7] Ibid, 198–199.

[8] Masunaga, 1977, 44.

[9] Masunaga, 1987, 199

[10] General References
The Illustrated Encyclopedia of the Human Body, 1984, 70–75.
The Rand McNally Atlas of the Body, 1980, 52, 53.

[11] General References
The Human Body, 1984, 53–55.
The Atlas of the Body, 1980, 50–51.

[12] *The Human Body*, 1984, 55.

[13] Michio Kushi, *How to See Your Health*, 1980, 88–90.
Michio Kushi and Alex Jack, *Diet for a Strong Heart* (New York: St. Martin's Press, 1984), 162–182.

[14] Michio Kushi, 1985, 245–258.

[15] General References
Mann, 1964, 61–63.
Omura, 1982, 28.

[16] Omura, 1982, 28.

[17] Mann, 1964, 61.

[18] General References
Omura, 1982, 28.
An Outline of Chinese Acupuncture, 1975, 131–137.

[19] Masunaga, 1987, 66–68.

[20] Ibid, 199.

[21] Masunaga, 1977, 44.
[22] Masunaga, 1987, 199–200.
[23] General References
The Human Body, 1984, 112–115.
Steen/Montagu, 1959, vol. 1, 155, 156, 180–181, 186–187.
[24] Ballentine, 1978, 342.
[25] The Complete Home Medical Guide, 1985, 515.
[26] Ibid, 515–518.
[27] Ballentine, 1978, 340–342.
[28] Ibid, 341.
[29] Kushi, How to See Your Health, 1980.
Bill Tims, The Intestines Bodyhealth: A Guide to Keeping Your Body Well (Boston: East West Books, 1985), 47–49.
[30] Omura, 1982, 28.
[31] Mann, 1964, 82.
[32] Omura, 1982, 91–94.
An Outline of Chinese Acupuncture, 1975, 161–166.
[33] Masunaga, 1987, 70–72.
[34] Ibid, 201.
[35] Masunaga, 1977, 46.
[36] Masunaga, 1987, 201–202.
[37] Omura, 1982, 28.
[38] Mann, 1964, 87.
[39] Omura, 1982, 28.
[40] Mann, 1964, 87.
[41] General References
Omura, 1982, 95–98.
An Outline of Chinese Acupuncture, 1975, 166–172.
[42] Masunaga, 1987, 70–72.
[43] Ibid, 202.
[44] Masunaga, 1977, 46.
[45] Masunaga, 1987, 202.

The Spleen and Stomach Meridians:
[1] Masunaga, 1987, 65.
[2] General References
Kaptchuk, 1983, 57–59.
Mann, 1964, 41, 48–50.
O'Connor and Bensky, 13, 14.
[3] Omura, 1982, 28.
[4] O'Connor and Bensky, 1987, 13.
[5] Kaptchuk, 1983, 57.
[6] Ibid, 59.
[7] Ibid, 58.
[8] Mann, 1964, 41.
[9] Omura, 1982, 64–69.
An Outline of Chinese Acupuncture, 1975, 120–127
[10] Masunaga, 1987, 64–66.
[11] Ibid, 198.
[12] Masunaga, 1977, 43.
[13] Masunaga, 1987, 198.
[14] General References
Ballentine, 1978, 324, 325.
Steen/Montagu, 1959, Vol. 1, 165–166, 188.
[15] Ballentine, 1978, 483–491.

Michio Kushi, *Macrobiotic Health Education Series: Diabetes and Hypoglycemia* (Tokyo and New York: Japan Publications, Inc., 1985).

John Mann, *The Pancreas Bodyhealth: A Guide to Keep Your Body Well* (Boston: East West Books, 1985), 59–63.

[16] Michio Kushi, *How to See Your Health*, 1980.

Michio Kushi and Alex Jack, *The Cancer Prevention Diet* (New York: St. Martin's Press, 1983), 281–282.

[17] Omura, 1982, 29.

Mann, 1964, 41–43.

[18] Omura, 1982, 28.

[19] Mann, 1964, 41.

[20] Mann, 1964, 42.

[21] Omura, 1982, 59–63.

[22] Masunaga, 1987, 64–66.

[23] Ibid, 197.

[24] Masunaga, 1977, 43.

[25] Masunaga, 1987, 197.

[26] General References

Ballentine, 1978, 318–322.

The Human Body, 1984, 105–107.

Steen/Montagu, 1959, 158–160, 189–190.

Kob Allanson, *The Stomach Bodyhealth: A Guide to Keeping Your Body Well* (Boston: East West Books, 1985), 27–30.

[27] Ibid, 28.

[28] *The Human Body*, 1984, 106.

[29] Ballentine, 1978, 319.

[30] Allanson, 1985, 29.

[31] Ballentine, 1978, 371.

[32] Michio Kushi, *The Cancer Prevention Diet*, 1983, 307–308.

Michio Kushi, *How to See Your Health*, 1980.

Bill Tims, *The Stomach Bodyhealth: A Guide to Keeping Your Body Well* (Boston: East West Books, 1985), 31–35.

[33] Michio Kushi, *The Cancer Prevention Diet*, 1983, 308–311.

The Lung and Large Intestine Meridians:

[1] General References

Kaptchuk, 1983, 55–57.

Mann, 1964, 25–32.

O'Connor and Bensky, 1981, 14

[2] Omura, 1982, 28.

[3] Mann, 1964, 25.

[4] Ibid, 27.

[5] O'Connor and Bensky, 1981, 14.

[6] Mann, 1964, 26.

[7] O'Connor and Bensky, 1981, 14.

[8] Omura, 1982, 51–53.

An Outline of Chinese Acupuncture, 1975, 95–100

[9] Masunaga, 1987, 63–64

[10] Ibid, 196.

[11] Masunaga, 1977, 42.

[12] Masunaga, 1987, 196.

[13] General References

Swami Rama et al, *Science of Breath* (Honesdale, Pennsylvania: The Himalayan International Institute of Yoga Science and Philosophy, 1981), 27–55, 64–65.

The Human Body, 1984, 88–94.
Atlas of the Body, 1980, 60–61.
14 Swami Rama et al, 1987, 67.
15 *The Human Body*, 1984, 89, 90.
Atlas of the Body, 1980, 58.
Swami Rama et al, 1981, 26–55.
16 Swami Rama et al, 1981, 44–45.
17 *Complete Home Medical Guide*, 1985, 455.
Michio Kushi, *Natural Healing through Macrobiotics*, 1978, 98.
18 *The Complete Home Medical Guide*, 1985, 454.
Michio Kushi, 1978, 97.
19 *The Complete Home Medical Guide*, 1985, 461–463.
Michio Kushi, 1978, 97.
20 Michio Kushi, *How to See Your Health*, 1980.
Michio Kushi, *The Cancer Prevention Diet*, 1983, 246–247.
Bill Tims, *The Lungs Bodyhealth: A Guide to Keeping Your Body Well* (Boston: East West Books, 1985), 25–26.
21 Michio Kushi, *The Cancer Prevention Diet*, 1983, 246–249.
22 Please refer to the following books:
Mike Sayama, *Samadhi: Self Development in Zen, Swordmanship, and Psychotherapy* (New York: State University of New York Press, 1986).
Sekida Katsuki, *Zen Training: Methods and Philosophy* (New York and Tokyo: Weatherhill, 1976).
23 General Reference
Mann, 1964, 35–38.
24 Omura, 1982, 28.
25 Mann, 1964, 35.
26 Omura, 1982, 55–57.
An Outline of Chinese Acupuncture, 1975, 100–106.
27 Masunaga, 1987, 63–64.
28 Ibid, 196.
29 Masunaga, 1977, 42.
30 Masunaga, 1987, 196–197.
31 *The Human Body*, 1984, 116–119.
Steen/Montagu, vol. 1, 158–160, 181.
Ballentine, 1978, 333–365.
Robert Gray, *The Colon Health Handbook* (Reno, Nevada: Emerald Publishing, 1985).
Bernard Jensen, *Tissue Cleansing through Bowel Management* (Bernerd Jensen, D. C., Route 1, Box 52, Escondido, CA 92025, 1981).
32 Ballentine, 1978, 333, 336.
33 Ibid, 334, 335.
34 For the most recent information on vitamin B_{12} please refer to: *East West Magazine*, May 1988; *Macromuse*, Spring 1988.
35 Ballentine, 1978, 344–346.
36 Ibid, 348.
37 Gray, April 1985, 15.
38 Ballentine, 1978, 357.
Rob Allanson, *The Intestines Bodyhealth: A Guide to Keeping Your Body Well* (Boston: East West Books, 1985), 45.
39 Gray, April 1985, 12.
Jensen, 1987, 38–42.
40 Michio Kushi, *How to See Your Health*, 1980.
Michio Kushi, *The Cancer Prevention Diet*, 1983.
41 Ibid, 199–201.

The Kidney and Bladder Meridians:
1 General References
   Kaptchuk, 1983, 62–65.
   Mann, 1964, 72–79.
2 Omura, 1982, 28.
3 Kaptchuk, 1983, 63.
4 Mann, 1964, 73.
5 Kaptchuk, 1983, 63.
6 Ibid, 65.
7 Omura, 1982, 87–91.
   An Outline of Chinese Medicine, 1975, 154–161.
8 Masunaga, 1987, 68–70.
9 Ibid, 200–201.
10 Masunaga, 1977, 45.
11 Masunaga, 1987, 201
12 *The Human Body*, 1984, 120–127.
   Atlas of the Body, 1980, 62–63.
   The Complete Home Medical Guide, 1985, 602–618.
13 Ibid, 604–607.
14 Ibid, 609–612.
15 Ibid, 614.
16 Omura, 1982, 28.
17 Omura, 1982, 77–85.
   An Outline of Chinese Acupuncture, 1975, 138–154.
18 Masunaga, 1987, 68–70.
19 Ibid, 200.
20 Masunaga, 1977, 45.
21 Masunaga, 1987, 68–70.
22 Steen/Montagu, 1959, Vol. 2, 6, 7.
   The Human Body, 1984, 126, 127.
23 *The Complete Home Medical Guide*, 1985, 758–759.
24 Ibid, 759.
25 Ibid, 754–755.
26 Michio Kushi, *How to See Your Health*, 1980.
   Michio Kushi, *The Cancer Prevention Diet*, 1983, 329–330.
   Bill Tims, *The Kidney Bodyhealth: A Guide to Keeping Your Body Well* (Boston: East West Books, 1985), 65–67.
27 Michio Kushi, *The Cancer Prevention Diet*, 1983, 332–333.

Chapter 5
1 A video of this exercise program is available.
   Contact:
> **David Sergel**
> The Arcade Building
> 318 Harvard Street #39
> Brookline, MA 02146 U.S.A.
> (617) 566–4416

Chapter 7
Masunaga's Shiatsu Meridian Chart is available through the Iokai Shiatsu Center in Tokyo. This chart is in color and comes in two sizes: 31 inches × 40 inches, approximately US$20, and 12 inches × 16 inches, approximately US$14 plus postage.
Contact:
> **The Iokai Shiatsu Center**
> 1–8–9 Higashiueno

Taito-ku, Tokyo 110
Japan
(03) 832–2983

Another highly recommended book on meridians is the following: Kinoshita, Haruto, *Illustration of Acupoints* (Tokyo: Ido-no-Nippon-Sha).

Bibliography

An Outline of Chinese Acupuncture. The Academy of Traditional Chinese Medicine. Peking: Foreign Language Press, 1975.

Arasaki, Seibin and Teruko. *Vegetables from the Sea: To Help You Look and Feel Better*. Tokyo and New York: Japan Publications, Inc., 1983.

Ballentine, Rudolph, M.D. *Diet and Nutrition: A Holistic Approach*. Honesdale, Pennsylvania: The Himalayan International Institute, 1982.

Blofeld, John. *Taoism: The Road to Immortality*. Boston: Shambhala, 1978.

Bodyhealth: A Guide to Keeping Your Body Well. An East West Journal Anthology. Boston: East West Books, 1985.

Chang, Chung-Yuan, Ph. D. *Creativity and Taoism: A Study of Chinese Philosophy, Art and Poetry*. Harper Torchbooks. New York: Harper & Row, Publishers, Inc., 1970.

Chu, Wen Kuan, Ph. D. *Tao and Longevity: Mind-Body Transformation*. Translated by Huai-Chin. Nan York Beach, Maine: Samuel Weiser, Inc., 1984.

The Columbia University College of Physicians and Surgeons Complete Home Medical Guide. New York: Crown Publishers, Inc., 1985.

Connelly, Dianne M., Ph.D., M.Ac. *Traditional Acupuncture: The Law of the Five Elements*. Columbia, Maryland: The Centre for Traditional Acupuncture, Inc., 1979.

Esko, Edward and Wendy. *Macrobiotic Cooking for Everyone*. Tokyo and New York: Japan Publications, Inc., 1980.

Esko, Wendy. *Aveline Kushi's Introducing Macrobiotic Cooking*. Tokyo and New York: Japan Publications, Inc, 1987.

Feng, Gia-Fu, and Jane English. *Chuang Tsu: Inner Chapters*. New York: Vintage Books, 1974.

Feuchtwang, Stephan D. R. *An Anthropological Analysis of Chinese Geomancy*. Vientiane, Laos: Editions Vithagra, 1974.

Franck, Frederick., ed. *The Buddha Eye: An Anthology of the Kyoto School*. New York: Crossroad Publishing Company, 1982.

Govinda, Lama Anagarika. *The Inner Structure of the I Ching: The Book of Transformation*. Tokyo and New York: Weatherhill, 1981.

Gray, Robert. *The Colon Health Handbook: New Health through Colon Rejuvenation*. Reno, Nevada: Emerald Publishing, 1985 (Rev. ed.).

Hashimoto, Keizo, M.D., with Yoshiaki Kawakami. *Sôtai: Balance and Health through Natural Movement*. Tokyo and New York: Japan Publications, Inc., 1983.

Hashimoto, M., Dr. *Japanese Acupuncture*. New York: Liveright Publishing Corporation, 1971.

Hung, Ying-Ming. *The Roots of Wisdom: Saikontan*. Translated by William Scott Wilson. Tokyo and New York: Kodansha International Ltd., 1984.

The Illustrated Encyclopedia of the Human Body. New York: Exeter Books, 1984.

Jensen Bernard D. C. *Tissue Cleansing through Bowl Management*. Route 1, Box 52 Escondido, CA 92025: Bernard Jensen D. C., 1981.

Kaptchuk, Ted J., O.M.D. *The Web That Has No Weaver: Understanding Chinese Medicine*. New York: Congdon & Weed, 1983.

Kinoshita, Haruto. *Illustration of Acupoints*. Tokyo: Ido-no-Nippon-Sha.

Kushi, Aveline. *How to Cook with Miso*. Tokyo and New York: Japan Publications, Inc., 1978.

————. *Macrobiotic Food and Cooking Series: Diabetes and Hypoglycemia; Allergies*. Tokyo and New York: Japan Publications, Inc., 1985.

————. *Macrobiotic Food and Cooking Series: Obesity, Weight Loss and Eating Disorders; Infertility and Reproductive Disorders*. Tokyo and New York: Japan Publications, Inc., 1987.

————. *Macrobiotic Food and Cooking Series: Stress and Hypertension; Arthritis*. Tokyo and New York: Japan Publications, Inc., 1988.

Kushi, Aveline, and Wendy Esko. *The Changing Seasons Macrobiotic Cookbook*. Wayne, N. J.: Avery Publishing Group, 1984.

Kushi, Michio. *The Book of Dō-in: Exercise for Physical and Spiritual Development*. Tokyo and New York: Japan Publiations, Inc., 1979.

————. *The Book of Macrobiotics: The Universal Way of Health, Happiness and Peace*. Tokyo and New York: Japan Publications, Inc., 1986 (Rev. ed.).

————. *Cancer and Heart Disease: The Macrobiotic Approach to Degenerative Disorders*. Tokyo and New York: Japan Publications, Inc., 1986 (Rev. ed.).

————. *Crime and Diet: The Macrobiotic Approach*. Tokyo and New York: Japan Publications, Inc., 1987.

————. *The Era of Humanity*. Brookline, Mass.: East West Journal, 1980.

————. *How to See Your Health: The Book of Oriental Diagnosis*. Tokyo and New York: Japan Publications, Inc., 1980.

————. *The Macrobiotic Approach to Cancer*. Wayne, N. J.: Avery Publishing Group., 1982.

————. *Macrobiotic Health Education Series: Diabetes and Hypoglycemia; Allergies*. Tokyo and New York: Japan Publications, Inc., 1985.

————. *Macrobiotic Health Education Series. Obesity, Weight Loss and Eating Disorders; Infertility and Reproductive Disorders*. Tokyo and New York: Japan Publications, Inc., 1987.

————. *Macrobiotic Health Education Series: Arthritis*. Tokyo and New York: Japan Publications, Inc., 1988.

————. *Natural Healing through Macrobiotics*. Tokyo and New York: Japan Publications, Inc., 1978.

————. *Your Face Never Lies*. Wayne, N. J.: Avery Publishing Group, 1983.

Kushi, Michio, and Alex Jack. *The Cancer Prevention Diet*. New York: St. Martin's Press, 1983.

————. *Diet for a Strong Heart*. New York: St. Martin's Press, 1984.

Kushi, Michio and Aveline. *Macrobiotic Pregnancy and Care of the Newborn*. Edited by Edward and Wendy Esko. Tokyo and New York: Japan Publications, Inc., 1984.

Kushi, Michio and Aveline, with Alex Jack. *Macrobiotic Diet*. Tokyo and New York: Japan Publications, Inc., 1985.

Liu, Da. *The Tao and Chinese Culture*. New York: Schocken Books, 1979.

Mann, Felix, *The Meridians of Acupuncture*. London: William Heinemann Medical Books, Ltd., 1964.

Masunaga, Shizuto, with Wataru Ohashi and the Shiatsu Education Center of America. *Zen Shiatsu: How to Harmonize Yin and Yang for Better Health*. Tokyo and New York: Japan Publications, Inc., 1977.

Masunaga Shizuto, with Stephen Brown. *Zen Imagery Exercises: Meridian Exercises for Wholesome Living*. Tokyo and New York: Japan Publications, Inc., 1987.

Ni, Hua-Ching. *Tao: The Subtle Universal Law and the Integral Way of Life*. Calif: The Shrine of the Eternal Breath of Tao, 1982.

O'Connor, John, and Dan Bensky. *Acupuncture: A Comprehensive Text*. Shanghai College of Traditional Medicine. Seattle: Eastland Press, 1981.

Ohsawa, George. *Zen Macrobiotics*. Calif.: George Ohsawa Macrobiotic Foundation, 1965.

Omura, Yoshiaki. *Acupuncture Medicine: Its Historical and Clinical Background*. Tokyo and New York: Japan Publications, Inc., 1982.

Perrin, Noel. *Giving Up the Gun: Japan's Reversion to the Sword, 1543–1879*. Boulder, Colorado: Shambhala, 1980.

Rama, Swami, Ballentine, Rudolph, M.D., Hymes, Alan, M.D. *Science of Breath: A Practical Guide*. Pennsylvania: The Himalayan International Institute of Yoga Science and Philosophy, 1981.

The Rand McNally Atlas of the Body. Chicago, New York, and San Francisco: Rand McNally and Company, 1980.

Sayama, Mike. *Samadhi: Self Development in Zen, Swordmanship, and Psychotherapy*. New York: State University of New York Press, 1986.

Sekida, Katsuki. *Zen Training: Methods and Philosophy*. New York and Tokyo: Weatherhill, 1976

Serizawa, Katsusuke, M.D. *Effective Tsubo Therapy: Simple and Natural Relief without Drugs*. Tokyo and New York: Japan Publications, Inc., 1984.

———. *Tsubo: Vital Points for Oriental Therapy*. Tokyo and New York: Japan Publications, Inc., 1976.

Serizawa, Katsusuke, with Mari Kusumi. *Clinical Acupuncture: A Practical Japanese Approach*. Tokyo and New York: Japan Publications, Inc., 1988.

Steen, Edwin B./Montagu, Ashley. *Anatomy and Physiology*. 2 vols. New York, Hagerstown, San Francisco, and London: Barnes and Noble Books, 1959.

Stiskin, Nahum. *The Looking Glass God: Shinto, Yin-Yang, and a Cosmology for Today*. Brookline, Mass.: Autumn Press, Inc., 1972.

Suzuki, Daisetsu T. *The Awakening of Zen*. Boulder, Colorado: Prajna Press, 1980.

———. *The Zen Doctrine of No Mind*. London, Melbourne, Sydney, Aukland, and Johannesburg: Rider, 1983.

———. *Studies in Zen*. Delta Books. New York: Dell Publishing Company, 1955.

———. *Zen and Japanese Culture*. Bollingen Series LXIV. New Jersey: Princeton University Press, 1973.

Takahashi, Masaru, and Stephen Brown. *Qigong for Health: Chinese Traditional Exercise for Cure and Prevention*. Tokyo and New York: Japan Publications, Inc., 1986.

Tara, William. *Macrobiotics and Human Behavior*. Tokyo and New York: Japan Publications, Inc., 1985.

Tohei, Koichi. *Ki in Daily Life*. Tokyo: Ki no Kenkyukai, 1978.

Wei, Henry. *The Guiding Light of Lao Tsu: A New Translation and Commentary on the Tao Teh Ching*. Illinois: Quest, The Theosophical Publishing House, 1985.

Yamamoto, Shizuko. *Barefoot Shiatsu*. Tokyo and New York: Japan Publications, Inc., 1979.

The Yellow Emperor's Classic of Internal Medicine. Translated by Ilza Veith. Berkeley: University of California Press, 1949.

Index